Heart Failure

Commissioning Editor: Thomas V. Hartman
Development Editor: Kate Newell
Production Editor: Cathryn Gates
Production Controller: Susan Shepherd

Heart Failure: Device Management

EDITED BY

Arthur M. Feldman, MD, PhD

Magee Professor and Chairman
Department of Medicine
Jefferson Medical College
Philadelphia, PA
USA

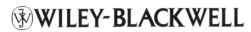

A John Wiley & Sons, Ltd., Publication

This edition first published 2010, © 2010 by Blackwell Publishing Ltd

Blackwell Publishing was acquired by John Wiley & Sons in February 2007. Blackwell's publishing program has been merged with Wiley's global Scientific, Technical and Medical business to form Wiley-Blackwell.

Registered office: John Wiley & Sons Ltd, The Atrium, Southern Gate, Chichester, West Sussex, PO19 8SQ, UK

Editorial offices: 9600 Garsington Road, Oxford, OX4 2DQ, UK
　　　　　　　　　The Atrium, Southern Gate, Chichester, West Sussex, PO19 8SQ, UK
　　　　　　　　　111 River Street, Hoboken, NJ 07030-5774, USA

For details of our global editorial offices, for customer services and for information about how to apply for permission to reuse the copyright material in this book please see our website at www.wiley.com/wiley-blackwell

Library of Congress Cataloging-in-Publication Data

　　Heart failure : device management / edited by Arthur M. Feldman.
　　　　p. ; cm.
　　Includes bibliographical references.
　　ISBN 978-1-4051-5258-7
　　1. Heart failure–Treatment.　2. Heart, Artificial.　I. Feldman, Arthur M. (Arthur Michael), 1949–
　　[DNLM: 1. Heart Failure–therapy.　2. Heart-Assist Devices. WG 370 H436305 2010]
　　RC685.C53H4347 2010
　　616.1′29–dc22

　　　　　　　　　　　　　　　　　　　　　　　　　　　　　　　　　　　　　2009018586

ISBN 978-1-4051-5258-7

A catalogue record for this book is available from the British Library.

Set in 9.5/12 pt. Minion by Aptara®, Inc., New Delhi, India
Printed and bound in Malaysia by Vivar Printing Sdn Bhd

1　2010

Contents

Contributors

Nisha Aggarwal, MD
Division of Cardiology
Department of Medicine
Jefferson Medical College
Philadelphia, PA
USA

Abbas Ardehali, MD
David Geffen School of Medicine
University of California
Los Angeles, CA
USA

Juan M. Bernal, MD
Division of Interventional Cardiology
Massachusetts General Hospital
Boston, MA
USA

Martin Borggrefe, MD
Fakultät für klinische
Medizin der Universität Heidelberg
Mannheim
Germany

Daniel Burkhoff, MD, PhD
Columbia University
New York, NY
USA; and
IMPULSE Dynamics USA
Orangeburg, NY
USA

Christian Butter, MD
Heart Center Brandenburg Bernau/Berlin
Bernau
Germany

Howard A. Cohen, MD
Lenox Hill Heart and Vascular Institute
New York, NY
USA

Maria Rosa Costanzo, MD
Midwest Heart Foundation
Edward Heart Hospital
Naperville, IL
USA

Mark H. Drazner, MD, MSc
Donald W. Reynolds Cardiovascular Clinical Research Center
Division of Cardiology
Department of Internal Medicine
University of Texas Southwestern Medical Center
Dallas, TX
USA

Arthur M. Feldman, MD, PhD
Department of Medicine
Jefferson Medical College
Philadelphia, PA
USA

Arnold J. Greenspon, MD
Division of Cardiology
Department of Medicine
Jefferson Medical College
Philadelphia, PA
USA

John Gorcsan III, MD
The Cardiovascular Institute
University of Pittsburgh
Pittsburgh, PA
USA

Reginald T. Ho, MD
Division of Cardiology
Department of Medicine
Jefferson Medical College
Philadelphia, PA
USA

Sandeep A. Kamath, MD
Donald W. Reynolds Cardiovascular Clinical Research Center
Division of Cardiology
Department of Internal Medicine
University of Texas Southwestern Medical Center
Dallas, TX
USA

Thomas J. Kiernan, MD
Division of Interventional Cardiology
Massachusetts General Hospital
Boston, MA
USA

William E. Lawson, MD
SUNY, Stony Brook
Stony Brook, NY
USA

Douglas L. Mann, MD
Winters Center for Heart Failure Research
Section of Cardiology
Department of Medicine and Department of
Molecular Physiology and Biophysics
Baylor College of Medicine
Houston, TX
USA

Daniel Marelli, MD
Division of Cardiothoracic Surgery
Department of Surgery
Jefferson Medical College
Philadelphia, PA
USA

Paul J. Mather, MD
Division of Cardiology
Department of Medicine
Jefferson Medical College
Philadelphia, PA
USA

Yuval Mika, PhD
IMPULSE Dynamics USA
Orangeburg, NY
USA

Suresh Mulukutla, MD
University of Pittsburgh Medical Center
Pittsburgh, PA
USA

Igor F. Palacios, MD
Division of Interventional Cardiology
Massachusetts General Hospital
Boston, MA
USA

Sunthosh V. Parvathaneni, MD
Harrington-McLaughlin Heart & Vascular Institute
Department of Internal Medicine
University Hospitals Case Medical Center
Case Western Reserve University
Cleveland, OH
USA; and
Louis Stokes Cleveland VA Medical Center
Cleveland, OH
USA

Ileana L. Piña, MD
Harrington-McLaughlin Heart & Vascular Institute
Department of Internal Medicine
University Hospitals Case Medical Center
Case Western Reserve University
Cleveland, OH
USA; and
Louis Stokes Cleveland VA Medical Center
Cleveland, OH
USA

Behzad Pavri, MD
Division of Cardiology
Department of Medicine
Jefferson Medical College
Philadelphia, PA
USA

Andra M. Popescu, MD
Department of Medicine
Jefferson Medical College
Philadelphia, PA
USA

Nicholas J. Ruggiero II, MD
Division of Interventional Cardiology
Massachusetts General Hospital
Boston, MA
USA

Hani N. Sabbah, PhD
Henry Ford Health System
Detroit, MI
USA

Lawrence Schneider, MBBS
Lenox Hill Heart and Vascular Institute
New York, NY
USA

Marc A. Silver, MD
Department of Medicine
Heart Failure Institute
Advocate Christ Medical Center
Oak Lawn, IL
USA; and
University of Illinois
Chicago, IL
USA

Louis Stein, MHS, PhD
Division of Cardiothoracic Surgery
Department of Surgery
Jefferson Medical College
Philadelphia, PA
USA

David J. Whellan, MD, MHS, FACC
Division of Cardiology
Department of Medicine
Jefferson Medical College
Philadelphia, PA
USA

Preface

Heart failure is a disease of epidemic proportions affecting over 5 million people in the United States and close to 30 million worldwide. Over the last three decades enormous strides have been made in our ability to improve symptoms and prolong life in patients with heart failure. In the previous volume of *Heart Failure* we discussed the traditional drug treatments available for heart failure patients as well as the many new and innovative pharmacologic therapies that have been or will shortly be added to our therapeutic armamentarium. In this volume of *Heart Failure* we will focus on the many new and novel "device" technologies that enhance our ability to care for patients with this progressive disease. For the purposes of this text the term "device" will be given a relatively liberal definition as it will apply to "equipment" or "technology" that is implanted within the patient to measure or enhance cardiac function, is attached to the patient for diagnostic information or therapeutic effects, or is used to evaluate the patient in a way that provides fundamental information in real time regarding the physiology of the heart—information that can then be utilized to modify therapy or to "tune" the effectiveness of an implanted device or pharmacologic therapy.

Drugs have been available for the treatment of heart failure since William Withering first discovered the salutary benefits of the foxglove plant (later recognized as digoxin) during the 1700s. By contrast, the first use of a "device" for the treatment of heart failure occurred on 4 February 1980 when Dr Levi Watkins implanted an automatic implantable defibrillator invented by Dr Michel Mirowski in the abdominal cavity of a patient at the Johns Hopkins Hospital. The hope was that the defibrillator would prevent sudden death in a patient with a history of ventricular tachycardia. This was an enormous leap forward in the treatment of patients with heart failure as 50% of them died suddenly, presumably secondary to a tachyarrhythmia. However, it would be nearly 25 years before the use of the device was shown to improve survival when used for either primary or secondary protection. Over the past 30 years, the size of the device has been decreased allowing it to be moved from the patient's abdomen to the subclavian position, leads can now be implanted percutaneously rather than being placed surgically on the epicardial surface of the heart, the battery life has been greatly extended, the devices can be interrogated telephonically to assess extensive information about both the device and cardiac function, and the defibrillator can be combined with a biventricular pacemaker.

Interestingly, the paradigm for the development of devices for the treatment of heart failure is quite different from the developmental paradigm for new drugs. With rare exceptions, pharmacologic agents developed for the treatment of heart failure undergo rigorous clinical evaluation in Phase I, Phase II, and Phase III clinical trials. The primary endpoint of most Phase III clinical trials (e.g. β-blockers, angiotensin-converting enzyme inhibitors, aldosterone antagonists) has been the effect of a pharmacologic agent either on the combined endpoint of hospitalization for worsening heart failure or death or on the single endpoint of all-cause mortality. By contrast, devices are often evaluated and approved based on their ability to effectively fulfill their proposed need in a safe and reliable manner. For example, ventricular pacemakers were not approved because they saved lives, but rather because they demonstrated the ability to initiate a signal that would effectively induce a contractile response in the presence of a block in the normal electromechanical signaling pathway. In some cases, the value of individual devices has come after, rather than before the approval of the device. One example is biventricular pacing, first approved on the basis of early studies demonstrating that resynchronization of the heart could improve heart failure symptoms, exercise tolerance, and quality of life in patients with heart failure. The role of resynchronization therapy in improving both survival and the combined endpoint of survival and hospitalization for worsening heart failure came in subsequent Phase IV studies. However, studies of resynchronization were surprising as they demonstrated that a device could actually enhance cardiac remodeling, alter the molecular biology of the heart, and improve survival. Thus, the long-held view that a "device" could not influence the biology of the heart was challenged not just by the results of a single study but by multiple studies in a variety of patient populations.

Another important difference between drugs and devices is that an individual physician can administer a drug to their patient. However, the use of a device often requires the collaboration of a multidisciplinary team. For example, the placement of an internal cardioverter defibrillator requires the collaboration of a cardiologist (or internist), an electrophysiologist, and occasionally a surgeon specializing in the thorascopic placement of leads on the epicardium of the heart. For other devices, there may only be a single physician at an institution that can implant a specific device. For example, some percutaneous devices require skills in transseptal procedures—a technology around which only some interventional cardiologists are skilled and one that requires the collaboration of heart failure specialists and interventionalists. Similarly, valve replacement or repair can be a critical feature in the treatment of a patient with heart failure—but one that also requires a multidisciplinary team approach to the patient.

The various chapters in this text can be subdivided based on the role of the device in the care of patients with heart failure. The first five chapters detail a group of devices that are chronically implanted to either improve cardiac function or increase survival (Cardiac Resynchronization Therapy and Implantable Cardioverter-Defibrillator Therapy), provide online and real-time monitoring of cardiac function (Chronic Implantable Monitoring), or new implantable devices that may have the ability to improve cardiac function or delay maladaptive cardiac remodeling (Impulse Therapy and Cardiac Restraint). The next three chapters describe external devices that have the potential to assess cardiac risk and/or the ability to help physicians titrate both drug and device therapy. These include The Role of Right Heart Catheterization in the Management of Patients with Heart Failure, the value of Bioimpedance for serial monitoring of heart failure patients, and the Use of Echocardiography in Evaluating the Heart Failure Patient and Response to Therapy. The final group of chapters provides a discussion of invasive technologies—both surgical and nonsurgical—that can provide urgent or chronic support in patients with severe left ventricular dysfunction, including Revascularization for Left Ventricular Dysfunction, the use of Minimally Invasive Treatment for Mitral Valve Disease, Percutaenous Mechanical Assist Devices in patients with acute cardiac decompensation or as a support device during high-risk revascularization, the use of Left Ventricular Assist Devices as a bridge to transplantation or a bridge to recovery, and the use of Counterpulsation and Ultrafiltration in patients with both acute and chronic heart failure.

The treatment of patients with heart failure is a continuously moving target as new devices are being developed. In this text we have focused on those technologies that in some cases are available at most hospitals that have programs in electrophysiology and cardiac surgery as well as new technologies that are available or undergoing late-stage investigation at quaternary hospitals with surgical and medical heart failure programs. With the increasing number of options available to physicians, there will be an increasing need to identify the right intervention for the right patient. Thus, we have tried to provide guidelines within each chapter that will help to define those patients that will be benefited the most by each of these different therapies. However, decisions regarding each of these new therapeutic options will in many cases be based on the presentation and needs of each individual patient. Unlike drug therapy where practice guidelines have defined both the list of optimal medications and the target therapeutic levels for heart failure medications, we will see that the use of device therapy is far less clear. Hopefully, future studies will better define the effectiveness of these various therapies and more clearly define their role in the care of heart failure patients.

This text would not have been possible without the contribution of the many experts who gave of their time and energy to address each of these complex technologies in a manner that will be useful for the cardiologist,the surgeon, and the general internist. Thanks go to Kate Newell at Wiley-Blackwell who has nursed this book through the editorial process. Special thanks go to Marianne LaRussa without whose editorial support this book would not have been possible.

Arthur M. Feldman

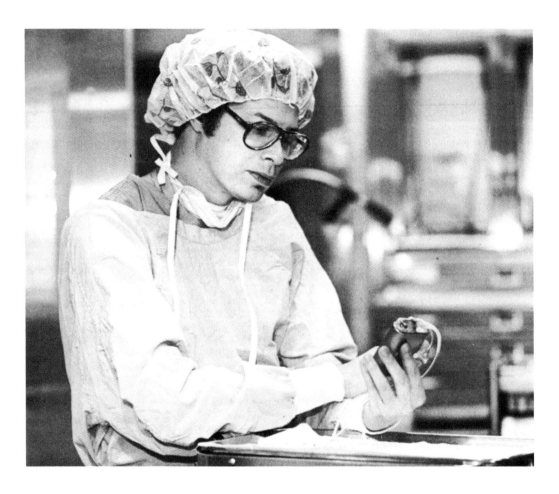

CHAPTER 1

Cardiac Resynchronization Therapy

Behzad Pavri, & Arthur M. Feldman

Jefferson Medical College, Philadelphia, PA, USA

History of cardiac resynchronization

Cardiac resynchronization therapy (CRT) was first described nearly 25 years ago. In 1983 at the 7th World Symposium on Cardiac Pacing, de Teresa et al. described a series of 4 patients with left bundle branch block (LBBB) who underwent aortic valve replacement [1]. An epicardial left ventricular (LV) lead was placed and attached to the ventricular port of a dual chamber pacemaker along with a right atrial lead. The atrioventricular (AV) delay was adjusted to allow for fusion between native conduction and LV pacing. There was a 25% increase in ejection fraction (EF) and improvement in dyssynchrony based on angioscintigraphy. The importance of these observations was unappreciated, and this report remained largely unnoticed for almost a decade.

Also the 1980s and early 1990s saw reports of echocardiography and angioscintigraphy in patients with widened QRS from either bundle branch block or pacing, which demonstrated dyssynchronous contraction [2,3]. However, little was known about the hemodynamic effects of such dyssynchronous contraction. Several investigators performed animal experiments involving pacing-induced models of dyssynchrony. Burkhoff et al. paced 8 dogs at several sites, including the epicardial atrium, LV apex, LV and RV free walls, and endocardial RV apex [4]. LV pressure was highest with atrial pacing and lowest with RV free wall pacing. They reported that LV pressure was negatively correlated with QRS width ($r = 0.971$). Park et al. paced dogs in the RV and demonstrated a rightward shift in LV end-systolic pressure–volume relation, with increasing QRS width indicating poorer LV pump function [5]. Lattuca et al. were the first to report experience with biventricular pacing [6]. Three dogs were paced in the RV, LV, or both. Marked improvement was seen in QRS duration, cardiac output, aortic pressure, and right atrial pressure when paced in both ventricles.

Further human experience with pacing therapy for heart failure did not occur until the early 1990s. Initial efforts were focused toward resynchronization of AV timing for heart failure. One initial study demonstrated benefit of AV sequential pacing [7] but subsequent studies either failed to duplicate success or demonstrated worsening outcomes [8–11]. Other studies examined the potential of alternative pacing sites in the RV for improvement in dyssynchrony [12–14].

The first report of CRT in heart failure was in 1994. Caqeau et al. reported a single patient with alcohol-induced dilated cardiomyopathy with LBBB, prolonged PR interval of 200 milliseconds, and New York Heart Association (NYHA) class IV congestive heart failure (CHF) symptoms who was clinically deteriorating despite maximal medical therapy [15]. M-mode echocardiography demonstrated significant delay between septal and posterior wall contraction. In an attempt to correct his conduction abnormalities, the authors implanted a four-chamber pacemaker. An epicardial LV lead

Heart Failure: Device Management. Edited by Arthur Feldman. © 2010 Blackwell Publishing.

was placed in addition to transvenously placed right atrial, right ventricular, and left atrial leads. Interestingly, the left atrial lead was placed in the distal coronary sinus. Both atrial leads and both ventricular leads were Y-adapted and connected to a dual chamber pacemaker. The patient experienced acute improvements in pulmonary capillary wedge pressure, cardiac output, and QRS duration. Six weeks after implantation the patient exhibited NYHA class II symptoms. In their conclusion, the authors predicted that resynchronization therapy might be beneficial in the short term but doubted that any long-term benefit would be realized. Shortly after this report, several other groups reported small case reports of the acute benefits of resynchronization [16–18]. All these initial reports involved epicardial lead placement. Transvenous insertion of an LV lead into a branch of the coronary sinus was first described in 1998 by Daubert et al. [19].

These initial small reports were the foundation for the larger clinical trials that followed. Initial feasibility studies were followed by prospective multicenter randomized trials. As a result of these efforts, in 2001 the Food and Drug Administration approved the Medtronic InSync Biventricular pacemaker for treating CHF. As clinical trials continued to report both acute and chronic improvement with resynchronization therapy with most recent trials demonstrating mortality benefits, the ACC/AHA guidelines include a class I recommendation for CRT for patients with EF ≤ 35%, sinus rhythm, NYHA class III or IV symptoms despite optimal medical therapy with dyssynchrony, and QRS width > 120 milliseconds [20]. CRT was incorporated into defibrillators, thereby increasing the therapeutic potential of these devices. We now recognize CRT as state-of-the-art treatment for selected patients with heart failure, and continued advancements are being reported in device technology, newer LV lead designs, coronary sinus delivery systems, ability to alter V–V timing, tools to track CHF, and imaging modalities to assist in patient identification and therapy titration.

Pathophysiology of dyssynchrony

Mechanical/structural dyssynchrony

As the heart fails, LV remodeling begins. This has been best studied in postinfarction LV dysfunction but has also been extended to cardiomyopathy due to other causes. There are numerous factors that contribute to the remodeling process. In myocardial infarction, remodeling starts within a few hours after the acute event. Initial events include myocyte slippage due to lengthening of cardiac myocytes, followed by thinning of the ventricular wall, expansion of the infraction, inflammation and necrotic zone resorption, ultimately resulting in scar formation. The infarction zone can expand and lead to LV deformation and dilatation. Unaffected regions of the heart show compensatory hypertrophy. In addition, the extracellular matrix, under the influence of metalloproteases, remodels with collagen accumulation. These changes are mediated by neurohormonal activation, and the remodeling leads to worsening cardiac function through elevated wall stress/hypertrophy, resulting in a vicious cycle leading to progressive decline.

Electrical dyssynchrony

In addition to these mechanical changes, the electrical system can develop disease. While conduction delay can occur in all parts of the electrical system, focus has been on the importance of AV synchrony and interventricular synchrony. As will be discussed further below, the loss of electrical synchrony in itself leads to further electrical, structural, physiologic, and molecular remodeling, which in turn contribute to the vicious downward spiral seen in heart failure patients.

AV dyssynchrony

AV nodal delay can occur because of intrinsic disease or because of medical therapy. When AV nodal conduction time increases, atrial contraction no longer contributes to late diastolic filling. Rather it occurs during passive early filling. With prolonged AV delays, left atrial pressure can fall below LV pressure late in diastole, leading to "presystolic" mitral regurgitation. Evidence from animal studies suggests that chronic AV block induces mechanical and electrical remodeling.

Infra-His dyssynchrony

Widening of the QRS is seen in up to 30% of patients with heart failure, most commonly in an LBBB pattern, and is associated with increased 1-year sudden and total mortality rate [21]. The effect of pacing-induced LBBB on the LV has been well studied in animals and correlated with humans. Tagged magnetic resonance imaging (MRI) studies in animals reveal that initial activation occurs in the interventricular septum [22]. This early septal activation occurs with lateral wall prestretch and is unable to mount sufficient pressure to effect mitral valve closure. Delayed activation of the lateral wall occurs after the septum has contracted. This contraction occurs against a higher pressure ventricle and a relaxing, noncompliant septum. This leads to paradoxical septal motion, which can worsen mitral regurgitation. Similar patterns have been also demonstrated in humans with dilated cardiomyopathy [23,24]. Tagged MRI studies also demonstrate increased myofiber workload in the late activated lateral wall. Positron emission tomographic scanning reveals differences in regional metabolism, with lateral walls exhibiting twice the septal metabolism, and there is evidence that local myocardial blood flow is altered [25–27]. Such differences in workload can also lead to altered mechanical stretch, which may affect calcium handling with resultant tachyarrhythmias [28].

Clinically, LBBB has been associated with higher event rates in patients with CHF [29] and also has been proposed as a risk factor for developing future CHF in asymptomatic patients [30]. One study suggested that LBBB may be responsible for a reversible form of idiopathic dilated cardiomyopathy [31]. There is animal evidence that electrical dyssynchrony, both within the AV node and with LBBB, can lead to adverse remodeling.

Spragg et al. studied the effects of different types of pacing-induced cardiomyopathy in 11 dogs [32]. Six dogs were paced at over 200 bpm in the right atrium and 5 were paced in the RV at the same rate; 4 dogs served as controls. Dogs were studied with MRI to document dyssynchrony. Both pacing groups resulted in similar degrees of cardiomyopathy. Atrially paced dogs demonstrated uniform LV activation while RV-paced dogs exhibited early septal contraction with concomitant lateral stretch followed by delayed lateral contraction and septal stretch. Western blot analysis of the RV-paced hearts revealed both transmural and interventricular gradients in myocardial protein expression, but these gradients were not seen in the atrial-paced or control groups. Thus, it appears that mechanical dyssynchrony rather than cardiomyopathy contributed to molecular remodeling. Prinzen et al. reported their studies in 8 dogs that underwent radiofrequency (RF) ablation of the left bundle [33]. After 16 weeks, there was a decrease in EF and an increase in LV cavity volume and LV mass. Both the septum and lateral walls demonstrated hypertrophy, but with an altered ratio. Spragg et al. reported experience with 9 dogs that underwent RF ablation of the left bundle [34]. One month later, tissue was examined from both early-activated anterior segments and late-activated lateral LV myocardial segments. They noted that the conduction velocity, action potential duration and refractory periods of late-activated lateral segments were significantly reduced compared to anterior segments. The distribution of connexin 43 was altered from intercalated disks to lateral myocyte membranes. In addition, the normal gradient in conduction velocity from epicardium to endocardium was reversed. In a pressure overload heart failure model of mice reported by Wang et al., failing hearts exhibited a loss of the normal transmural gradient in the action potential duration and prolongation of epicardial action potential duration [35]. The morphology of the action potential was also altered, with a significantly elevated plateau potential. In addition, increased pacing rates led to increased action potential duration and decreased critical conductance required to propagate the action potential. Wiegerinck et al. used a computer simulation in their rabbit model of pressure–volume overload heart failure [36]. They discovered that conduction velocity of the myocardium increased, but that myocardial cell size increased to a greater degree, leading to a widened QRS. Thus, there is evidence that AV block and LBBB lead to electrical remodeling.

Review of major CRT trials

The short-term clinical response to resynchronization therapy has been examined in numerous studies [37–40]. Consistently, these studies have shown that resynchronization therapy dramatically improves symptoms and functional capacity in patients with severe heart failure symptoms (NYHA class III–IV), LVEF < 35%, and widened QRS (see Table 1.1) [1–43].

Table 1.1 Major cardiac resynchronization therapy trials.

Trial design	Number of patients	Age (years)	Follow up	NYHA class	QRS width	Significant endpoints (all $p < 0.05$)
Clinical improvement						
CONTAK CD [37]	490	66	3–6 mo	II–IV	158	Composite of all-cause mortality, heart failure hospitalization, and ventricular tachycardia requiring ICD intervention
InSync ICD [38]	554	66	6 mo	II–IV	165	QoL score, NYHA functional class, and 6-min hall walk distance
MUSTIC [39]	58	63	6 mo	III	176	Improved 6-min walk, QoL score, and Vo_2max
MIRACLE [40]	532	64	3–6 mo	III–IV	166	Improved 6-min walk, QoL score, and NYHA functional class
Mortality						
Meta-analysis [41]	1634	63–66	3–6 mo	II–IV	158–176	OR 0.49, death from CHF (95% CI 0.25–0.93)
						OR 0.71, overall mortality (95% CI 0.51–1.18)
COMPANION [42]	1520	65	12 mo	III–IV	158	OR 0.66, death or CHF hospitalization (95% CI 0.53–0.87)
						OR 0.76, overall mortality (95% CI 0.58–1.01)
CARE-HF [43]	813	66	29.4 mo	III–IV	160	HR 0.54, death or CHF hospitalization (95% CI 0.43–0.68)
						HR 0.64, overall mortality (95% CI 0.48–0.85)

CHF, congestive heart failure; ICD, implantable cardioverter-defibrillator; QoL, quality of life scores (Minnesota Living with Heart Failure questionnaire); OR, odds ratios; HR, hazard ratios.

The MIRACLE study was the first large randomized, double-blinded study comparing optimal medical management and resynchronization therapy in 453 patients. Over a 6-month follow-up, the MIRACLE investigators found significant improvement in NYHA functional class, 6-minute walk distances, and quality of life scores in patients randomized to CRT. Furthermore, patients randomized to CRT had significantly greater improvement in EF, increase in measured Vo_2max, decrease in mitral regurgitant jet area, and decrease in LV end-diastolic dimensions. These responses to CRT were seen as early as 1-month postimplant in the majority of patients, and were maintained at 6-month and 1-year follow-up.

While earlier studies were underpowered to detect changes in mortality over their relatively short follow-up periods, the COMPANION [42] and CARE-HF [43] trials were designed specifically for this purpose. The largest study to date, COMPANION, randomized 1520 patients with severe heart failure and wide QRS to CRT (biventricular pacing only), CRT-D (defibrillator with biventricular pacing capability), and optimal medical management [42]. Over a follow-up period of approximately 12 months, both the CRT and CRT-D arms showed a comparable and statistically significant improvement in the primary endpoint, a composite of death or hospitalization for any cause. While CRT alone did not reach a statistically significant reduction in death ($p = 0.06$), the addition of defibrillation therapy achieved an incremental and significant improvement, likely due to reduction in sudden death events. Kaplan–Meier curves for the primary and

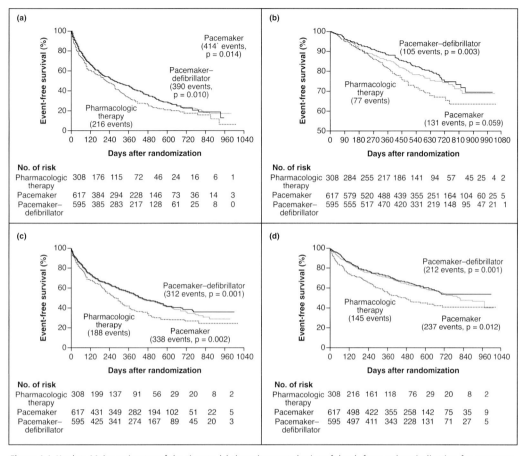

Figure 1.1 Kaplan–Meier estimates of the time to (a) the primary endpoint of death from or hospitalization for any cause, (b) the time to the secondary endpoint of death from any cause, (c) the time to death from or hospitalization for cardiovascular causes and (d) the time to death from or hospitalization for heart failure. (Reproduced with permission from [42]. Copyright © 2004 Massachusetts Medical Society. All Rights Reserved.)

secondary endpoints separated early and continued to diverge throughout the 12-month follow-up (see Figure 1.1).

The recently published CARE-HF trial [43] compared CRT (biventricular pacing without a defibrillator) and optimal medical management in 813 patients for a mean duration of 29.4 months. CARE-HF was the first trial to demonstrate a significant reduction of death of 36% ($p = 0.003$) with CRT compared with medical management. Furthermore, this study supported and extended the findings of COMPANION with regard to reduction in hospitalization for cardiac causes over an extended period of follow-up. Both COMPANION and CARE-HF reproduced prior study findings of a significant improvement in clinical symptoms and

evidence of the ability of resynchronization to cause reverse remodeling.

Effects of CRT

Improvements in cardiac hemodynamics are often seen shortly after the initiation of CRT. Several studies in which invasive hemodynamic monitoring was performed during CRT device implantation have demonstrated acute improvements in systolic blood pressure, cardiac output, peak dP/dT, EF, accompanied by a decline in pulmonary capillary wedge pressures [44–49].

Proposed mechanisms for this abrupt improvement in cardiac function include changes in loading conditions, reduced mitral regurgitation, and enhanced contractile function. Coordinated contraction of the septum and the LV free wall improve ejection efficiency, which can be seen in pressure–volume tracings by an increase in stroke volume and stroke work and decrease in end-systolic volume [49]. These changes occur without an increase in myocardial oxygen consumption, suggesting improved cardiac efficiency as the predominant acute effect of cardiac resynchronization [50].

Numerous studies have reported decreases in functional mitral regurgitation with the initiation of resynchronization therapy [39,40,43,51]. Breithardt et al. have shown that the change in LV dP/dT after initiation of CRT directly correlated with the reduction in effective regurgitant orifice area, suggesting that improved contractile function resulted in an increase in the transmitral pressure gradient and earlier mitral valve closure [52]. Subsequent studies have suggested that the restoration of coordinated papillary muscle activation is another beneficial response to CRT that contributes to reduced regurgitant volumes. Late improvements in mitral regurgitation may occur due to the effects of delayed LV remodeling, associated with a decrease in the sphericity index and reduction in mitral annular dilatation [52–54]. However, patient with significant mitral regurgitation (regurgitant orifice area ≥ $0.20 \, cm^2$) prior to CRT may not show improvement [55]. An important benefit may be the observation that CRT attenuates the worsening of functional mitral regurgitation during exercise [56].

While many patients demonstrate improvements in noninvasive indices of diastolic function after CRT initiation, a direct effect on ventricular relaxation has been more difficult to prove. In patients with elevated filling pressures and a "pseudonormalized" mitral filling pattern, the E wave/Em septal and E/FP ratios have been noted to improve shortly following resynchronization [57]. However, in patients with normal baseline filling patterns, acute effects of CRT fail to improve these noninvasive diastolic indices. This absence of effect suggests that measured changes in LV diastolic filling are caused primarily by a reduction in ventricular volumes and are not in fact due to fundamental changes in myocardial lusitropic properties [57]. Similarly, recent studies have reported a beneficial effect on atrial systolic function, atrial compliance, and atrial dimensions [58].

Cardiac resynchronization also has been shown to have significant effects on the maladaptive neurohormonal responses seen in CHF. Early studies failed to show significant reduction in norepinephrine, dopamine, endothelin, and brain natriuretic peptide levels, possibly due to their small size, short follow-up periods, or methodological limitations [59]. More recently, data have emerged to suggest that sympathetic nerve activity is reduced with CRT, above and beyond the effects of optimal pharmacologic treatment [60]. Furthermore, CARE-HF demonstrated a large reduction in N-terminal BNP, which was not evident until the end of the follow-up period [43]. CRT is associated with long-term improvements in cardiac sympathetic nerve activity, as reflected by improvements in cardiac ^{123}I-MIBG uptake [61]. Several studies have also shown significant improvement in heart rate variability and heart rate profiles after initiation of CRT, which further supports the hypothesis that the neurohormonal balance is shifted away from the sympathetic excess that is ubiquitous in CHF [62].

The application of CRT to a growing population of patients with CHF has also lead to numerous observations beyond improvement in LV systolic function. In particular, improvements in sleep disordered breathing [63], pulmonary hypertension [64], RV function and tricuspid regurgitation [65,66], and the frequency of atrial fibrillation (AF) events [67] are examples of the global cardiac benefit due to the elimination of ventricular dyssynchrony. Occasional case reports of increased ventricular tachycardia burden (proarrhythmia) have been described [68,69], and proximity of LV pacing site to the culprit reentrant circuit has been postulated as the possible explanation.

Patient selection--responders and nonresponders

The cumulative results of the above-referenced trials have lead to CRT receiving a class IIa indication in the 2002 ACC/AHA/NASPE guidelines for cardiac pacing [70], and a class I indication in the 2005 HFSA guidelines [71] for patients with NYHA class III–IV CHF, EF < 35%, and QRS width > 120 milliseconds. Despite the impressive results of these studies, it has become clear that the benefits of CRT are not uniform within this patient population.

Table 1.2 Causes for failure of or "nonresponse" to cardiac resynchronization therapy.

Factors related to patient selection
    Absence of dyssynchrony
    Posterolateral wall scarred or hibernating
Factors related to individual patient
    Atrial anatomic distortion leading to nonengageable coronary sinus
    Lack of suitable posterolateral venous branch (anatomy, diaphragm stimulation), leading to nonplacement of LV
        lead or placement in suboptimal location
    High LV pacing threshold leading to loss of consistent LV capture
    High burden of AF with rapid ventricular response
    Conduction delay from LV pacing site (marked latency)
Factors related to device programming
    Failure to adjust AV delay to optimize AV blood flow
    Failure to adjust V–V timers (when available) to compensate for suboptimal lead LV location
    Failure to adjust LV output to accommodate high LV capture threshold

AF, atrial fibrillation; AV, atrioventricular; LV, left ventricular.

Table 1.2 lists potential reasons for the lack of response to CRT.

As many as one-third of patients receiving CRT are considered "nonresponders." The definition of a "nonresponder" has not been uniform in the multitude of studies published to date, which adds to the confusion regarding what endpoints ought to be considered appropriate measures of treatment success. There are three primary categories of responses: *hemodynamic* (both acute and chronic measurements), *clinical* (includes quality of life scores, 6-min walk times, and functional classification), and *volumetric* (changes in ventricular volumes or EF). More strict definitions of response, such as improvement in volumetric changes, increase the percentage of nonresponders to 36–43%; accurate recognition of patients who will benefit most from CRT continues to be a primary goal [72].

Measurement of the hemodynamic responses to CRT requires invasive monitoring and is not practical for long-term follow-up. Defining responders by clinical measures is confounded by the strong placebo effect seen in the large clinical studies such as MIRACLE, where 39% of the control arm were considered to have improved by one or more clinical endpoints [40]. Yu et al. recently have shown that a reduction in LV end-systolic volume by >10% predicted a significant decease in morbidity and mortality, while standard clinical measures of response failed to do so. In light of this information it appears that volumetric response may be a more robust measure of success [73].

Current practice involves patient selection on the basis of QRS width and morphology, using both as indirect markers of ventricular dyssynchrony. However, the degree of mechanical dyssynchrony is not always reflected in the QRS width, and this may explain some of the observed variability in response to CRT. In patients with severe heart failure, as many as one-third of patients who meet standard criteria for CRT implant may have little or no demonstrable dyssynchrony, while in one-third of patients with RBBB or narrow QRS, significant dyssynchrony may be present [74,75]. As a treatment modality aimed at restoring ventricular synchrony, it is not surprising to note that the strongest independent predictor of response to CRT is the presence of dyssynchrony at baseline. Neither baseline QRS width nor morphology was accurate predictors of response, in keeping with the growing recognition that QRS duration is a poor surrogate for the presence or absence of mechanical dyssynchrony [76]. Achilli et al. have shown that in patients with significant dyssynchrony, clinical and volumetric responses were seen to an equal degree in patients with both wide and narrow QRS morphologies [77]. Under current guidelines, however, CRT would not be offered to patients with LV dyssynchrony and narrow QRS complexes. It should be noted that there is some controversy about the importance of mechanical dyssynchrony as a predictor of response, and some have correctly pointed out that randomized trials need to be conducted before current guidelines can be changed [78].

Simply stated, the best modality to define dyssynchrony has yet to be validated. Imaging modalities including the echocardiogram, tissue Doppler, tissue strain imaging, speckle tracking, nuclear imaging, and MRI have been employed (Table 1.3). Echocardiography with tissue Doppler imaging is currently the methodology most likely to replace QRS duration [79]. In small studies, each of these methods of defining dyssynchrony has shown promising ability in predicting responders. The PROSPECT study [80] will individually and prospectively evaluate the prognostic accuracy of a variety of echocardiographic and tissue Doppler imaging parameters in an effort to determine the best method to diagnose dyssynchrony.

Demographic factors such as age, sex, baseline EF, or the presence of AF have shown little or no prognostic significance [81]. On the other hand, the etiology of the patient's cardiomyopathy has been shown to predict response [82]. Patients with idiopathic dilated cardiomyopathies seem to have a greater, more homogenous response to CRT than patients with ischemic heart disease. This may be related to the progressive nature of coronary artery disease, or (more likely) due to the presence of scar in the region of the LV targeted for pacing. In this population, the amount of viable myocardium, both globally and in the lateral wall, has been shown to predict response to CRT [83,84]. End-stage heart failure (NYHA class IV), severe mitral regurgitation and LV end-diastolic dimensions greater than 75 mm all were independent predictors of non-response [85]. In the CARE-HF trial [43], the effect of CRT on progression to heart transplantation was not significant. The resynchronization arm of CARE-HF had fewer emergent heart transplants (1 vs 3), but the same number of transplanted patients overall. However, in one report of 34 patients enrolled in the CRT arm of a major clinical study and who met indications for heart transplantation, only 2 still met criteria after 6 months [86]. In these patients being considered for heart transplantation, the duration of response is not known, and concerns remain that CRT may simply delay the need for heart transplantation, ultimately disqualifying some patients from transplant eligibility due to advanced age.

Special populations

Patients with AF

AF is a common occurrence with heart failure. However, most of the major clinical trials on cardiac resynchronization excluded patients with AF. Most of the smaller trials on patients with AF included mostly patients who had previously undergone AV node ablation for difficulty in rate control or patients who had combined AF and bradycardia [87,88]. The PAVE trial [89] enrolled patients with chronic (>30 days) AF who had undergone AV junction ablation and pacemaker implantation for rate control, and limited exercise capacity in spite of medical therapy. EF was not an inclusion criteria and the average EF was 46%. CRT resulted in improved 6-minute walk distance and higher LVEF at 6 months, compared to RV pacing. These benefits were limited to patients with EF $\leq$ 45% and NYHA class $\geq$II. At 6 months of follow-up, patients with CRT had a significantly higher EF than patients with RV leads only (46% vs 41%, $p = 0.03$). There was no significant difference in mortality or in complications.

Few data are available on the effects of resynchronization in patients with AF without a standard pacing indication. In one study, clinical response to CRT was not different in sinus rhythm versus AF [90], about half of whom had undergone AV nodal ablation. It is not the irregularity of R–R intervals but the rapidity of the heart rate in AF that impacts most on LVEF [91]. Therefore, even with the use of cardiac resynchronization in patients with heart failure and AF, rate control remains extremely important. Features available in many CRT devices designed to provide biventricular pacing even during rapid rates in AF (such as "sense assurance," "conducted AF response," and "rate regulation") have not been proven to be of clinical benefit. The positive effects of CRT in patients with AF continue for at least 12 months [92]. Although left atrial remodeling after CRT in patients with chronic AF has been described, it is a small minority of patients who will show spontaneous conversion to sinus rhythm [93].

Patients with LV dysfunction and standard pacing indications

The detrimental effects of RV pacing-induced dyssynchrony are now firmly established, as

Table 1.3 Criteria for dyssynchrony and response.

Author (year)	N	Definition of responders	Follow-up	Modality	Criteria	Cutoff	Methodology of cutoff	Sensitivity (%)	Specificity (%)
Pitzalis M (2002)	20	↓LVVs index ≥ 15%	1 mo	M-mode at short-axis view	Septoposterior delay in systole	130 ms	Derived from ROC curve of study population	100	63
Bax JJ (2003)	25	Absolute ↑EF ≥ 5%	1 day	TDI	Septolateral delay in Ts (ejection phase)	60 ms	Derived from study population	76	87.5
Yu CM (2003)	30	↓LVVs > 15%	3 mo	TDI	Ts-SD of six basal, six mid-LV segments	32.6 ms	+2 SD from mean of 88 normal controls	100	100
Yu CM (2004)	54	↓LVVs > 15%	3 mo	TDI		31.4 ms	Derived from ROC curve of study population	96	78
Penicka M (2004)	49	Relative ↑EF ≥ 25%	6 mo	TDI	Ts (onset) of BS, BL, BP, and BRV by summation of inter- and intraventricular delay	102 ms	Derived from study population	96	71
Nortabartolo D (2004)	49	↓LVVs > 15%	3 mo	TDI	Maximal difference in Ts in six basal segments (both ejection phase and postsystolic shortening)	110 ms	Derived from study population	97	55

(Cont.)

Table 1.3 (*Continued*)

Author (year)	N	Definition of responders	Follow-up	Modality	Criteria	Cutoff	Methodology of cutoff	Sensitivity (%)	Specificity (%)
Gorcsan J III (2004)	29	↑Stroke volume ≥ 25%	Acute (within 48 h)	TSI	Septoposterior delay (both ejection phase and postsystolic shortening)	65 ms	Derived from 15 pilot patients	87	100
Yu CM (2005)	56	↓LVVs > 15%	3 mo	TSI	(1) Lateral wall delay	(1) Qualitative	(1) Qualitative	47	89
					(2) Ts-SD of six basal, six mid-LV segments	(2) 34.4 ms	(2) Derived from ROC curve of study population	87	81

BS, basal septal; BL, basal lateral; BP, basal posterior; BRV, basal right ventricular; EF, ejection fraction; LV, left ventricular; LVVs, left ventricular end-systolic volume; ROC, receiver operating curve; TDI, tissue Doppler imaging; TSI, tissue synchronization imaging; Ts, time to peak myocardial systolic velocity; Ts(onset), time to onset of myocardial systolic velocity; Ts-SD, standard deviation of time to peak myocardial systolic velocity.
Reproduced with permission from [72].

reported in the DAVID [94] and other trials. The HOBIPACE trial [95] examined CRT in patients with CHF and standard pacing indications using a randomized, crossover study design. Compared to RV pacing, CRT led to significant improvements in the study's primary (LV end-systolic volume, LVEF, and Vo$_2$max) and secondary (NT-proBNP, NYHA class, quality of life, and exercise capacity) endpoints.

Patients with class I–II CHF

Subgroup analysis of CRT trials suggested that in patients with mild heart failure symptoms with a wide QRS complex and an implantable cardioverter-defibrillator (ICD) indication, CRT did not alter exercise capacity but did result in significant improvement in cardiac structure and function and composite clinical response over 6 months [96]. Based on such observations, the role of resynchronization therapy in patients with class I–II CHF is currently being examined with several ongoing clinical trials, most notably the MADIT-CRT trial [97], where patients with NYHA class I or II heart failure are being randomly assigned to treatment with CRT-D versus dual chamber defibrillators.

Patients with narrow QRS

Recognizing that the QRS duration may be a poor surrogate for mechanical dyssynchrony, data are accumulating from a few studies that have specifically examined the effect of resynchronization therapy on patients with narrow QRS complexes, but with mechanical dyssynchrony by echocardiogram. In one study, there was similar and significant improvement in NYHA class, LVEF, LV end-diastolic volume, mitral regurgitation area, deceleration time, interventricular delay in all patients, irrespective of baseline QRS duration [77]. Similarly, preliminary reports from a multicenter study [98] and other studies [99,100] suggest that about half of the patients with a narrow QRS complex will benefit from CRT, and baseline QRS duration does not predict favorable response.

Patients with RBBB as the qualifying wide QRS

The majority of patients enrolled in major CRT trials (>85%) had either LBBB or nonspecific intraventricular conduction delay on the initial echocardiogram. Patients with RBBB, therefore, were clearly underrepresented in these trials, and it would seem intuitively obvious that delayed RV activation with preserved LV activation would be unlikely to benefit from the placement of an LV pacing lead. In keeping with this, a recent meta-analysis suggested that except for NYHA functional class, patients with RBBB as the qualifying wide QRS did not show any improvement in objective measurements (VO$_2$, 6-min walk distance, LVEF, and norepinephrine levels) studied at 3 or 6 months [101]. However, as discussed above, the presence of an RBBB pattern on the echocardiogram does not mean that left bundle conduction is normal and that intraventricular conduction delays are often present in the failing LV. This is why some have argued that until prospective data are available, all patients with wide QRS complexes should be offered CRT according to current guidelines.

Limitations and complications

Clinically, the success rate of transvenous LV lead placement is approximately 90% [102], although distortion of right atrial anatomy and severe tricuspid dilation/regurgitation from long-standing CHF can lead to difficulty in cannulation of the ostium of the coronary sinus (see Table 1.2). Vein branch size, presence of valves, venous tortuosity, or phrenic nerve stimulation may complicate or prevent LV lead deployment. Complications include infection, pneumothorax, bleeding, lead dislodgement, and dissection or perforation of the coronary venous system [103]. Coronary sinus or venous trauma is usually of little consequence, especially in patients with prior open heart surgery where the pericardial space is often obliterated, and usually allows successful completion of the procedure. Tamponade and death are rare [104].

Epicardial LV pacing, by reversing the normal endocardium-to-epicardium depolarization sequence, has raised theoretical concerns about proarrhythmia [105]. The QT interval, dispersion of refractoriness, and ventricular premature depolarization frequency were increased in one study with LV epicardial and biventricular pacing compared to RV pacing [106], and case reports have described torsade de pointes after CRT. However, other studies have demonstrated that

CRT is beneficial in reducing the dispersion of refractoriness compared to LV pacing alone [107]. In addition, analysis of the CONTAK CD and InSync ICD studies demonstrated no increase in polymorphic ventricular tachycardia in CRT patients [108]. Recent data from body surface mapping suggest that CRT improves transmural dispersion of repolarization [109].

Cost-effectiveness of CRT

To understand the cost-effectiveness of resynchronization therapy, intent-to-treat data from the COMPANION trial were modeled to estimate the cost-effectiveness of CRT-D and CRT-P relative to optimal pharmacological therapy over a 7-year base-case treatment episode [110]. Exponential survival curves were derived from trial data and adjusted by quality-of-life trial results to yield quality-adjusted life years (QALYs). For the first 2 years, follow-up hospitalizations were based on trial data. The model assumed equalized hospitalization rates beyond 2 years. Initial implantation and follow-up hospitalization costs were estimated using Medicare data.

Over 2 years, follow-up hospitalization costs were reduced by 29% for CRT-D and 37% for CRT-P. Extending the cost-effectiveness analysis to a 7-year base-case time period, the ICER (incremental cost-effectiveness ratio) for CRT-P was $19,600 per QALY and the ICER for CRT-D was $43,000 per QALY relative to optimal pharmacological therapy. These results were slightly lower but consistent with data derived by Sanders et al. looking at eight studies of implantable cardioverter-defibrillation [111].

Thus, the use of CRT-P and CRT-D was associated with a cost-effectiveness ratio below generally accepted benchmarks for therapeutic interventions of $50,000 per QALY to $100,000 per QALY. This suggests that the clinical benefits of CRT-P and CRT-D can be achieved at a reasonable cost.

Recent advances, future directions, and conclusions

Newer generations of CRT devices also provide important information regarding a patient's heart failure status. Indices such as average nighttime vs daytime heart rates and heart rate variability offer clues to a patient's clinical status. In addi-

tion, measurement and trending of transthoracic impedance (resistance to current flow between the device and the RV lead) may be reasonably reflective of "lung wetness" [112]. Some devices have proprietary algorithms that may be useful in alerting physicians about impending worsening of heart failure, although preliminary data suggest that unfiltered shock impedance trends may also provide similar information [113].

As many as 40% of patients referred to heart failure and transplant clinicians meet the 2002 ACC/AHA/NASPE guidelines for biventricular pacing [114]. In the past 12 years, CRT has been convincingly shown to improve both the functional and symptomatic consequences of heart failure and also to effect beneficial structural changes in the failing ventricle. The mortality benefit accrued from CRT rivals that from proven pharmacologic interventions such as beta-blockade and ACE-inhibition [59]. The addition of defibrillation therapy provides an incremental improvement in survival, likely due to the reduction in sudden arrhythmic deaths. In the absence of optimal medical management the beneficial effects of resynchronization and defibrillation are blunted, highlighting the importance on continued optimal medical therapy [42]. Better tools are needed to identify which patients with heart failure have significant dyssynchrony. An effective method will allow for the recognition of patients with a "normal" QRS who would also benefit from CRT, and possibly guide electrophysiologists in selecting optimal LV pacing sites, as being studied in the RETHINQ trial [115]. When endovascular choices for lead positioning are limited by patient-specific anatomy, venoplasty or surgical epicardial lead placement remains an effective alternative [116]. Optimization of the AV interval and sequential LV–RV timing may improve the overall rate and degree of response.

The future is likely to see continued broadening of the patient populations selected for resynchronization therapy. It is hoped that QRS duration will be replaced by echocardiographic parameters of dyssynchrony as qualifying criteria for patient selection for resynchronization therapy. Initiation of resynchronization therapy at earlier stages of CHF may, by ending the negative cascade of events caused by electrical and mechanical dyssynchrony, prevent progression of disease.

In conclusion, the assessment of ventricular dyssynchrony should be part of the initial evaluation of patients presenting with systolic LV dysfunction. Patients with dyssynchrony should be offered CRT as an important adjunct to medical management, both for symptomatic improvement and for mortality benefit. Evidence of volumetric response, including improvement in EF and reduction of LV end-systolic volumes by >10%, should be considered as the primary goal of the treatment. With the improvement in operator experience and implantation tools, CRT can be safely performed percutaneously in nearly 95% of patients, and conservative estimates of its cost-effectiveness are on par with other lifesaving medical treatments such as hemodialysis.

References

1. de Teresa E, Chamorro JL, Pulpon A, *et al.* An even more physiological pacing: changing the sequence of ventricular activation. In: Steinbach K, editor. Cardiac Pacing: Proceedings of the 7th World Symposium on Cardiac Pacing, Vienna. Darmstadt, Germany: Dr Dietrich Steinkopff Verlag, GmbH & Co. K.G.; 1983:395–401.

2. Rosenbush S, Ruggie N, Turner D, *et al.* Sequence and timing of ventricular wall motion in patients with bundle branch block: assessment by radionuclide cineangiography. Circulation 1982;66:1113–1119.

3. Xiao HB, Brecker SJ, Gibson DG. Differing effects of right ventricular pacing and left bundle branch block on left ventricular function. Br Heart J 1993;69:166–173.

4. Burkhoff D, Oikawa RY, Sagawa K. Influence of pacing site on canine left ventricular contraction. Am J Physiol 1986;251:H428–H435.

5. Park RC, Little WC, O'Rourke RA. Effect of alteration of the left ventricular activation sequence on the left ventricular end-systolic pressure–volume relation in closed-chest dogs. Circ Res 1985;57:706–717.

6. Lattuca JJ, Cohen TJ, Mower MM. Biventricular pacing to improve cardiac hemodynamics. Clin Res 1990;38:882A.

7. Hochleitner M, Hortnogl H, Ng CK, *et al.* Usefulness of physiologic dual-chamber pacing in drug-resistant idiopathic dilated cardiomyopathy. Am J Cardiol 1990;66:198–202.

8. Hochleitner M, Hortnagl H, Hortnagl H, Fridrich L, Gschnitzer F. Long-term efficacy of physiologic dual-chamber pacing in the treatment of end-stage idiopathic dilated cardiomyopathy. Am J Cardiol 1992;15:1320–1325.

9. Lindle C, Gadler F, Edner M, *et al.* Results of atrioventricular synchronous pacing with optimized delay in patients with severe congestive heart failure. Am J Cardiol May 1, 1995;75:919–923.

10. Innes D, Leitch JW, Fletcher PJ. VDD pacing at short atrioventricular intervals does not improve cardiac output in patients with dilated heart failure. Pacing Clin Electrophysiol 1994;17:959–965.

11. Gold MR, Feliciano Z, Gottlieb SS, *et al.* Dual chamber pacing with a short atrioventricular delay in congestive hear failure: a randomized study. J Am Coll Cardiol 1995;26:967–973.

12. Gold MR, Shorofsky SR, Metcalf MD, *et al.* The acute hemodynamic effects of right ventricular septal pacing in patients with congestive heart failure secondary to ischemic or idiopathic dilated cardiomyopathy. Am J Cardiol 1997;79:679–681.

13. De Cock CC, Giudici MC, Twisk JW. Comparison of the haemodynamic effects of right ventricular outflow-tract pacing with right ventricular apex pacing: a quantitative review. Europace 2003;5:275–278.

14. Occhetta E, Bortnik M, Magnani A, *et al.* Prevention of ventricular desynchronization by permanent para-hisian pacing after atrioventricular node ablation in chronic atrial fibrillation. J Am Coll Cardiol 2006;47:1938–1945.

15. Caqeau S, Ritter P, Bakdach H, *et al.* Four chamber pacing in dilated cardiomyopathy. Pacing Clin Electrophysiol 1994;17:1974–1979.

16. Foster AH, Gold MR, McLaughlin JS. Acute hemodynamic effects of atrio-biventricular pacing in humans. Ann Thorac Surg 1995;59:294–300.

17. Leclercq C, Cazeau S, Le Breton H, *et al.* Acute hemodynamic effects of biventricular DDD pacing in patients with end stage heart failure. J Am Coll Cardiol 1998;32:1825–1831.

18. Blanc JJ, Etienne Y, Gilard M, *et al.* Evaluation of different ventricular pacing sites in patients with severe heart failure: results of an acute hemodynamic study. Circulation 1997;96:3273–3277.

19. Daubert JC, Ritter P, Le Breton H, *et al.* Permanent left ventricular pacing with transvenous leads inserted into the coronary veins. Pacing Clin Electrophysiol 1998;21:239–245.

20. Hunt SA, Abraham WT, Chin MH, *et al.* ACC/AHA 2005 guideline update for the diagnosis and management of chronic heart failure in the adult: a report of the American College of Cardiology/American Heart Association Task Force on Practice Guidelines. Circulation 2005;112:e154–e235.

21. Baldasseroni S, Opasich C, Gorini M, *et al.* Left bundle branch-block is associated with increased 1-year sudden and total mortality rate in 5517 outpatients

with congestive heart failure: a report from the Italian network on congestive heart failure. Am Heart J 2002;143:398–405

22. Prinzen FW, Hunter WC, Wyman BT, *et al.* Mapping of regional myocardial strain and work during ventricular pacing: experimental study using magnetic resonance tagging. J Am Coll Cardiol 1999;33:1735–1742.

23. Curry CW, Nelson GS, Wyman BT, *et al.* Mechanical dyssynchrony in dilated cardiomyopathy with intraventricular conduction delay as depicted by 3D tagged magnetic resonance imaging. Circulation 2000;101:e2

24. Nelson GS, Curry C, Wyman B, *et al.* Predictors of systolic augmentation from left ventricular pre-excitation in patients with dilated cardiomyopathy and intraventricular conduction delay. Circulation 2000;101:2703–2709.

25. Vernooy K, Verbeek X, Peschar M, *et al.* Left bundle branch block induces ventricular remodeling and functional septal hypoperfusion. Euro Heart J 2004;26:91–98.

26. Nowak B, Sinha A, Schaefer W, *et al.* Cardiac resynchronization therapy homogenizes myocardial glucose metabolism and perfusion in dilated cardiomyopathy and left bundle branch block. J Am Coll Cardiol 2003;41:1523–1528.

27. Ukkonen H, Beanlands R, Burwash I, *et al.* Effect of cardiac resynchronization on myocardial efficiency and regional oxidative metabolism. Circulation 2003;107:28–31.

28. Sarubbi B, Ducceschi V, Santangelo L, *et al.* Arrhythmias in patients with mechanical ventricular dysfunction and myocardial stretch: roles of mechano-electric feedback. Can J Cardiol 1998;14:245–252

29. Aaronson KD, Schwartz JS, Chen TM, *et al.* Development and prospective validation of a clinical index to predict survival in ambulatory patients referred for cardiac transplant evaluation. Circulation 1997;95:2597–2599.

30. Dhingra R, Pencina M, Wang T, *et al.* Electrocardiographic QRS duration and the risk of congestive heart failure. Hypertension 2006;47:861–867.

31. Blanc JJ, Fatemi M, Bertault V, Baraket F, Etienne Y. Evaluation of left bundle branch block as a reversible cause of non-ischaemic dilated cardiomyopathy with severe heart failure: a new concept of left ventricular dyssynchrony-induced cardiomyopathy. Europace 2005;7:604–610.

32. Spragg DD, Leclercq C, Loghmani M, *et al.* Regional alterations in protein expression in the dyssynchronous failing heart. Circulation 2003;108:929–932.

33. Prinzen FW, Cheriex EC, Delhaas T, *et al.* Asymmetric thickness of the left ventricular wall resulting from asynchronous electric activation: a study in dogs with ven-

tricular pacing and in patients with left bundle branch block. Am Heart J 1995;130:5:1045–1053.

34. Spragg DD, Akar FG, Helm RH, *et al.* Abnormal conduction and repolarization in late-activated myocardium of dyssynchronously contracting hearts. Cardiovasc Res 2005;67:77–86.

35. Wang Y, Cheng J, Joyner R, Wagner M, Hill J. Remodeling of early-phase repolarization: a mechanism of abnormal impulse conduction in heart failure. Circulation 2006;113:1849–1856.

36. Wiegerinck R, Verkerk A, Belterman C, *et al.* Larger cell size in rabbits with heart failure increases myocardial conduction velocity and QRS duration. Circulation 2006;113:806–813.

37. Higgins SL, Hummel JD, Niazi IK, *et al.* Cardiac resynchronization therapy for the treatment of heart failure in patients with intraventricular conduction delay and malignant ventricular tachyarrhythmias. J Am Coll Cardiol 2003;42:1454–1459.

38. Abraham WT, Young JB, Leon AR. Medtronic InSync ICD cardiac resynchronization system (draft sponsor presentation). US Food and Drug Administration Center for Devices and Radiological Health Circulatory System Devices Advisory Panel Meeting, Gaithersburg, MD, March 5, 2002. Available at: http://www.fda.gov/ohrms/dockets/ac/02/briefing/3843b2.htm.

39. Cazeau S, Leclercq C, Lavergne T, *et al*, for the MUSTIC Study Investigators. Effects of multisite biventricular pacing in patients with heart failure and intraventricular conduction delay. N Engl J Med 2001;344:873–880.

40. Abraham WT, Fisher EG, Smith AL, *et al.* Cardiac resynchronization in chronic heart failure. N Engl J Med 2002;346:1845–1853.

41. Bradley DJ, Bradley EA, Baughman KL, *et al.* Cardiac resynchronization and death from progressive heart failure: a meta-analysis of randomized controlled trials. JAMA 2003;289:730–740.

42. Bristow MR, Saxon LA, Boehmer J, *et al.* Cardiac resynchronization therapy with or without an implantable defibrillator in advanced heart failure. N Engl J Med 2004;350:2140–2150.

43. Cleland JGF, Daubert C, Erdmann E, *et al.* The effect of cardiac resynchronization on morbidity and mortality in heart failure. N Engl J Med 2005;352:1539–1549.

44. Wing-Hong Fung J, Yu C, Yat-Sun Chan J, *et al.* Effects of cardiac resynchronization therapy on incidence of atrial fibrillation in patients with poor left ventricular systolic function. Am J Cardiol 2005;96:728–731.

45. Sinha, A, Skobel, EC, Breithardt O, *et al.* Cardiac resynchronization improves central sleep apnea and Cheyne–Stokes respiration in patients with chronic heart failure. J Am Coll Cardiol 2004;44:68–71.

46. Healey JS, Davies RA, Tang ASL. Improvement of apparently fixed pulmonary hypertension with cardiac resynchronization therapy. J Heart Lung Transplant 2004;23:650–652.

47. Janousek J, Tomek V, Chaoupecky V, et al. Cardiac resynchronization therapy: a novel adjunct to the treatment and prevention of right ventricular failure. J Am Coll Cardiol 2004;44:1927–1931.

48. Bleeker GB, Shalij MJ, Nihoyannopoulos P, et al. Left ventricular dyssynchrony predicts right ventricular remodeling after cardiac resynchronization therapy. J Am Coll Cardiol 2005;46:2264–2269.

49. Kass DA, Chen C, Curry, C, et al. Improved left ventricular mechanics from acute VDD pacing in patients with dilated cardiomyopathy and ventricular conduction delay. Circulation 1999;99:1567–1573.

50. Nelson GS, Berger RD, Fetics BJ, Talbot M, Hare JM, Soinelli JCKDA. Left ventricular or biventricular pacing improves cardiac function at diminished energy cost in patients with dilated cardiomyopathy and left bundle-branch block. Circulation 2000;102:3053–3059.

51. Young JB, Abraham WT, Smith AL, et al. Combined cardiac resynchronization and implantable cardioversion defibrillation in advanced chronic heart failure: the MIRACLE ICD Trial. JAMA 2003;289:2694.

52. Breithardt OA Sinha AM, Schwammenthal E et al. Acute effects of cardiac resynchronization therapy on functional mitral regurgitation in advanced systolic heart failure. J Am Coll Cardiol 2003;41:765–770.

53. Kanzaki H, Bazaz R, Schwartzman D, Dohi K, Sade LE, Gorcsan J. A mechanism for immediate reduction in mitral regurgitation after cardiac resynchronization therapy: insights from mechanical activation strain mapping. J Am Coll Cardiol 2004;44:1619–1625.

54. Lancelloti P, Melon P, Sakalihasan N, et al. Effect of cardiac resynchronization therapy on functional mitral regurgitation in heart failure. Am J Cardiol 2004;94:1462–1465.

55. Cabrera-Bueno F, Garcia-Pinilla JM, Pena-Hernandez J, et al. Repercussion of functional mitral regurgitation on reverse remodelling in cardiac resynchronization therapy [online]. Europace June 15, 2007; eum122v1.

56. Ennezat P-V, Gal B, Kouakam C, et al. Cardiac resynchronisation therapy reduces functional mitral regurgitation during dynamic exercise in patients with chronic heart failure: an acute echocardiographic study. Heart August 1, 2006;92(8):1091–1095.

57. Waggoner AD, Faddis MN, Gleva MJ, et al. Cardiac resynchronization therapy acutely improves diastolic function. J Am Soc Echocardiogr 2005;18:216–220.

58. Yu C-M, Fang F, Zhang Q et al. Improvement of atrial function and atrial reverse remodeling after cardiac resynchronization therapy for heart failure. J Am Coll Cardiol 2007;50:778–785.

59. Ellenbogen KA, Wood MA, Klein HU. Why should we care about CARE-HF? J Am Coll Cardiol 2005;46:2199–2203.

60. Grassi G, Vincenti A, Brambilla R, et al. Sustained sympathoinhibitory effects of cardiac resynchronization therapy in severe heart failure. Hypertension 2004;44:L727–L731.

61. Gould PA, Kong G, Kalff V, et al. Improvement in cardiac adrenergic function post biventricular pacing for heart failure [online]. Europace May 21, 2007; eum081v1.

62. Fantoni C, Raffa S, Regoli F, et al. Cardiac resynchronization therapy improves heart rate profile and heart rate variability with moderate to severe heart failure. J Am Coll Cardiol 2005;46:1875–1882.

63. Sinha AM, Skobel EC, Breithardt OA, et al. Cardiac resynchronization therapy improves central sleep apnea and Cheyne–Stokes respiration in patients with chronic heart failure. J Am Coll Cardiol 2004;44:68–71.

64. Healey JS, Davies RA, Tang ASL. Improvement of apparently fixed pulmonary hypertension with cardiac resynchronization therapy. J Heart Lung Transplant 2004;23:650–652.

65. Bleeker GB, Schalij MJ, Nihoyannopoulos P et al. Left ventricular dyssynchrony predicts right ventricular remodeling after cardiac resynchronization therapy. J Am Coll Cardiol 2005;46:2264–2269.

66. Janousek J, Tomek V, Chaloupecky V, et al. Cardiac resynchronization therapy: a novel adjunct to the treatment and prevention of systemic right ventricular failure. J Am Coll Cardiol 2004;44:1927–1931.

67. Fung J, Yu C, Chan J, et al. Effects of cardiac resynchronization therapy on incidence of atrial fibrillation in patients with poor left ventricular systolic function. Am J Cardiol 2005;96:728–731.

68. Mykytsey A, Maheshwari P, Dhar G, et al. Ventricular tachycardia induced by biventricular pacing in patient with severe ischemic cardiomyopathy. J Cardiovasc Electrophysiol 2005;16(6):655–658.

69. Shukla G, Chaudhry G, Orlov M, Hoffmeister P, Haffajee C. Potential proarrhythmic effect of biventricular pacing: fact or myth? Heart Rhythm 2; 9: 951–956.

70. Gregoratos G, Abrams J, Epstein AE, et al. ACC/AHA/NASPE 2002 Guideline update for implantation of cardiac pacemakers and antiarrhythmia devices— summary article. A report of the American College of Cardiology/American Heart Association Task Force on Practice Guidelines (ACC/AHA/NASPE Committee to Update the 1998 Pacemaker Guidelines). Circulation 2002;106(16):2145–2161.

71. Hunt SA, Abraham WT, Chin MH, *et al*. ACC/AHA 2005 Guideline update for the diagnosis and management of chronic heart failure in the adult—summary article. A report of the American College of Cardiology/American Heart Association Task Force on Practice Guidelines (Writing Committee to Update the 2001 Guidelines for the Evaluation and Management of Heart Failure): developed in collaboration with the American College of Chest Physicians and the International Society for Heart and Lung Transplantation: endorsed by the Heart Rhythm Society. Circulation September 20, 2005;112(12):1825–1852.

72. Yu C, Wing-Hong Fung J, Zhang Q, Sanderson JE. Understanding nonresponders of cardiac resynchronization therapy—current and future perspectives. J Cardiovasc Electrophysiol 2005;16:1117–1124.

73. Yu C, Bleeker GB, Wing-Hong Fung J, *et al*. Left ventricular reverse remodeling but not clinical improvement predicts long-term survival after cardiac resynchronization therapy. Circulation 2005;112:1580–1586.

74. Bleeker GB, Schalij MJ, Molhoek SG, *et al*. Frequency of left ventricular dyssynchrony in patients with heart failure and a normal QRS complex. Am J Cardiol 2005;95:140–142.

75. Ghio S, Constantin C, Klersey C, *et al*. Interventricular and intraventricular dyssynchrony are common in heart failure patients regardless of QRS duration. Eur Heart J 2004;25:571–578.

76. Bax JJ, Marwick TH, Molhoek SG, *et al*. Left ventricular dyssynchrony predicts benefit of cardiac resynchronization in patients with end-stage heart failure before pacemaker implantation. Am J Cadiol 2003;92:1238–1240.

77. Achilli A, Sassara M, Ficili S, *et al*. Long-Term effectiveness of cardiac resynchronization therapy in patients with refractory heart failure and "narrow" QRS. J Am Coll Cardiol 2003;42:2117–2124.

78. Hawkins NM, Petrie MC, MacDonald MR, Hogg KJ, McMurray JJV. Selecting patients for cardiac resynchronization therapy: electrical or mechanical dyssynchrony? Eur Heart J 2006;27:1270–1281.

79. Bax JJ, Ansalone G, Breithardt OA, *et al*. Echocardiographic evaluation of cardiac resynchronization therapy: ready for routine clinical use? A critical appraisal. J Am Coll Cardiol 2004;44:1–9.

80. Yu CM, Abraham WT, Bax J, *et al*. Predictors of response to cardiac resynchronization therapy (PROSPECT)—study design. Am Heart J 2005;149:600–605.

81. Yu C, Fung W, Lin H, Zhang Q, Sanderson JE, Lau C. Predictors of left ventricular remodeling after cardiac resynchronization therapy for heart failure secondary to idiopathic dilated or ischemic cardiomyopathy. Am J Cardiol 2002;91:684–668.

82. St John Sutton MG, Plappert T, Hilpisch KE, Abraham WT, Hayes DL, Chinchoy E. Sustained reverse left ventricular structural remodeling with cardiac resynchronization at one year is a function of etiology: quantitative Doppler echocardiographic evidence from the Multicenter InSync Randomized Clinical Evaluarion (MIRACLE). Circulation 2006;113:266–272.

83. Hummell JP, Linder JR, Belcik JT, *et al*. Extent of myocardial viability predicts response to biventricular pacing in ischemic cardiomyopathy. Heart Rhythm 2005;2:1211–1217.

84. Bleeker GB, Kaandorp TAM, Lamb JH, *et al*. Effect of posterolateral scar tissue on clinical and echocardiographic improvement after cardiac resynchronization therapy. Circulation 2006;113:969–976.

85. Diaz-Infante E, Mont L, Lea J, *et al*. Predictors of lack of response to resynchronization therapy. Am J Cardiol 2005;95:1436–1440.

86. Greenberg, J, Leon AR, Book WM, *et al*. Benefits of cardiac resynchronization therapy in outpatients with indications for heart transplantation. J Heart Lung Transplant 2003;22:1134–1140.

87. Hay I, Melenovsky V, Fetics BJ, *et al*. Short-term effects of right-left heart sequential cardiac resynchronization in patients with heart failure, chronic atrial fibrillation, and atrioventricular nodal block. Circulation 2004;110:3404–3410.

88. Valls-Bertault V, Fatemi M, *et al*. Assessment of upgrading to biventricular pacing in patients with right ventricular pacing and congestive heart failure after atrioventricular junctional ablation for chronic atrial fibrillation. Europace 2004;6(5):438–443.

89. Doshi RN, Daoud E, Fellows C, *et al*. Left ventricular-based cardiac stimulation post AV nodal ablation evaluation. J Cardiovasc Electrophysiol 2005;16:1160–1165.

90. Molhoek S, Bax JJ, Bleeker G, *et al*. Comparison of response to cardiac resynchronization therapy in patients with sinus rhythm versus chronic atrial fibrillation. Am J Cardiol 2004;94:1506–1509.

91. Melenovsky V, Hay I, Fetics B, *et al*. Functional impact of rate irregularity in patients with heart failure and atrial fibrillation receiving cardiac resynchronization therapy. Eur Heart J 2005;26:705–711.

92. Leclercq C, Crocq C, De Place C, *et al*. Long term effects of cardiac resynchronization therapy on atrial and ventricular remodeling in advanced heart failure patients with permanent atrial fibrillation and atrioventricular node ablation. Heart Rhythm 2006;3:S293–S293.

93. Kiès P, Leclercq C, Bleeker GB, *et al*. Cardiac resynchronisation therapy in chronic atrial fibrillation: impact on left atrial size and reversal to sinus rhythm. Heart 2006;92:490–494.

94. Wilkoff BL, Cook JR, Epstein AE, *et al.* Dual-chamber pacing or ventricular backup pacing in patients with an implantable defibrillator: the Dual Chamber and VVI Implantable Defibrillator (DAVID) Trial. JAMA 2002;288:3115–3123.

95. Fung J, Yu, CM, Chan JY, *et al.* Effect of cardiac resynchronization therapy on incidence of atrial fibrillation in patients with poor left ventricular systolic function. Am J Cardiol 2005;96:728–731.

96. Abraham WT, Young JB, León AR, *et al.* Effects of cardiac resynchronization on disease progression in patients with left ventricular systolic dysfunction, an indication for an implantable cardioverter-defibrillator, and mildly symptomatic chronic heart failure. Circulation 2004;110:2864–2868.

97. Moss AJ, Brown MW, Cannom DS, *et al.* Multicenter Automatic Defibrillator Implantation Trial–Cardiac Resynchronization Therapy (MADIT-CRT): design and clinical protocol. Ann Noninvasive Electrocardiol 2005;10:34–43.

98. Cazeau S, Leclercq C, Paul V, *et al.* Identification of potential CRT responders in narrow QRS using simple echo dyssynchrony parameters: preliminary results of the DESIRE study. Heart Rhythm 2006;3:S90.

99. Yu C, Chan Y, Zhang Q, *et al.* Benefits of cardiac resynchronization therapy for heart failure patients with narrow QRS complexes and coexisting systolic asynchrony by echocardiography. J Am Coll Cardiol 2006;48:2251–2257.

100. Bleeker GB, Holman ER, Steendijk P, *et al.* Cardiac resynchronization therapy in patients with a narrow QRS complex. J Am Coll Cardiol 2006;48:2243–2250.

101. Egoavil CA, Ho RT, Greenspon AJ, Pavri BB. Cardiac resynchronization therapy in patients with right bundle branch block: analysis of pooled data from MIRACLE and ContakCD trials. Heart Rhythm 2005: 2:611–615.

102. McAlister FA, Ezekowitz JA, Wiebe N, *et al.* Systematic review: cardiac resynchronization in patients with symptomatic heart failure. Ann Intern Med 2004;141:381–390.

103. Ellery S, Paul V. Complications of biventricular pacing. Eur Heart J Suppl 2004;6:D117–D121.

104. Leon AR, Abraham WT, Curtis AB, *et al.* Safety of transvenous cardiac resynchronization system implantation in patients with chronic heart failure: combined results of over 2000 patients from a multicenter program. J Am Coll Cardiol 2005;46:2348–2356.

105. Fish J, Brugada J, Antzelevitch C. Potential proarrhythmic effects of biventricular pacing. J Am Coll Cardiol 2005;46:2340–2347.

106. Medina-Ravell VA, Lankipalli RS, Yan G-X, *et al.* Effect of epicardial biventricular pacing to prolong QT interval and increase transmural dispersion of repolarization. Does resynchronization therapy pose a risk for patients predisposed to long QT or torsade de pointes? Circulation 2003;107:740–746.

107. Harada M, Osaka T, Yokoyama E, *et al.* Biventricular pacing has an advantage over left ventricular epicardial pacing alone to minimize proarrhythmic perturbation of reporlarization. J Cardiovasc Electrophysiol 2006;17:151–156.

108. Mcswain R, Schwartz R, Delurgio D, *et al.* The impact of cardiac resynchronization on ventricular tachycardia/fibrillation: an analysis from the combined Contak-CD and InSync-ICD studies. J Cardiovasc Electrophysiol 2005;16:1168–1171.

109. Pastore CA, Douglas RA, Samesima N, *et al.* Repercussions of cardiac resynchronization therapy on the ventricular repolarization of heart failure patients as assessed by body surface potential mapping. J Electrocardiol 2007;7(Suppl 1):79–81.

110. Feldman, AM, de Lissovoy, G, Bristow, MR, *et al.* Cost effectiveness of cardiac resynchronization therapy in the Comparison of Medical Therapy, Pacing, and Defibrillation in Heart Failure (COMPANION) Trial. J Am Coll Cardiol 2005;46:2311–2321.

111. Sanders, GD, Hlatky, MA, Owens, DK. Cost-effectiveness of implantable cardioverter-defibrillators. N Engl J Med 2005: 353:1471–1480.

112. Yu C-M, Wang L, Chau E, *et al.* Intrathoracic impedance monitoring in patients with heart failure: correlation with fluid status and feasibility of early warning preceding hospitalization. Circulation 2005;112:841–848.

113. Wicks TM, Hesser R, Pavri BB. Shock impedance trends provide information on heart failure. Heart Rhythm 2007;4: S107.

114. Pedone C, Grigoni F, Boriani G, *et al.* Implications of cardiac resynchronization therapy and prophylactic defibrillator implantation among patients eligible for heart transplantation. Am J Cardiol 2004;93:371–373.

115. St. Jude Medical. Resynchronization Therapy in Normal QRS (RethinQ) Clinical Investigation. Available at: http://clinicaltrials.gov/show/NCT00132977.

116. Leon AR, Delurgio DB, Mera F. Practical approach to implanting left ventricular pacing leads for cardiac resynchronization. J Cardiovasc Electrophysiol 2005;16:100–105.

CHAPTER 2

Implantable Cardioverter-Defibrillator Therapy

Reginald T. Ho, & Arnold J. Greenspon
Jefferson Medical College, Philadelphia, PA, USA

Introduction

Cardiac arrests account for more than 300,000 deaths annually in the United States. Ventricular tachyarrhythmias account for approximately 75% of these cases [1,2]. Rapid defibrillation is the most important determinant of survival for victims of sudden cardiac death (SCD). It is estimated that for every minute of delay in rescue defibrillation an additional 7–10% of lives are lost [3]. Even with resuscitation, survival is poor with less than 20% of patients able to leave the hospital alive [4]. Despite this knowledge, between 1989 and 1998 the percentage of cardiovascular deaths attributed to sudden death in the USA actually increased from 38 to 47% despite an overall decrease in cardiovascular mortality during that same time period [5]. By providing rapid defibrillation of malignant arrhythmias, the implantable cardioverter-defibrillator (ICD) has become the treatment of choice for sudden death protection. The purpose of this chapter is to discuss the (1) history of the ICD, (2) primary prevention ICD trials, (3) secondary prevention ICD trials, and (4) future directions of the ICD.

History of the ICD

The first human ICD implantation was performed in 1980 [6]. It required surgical implantation of epicardial pacing leads and defibrillator patches tunneled subcutaneously to an ICD generator, which,

because of its large size, had to be inserted into the abdomen. Significant morbidity and mortality associated with the procedure and the experimental nature of the clinical investigation required that consenting individuals be actual survivors of two sudden death episodes. Development of percutaneously implanted endovascular leads having both high-voltage coils for defibrillation and distal electrodes for rate sensing and pacing (1989) replaced the epicardial system and need for open thoracotomy but a surgeon was still required to create an abdominal pocket [7]. The use of a biphasic waveform for defibrillation along with advances in capacitor design allowed for the development of smaller pulse generators, which could be implanted in the pectoral region (1993). The number of ICD implantations increased dramatically because cardiologists in addition to surgeons could implant them. Dual chamber ICD for patients with bradycardia pacing indications and biventricular ICD for patients requiring resynchronization therapy became available in 1997 and 2000, respectively.

The current ICD generator consists of batteries, capacitors, and sensing and output circuitry hermetically sealed in a titanium can. The capacitors are arranged serially to store energy for defibrillation. Electrical signals from the ICD lead are filtered and amplified for accurate determination of ventricular rate, which when exceeding detection parameters activates device therapy. The ICD generators serve as an active electrode ("hot can") in the shocking vector and therefore are generally implanted in the left pectoral region (Figure 2.1). Use of an active can has significantly lowered the energy requirement for successful defibrillation.

Heart Failure: Device Management. Edited by Arthur Feldman. © 2010 Blackwell Publishing.

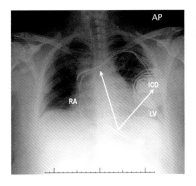

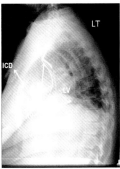

Figure 2.1 Chest radiograph of a biventricular defibrillator system with leads in the right atrium (RA), right ventricle (RV), and epicardial posterolateral left ventricular (LV) vein. Arrows denote the defibrillation vector. ICD, implantable cardioverter-defibrillator generator; AP, Anterior-Posterior; LT, Lateral.

The defibrillator lead contains either one or two high-voltage coils through which the shock energies are delivered and is typically positioned at the right ventricular apex. Distal bipolar electrodes are used for ventricular sensing and pacing. The ICD has programmable zones (also called tiered therapy) allowing selected therapies for different arrhythmias (ventricular tachycardia/ventricular fibrillation, VT/VF). Therapies include (1) anti-tachycardia pacing (ATP) (2) low-energy cardioversion, and (3) high-energy defibrillation (Figures 2.2 and 2.3). During ATP, short bursts of high-output pacing are delivered in an attempt to interrupt VT. Both ATP and low-energy cardioversion can be proarrhythmic and cause acceleration or degeneration of VT to VF. The energy of the first shock in the VF zone is programmed at least 10 J above the defibrillation threshold, which is the lowest amount of energy needed to successfully terminate VF. Subsequent shock energies are usually maximized.

A number of large-scale, multicenter trials have been performed evaluating the effectiveness of ICD on improving survival in patients at high risk for sudden death. These trials can be divided into primary prevention trials (trials studying asymptomatic patients having multiple-risk factors for malignant arrhythmias) and secondary prevention trials (trials studying symptomatic patients who survived a malignant arrhythmia).

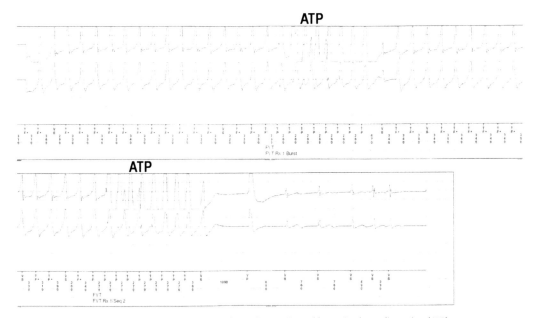

Figure 2.2 Episode of monomorphic ventricular tachycardia terminated by antitachycardia pacing (ATP).

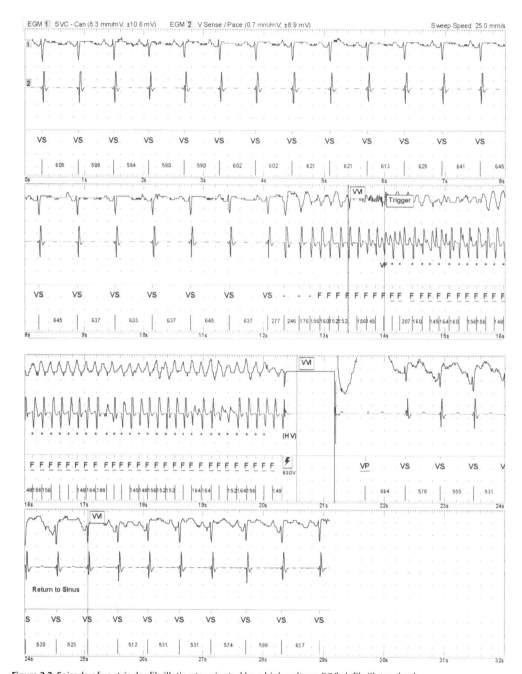

Figure 2.3 Episode of ventricular fibrillation terminated by a high-voltage (HV) defibrillator shock.

Primary prevention ICD trials

Survivors of cardiac arrest are at significant risk for recurrent arrhythmia but represent only a small fraction of the 300,000 sudden deaths per year [8]. There are many more high-risk patients who have not yet had a cardiac arrest. Patients with symptomatic heart failure represent such a high-risk group. In the Framingham study, the sudden death rate for patients with heart failure was seven times that of the general age-adjusted population [9]. In an analysis of 14 studies comprising 1432 patients with cardiomyopathy, the mean mortality rate after follow-up of 4 years was 42%, with 28% of deaths classified as sudden [10]. Intensive medical therapy with angiotensin-converting enzyme inhibitors, β-blockers, and aldosterone antagonists has improved survival by reducing pump failure [11–13]. However, newly diagnosed patients with heart failure still have a 20–25% risk of dying within the first 2.5 years of diagnosis [13]. Approximately half of these deaths are due to malignant ventricular arrhythmias. A primary prevention strategy, directed at these high-risk patients with heart failure, will have a greater impact in terms of preventing sudden death in the population as a whole since this subgroup accounts for a large proportion of the 300,000 who die suddenly [8].

Over the past decade, seven major randomized trials have evaluated the role of the ICD in primary prevention in patients with reduced left ventricular function (Table 2.1). These trials include the Multicenter Automatic Defibrillator Trials (I and II), the Coronary Artery Bypass Graft (CABG) Patch Trial, the Multicenter Unsustained Tachycardia Trial (MUSTT), the Sudden Cardiac Death in Heart Failure Trial (SCD-HeFT), the Defibrillators in Nonischemic Cardiomyopathy Treatment Evaluation (DEFINITE), and the Defibillator in Acute Myocardial Infarction Trial (DINAMIT). These studies demonstrated the superiority of the ICD over antiarrhythmic drugs, principally amiodarone, in preventing SCD in high-risk populations.

The first two large clinical trials to evaluate the effectiveness of the ICD in a high-risk population studied patients with coronary artery disease, prior myocardial infarction, and left ventricular dysfunction who had not yet had a life-threatening arrhythmia. This particular group was targeted because it is estimated that half of the deaths in this population were due to lethal ventricular arrhythmias [14,15]. These two studies, the Multicenter Automatic Defibrillator Implantation Trial (MADIT I) and Multicenter Unsustained Tachycardia Trial (MUSTT), required that patients have both documented spontaneous nonsustained VT as well as sustained VT/VF induced by programmed electrical stimulation (PES). MADIT I was the first large study to evaluate the effectiveness of the ICD versus antiarrhythmic drug [16]. A total of 196 patients with prior myocardial infarction, left ventric-

ular ejection fraction (LVEF) less than 35%, spontaneous nonsustained VT, and inducible, nonsuppressible sustained VT were assigned to receive either an ICD or conventional medical therapy. Conventional medical therapy consisted of amiodarone in 80%, though 46% of these patients ultimately discontinued the drug. During a mean follow-up of 27 months, total mortality was reduced from 34% in the conventional group to 16% in the ICD group (hazard ratio 0.46, 95% CI 0.26–0.82, $p = 0.009$).

A total of 2202 patients were enrolled in the MUSTT study, which was designed to test the hypothesis that antiarrhythmic drug therapy, guided by the results of PES, would reduce sudden death [17]. Patients whose inducible ventricular arrhythmia could not be suppressed with drugs could receive an ICD. There were 767 of 2202 patients (35%) with inducible ventricular arrhythmias of whom 704 were randomized to PES-guided drug therapy or no antiarrhythmic drug therapy. In the drug therapy group, 58% of patients had an ICD at the last follow-up. Improved survival was demonstrated in the antiarrhythmic therapy group. Overall, there was a 7% absolute reduction in the 5-year risk of cardiac arrest or death (hazard ratio 0.73, 95% CI 0.53–0.99, $p < 0.001$). All the survival benefit was due to the ICD and not antiarrhythmic drugs. Antiarrhythmic drug therapy had no effect on survival. In the group of patients receiving the ICD, the 5-year risk of death from all causes was lowered from 55 to 24% (hazard ratio 0.40, 95% CI 0.27–0.59, $p < 0.001$).

A substudy of MADIT Ishowed that patients with an LVEF of 26–35% did not benefit from the ICD while those with a lower EF showed improved survival [18]. These data suggest that those patients with the lowest EF are at the highest risk and the most likely to benefit from the ICD. The second Multicenter Automatic Defibrillator Implantation Trial (MADIT II) used an EF < 30% at least 1 month following an acute myocardial infarction as the sole inclusion criteria [19]. Spontaneous nonsustained ventricular arrhythmias or electrophysiologic studies were not required. Among 1232 patients, the ICD lowered all-cause mortality by 31% (hazard ratio 0.69, 95% C.I. 0.51–0.93, $p = 0.016$).

The three previous randomized clinical trials did not require patients to have a diagnosis of congestive heart failure upon entry into the trial. However,

Table 2.1 Summary of primary prevention ICD trials.

ICD trial	# of patients and Rx arms	Inclusion criteria	Ejection fraction	% CAD	β-blockers	Follow-up and results
MADIT I	$n = 196$ ICD Rx: 95 Conventional Rx: 101	Prior MI EF ≤ 35% NSVT inducible, nonsuppressible ventricular arrhythmias	ICD Rx: 27% Conventional Rx: 25%	100%	ICD Rx: 28% Conventional Rx: 9%	Mean f/u 27 mo: Deaths in ICD Rx: 15 Conventional Rx: 39 ($p = 0.009$)
CABG-Patch	$n = 900$ ICD Rx: 446 Control Rx: 454	Elective CABG EF ≤ 35% Abnormal SAEKG	ICD Rx: 27% Control Rx: 27%	100%	ICD Rx: 18% Control Rx: 24%	Mean f/u 32 mo: Deaths in ICD Rx: 101 Control Rx: 95 ($p = 0.64$)
MUSTT	$n = 704$ EP-guided Rx: drug or ICD No Rx	CAD EF ≤ 40% NSVT	EP-guided Rx: 30% No Rx: 29%	100%	EP-guided Rx: 29% No Rx: 51%	5-yr mortality: ICD Rx: 24% Non-ICD Rx: 55% ($p < 0.001$)
MADIT II	$n = 1232$ ICD Rx: 742 Conventional Rx: 490	Prior MI EF ≤ 30%	ICD Rx: 23% Conventional Rx: 23%	100%	ICD Rx: 70% Conventional Rx: 70%	Mean f/u 20 mo: Mortality rate in ICD Rx: 14.2% Conventional Rx: 19.8% ($p = 0.016$)
SCD-HeFT	$n = 2521$ Conventional Rx + placebo: 847 Conventional Rx + amiodarone: 845 Conventional Rx + ICD: 829	NYHA II or III CHF EF ≤ 35%	Placebo Rx: 25% Amiodarone Rx: 25% ICD Rx: 24%	52%	At enrollment: Placebo Rx: 69% Amiodarone Rx: 69% ICD Rx: 69%	Medial f/u 45.5 mo: Deaths in placebo Rx: 244 Amiodarone Rx: 240 ICD Rx: 182 ICD but not amiodarone reduced risk of death ($p = 0.007$)
DEFINITE	$n = 458$ Medical Rx: 229 Medical Rx + ICD: 229	Nonischemic cardiomyopathy symptomatic CHF EF ≤ 35% PVC's or NSVT	Medical Rx: 22% Medical Rx + ICD: 21%	0%	Medical Rx: 84% Medical Rx + ICD: 86%	Mean f/u 29 mo: Deaths in medical Rx: 40 Medical Rx + ICD: 28 ($p = 0.08$)
DINAMIT	$n = 674$ Non-ICD Rx: 342 ICD Rx: 332	6–40 days post-MI EF ≤ 35% Abnormal autonomic function	Non-ICD Rx: 28% ICD: 28%	100%	Non-ICD Rx: 87% ICD Rx: 87%	Mean f/u 30 mo: Deaths in non-ICD Rx: 58 ICD Rx: 62 ($p = 0.66$)

CAD, coronary artery disease; CABG, coronary artery bypass grafting; CHF, congestve heart failure; EP, electrophysiologic; EF, ejection fraction; f/u, follow-up; ICD, implantable cardioverter-defibrillator; MI, myocardial infarction; PVC, premature ventricular contraction; NSVT, non-sustained ventricular tachycardia; Rx, treatment; SAEKG, signal-averaged electrocardiogram.

approximately two-thirds of patients in these trials were New York Heart Association (NYHA) class II–IV (MADIT I = 65%, MUSTT = 63%, MADIT II = 65%). The Sudden Cardiac Death in Heart Failure Trial (SCD-HeFT) was designed to evaluate the effectiveness of the ICD in improving survival in patients with clinical heart failure [20]. Unlike the previous clinical trials, patients with both ischemic and nonischemic cardiomyopathy were included. Patients with an LVEF < 35% and NYHA class II or III and symptoms for at least 3 months were included. A total of 2521 patients were randomly assigned to the ICD, amiodarone, or placebo. The median duration of follow-up was 45.5 months. The mortality rate in the ICD group was reduced by 23% (hazard ratio 0.77, 95% CI 0.62–0.96, $p = 0.007$). Patients with both ischemic and nonischemic cardiomyopathy benefited though patients with NYHA class II appeared to show more benefit than class III patients.

The Defibrillators in Non-Ischemic Cardiomyopathy Treatment Evaluation (DEFINITE) enrolled 458 patients with nonischemic cardiomyopathy, EF < 35%, and a history of congestive heart failure [21]. Patients were also required to have spontaneous ventricular ectopy. These patients were randomly assigned to standard medical therapy or an ICD. The 2-year mortality in the control group was 14.1%, which was lowered to 7.9% in the ICD group (hazard ratio 0.65, 95% CI 0.40–1.06, $p = 0.08$). Almost all the difference in death was due to a decrease in arrhythmic death. A meta-analysis of all the primary prevention studies focused on the 1854 patients with nonischemic cardiomyopathy [22]. This study concluded that ICD therapy contributed to a 31% reduction in overall mortality. Although these data are pooled from studies with different entry criteria, this meta-analysis concludes that ICD therapy also significantly improves mortality in patients with nonischemic cardiomyopathy.

Two clinical trials failed to show a survival benefit for the ICD. The Coronary-Artery Bypass Graft-Patch Trial (CABG-Patch) studied the effect of a prophylactic ICD on survival in high-risk patients undergoing coronary artery bypass surgery [23]. Epicardial systems were implanted in 900 patients over a 7-year enrollment period (1990–1997). Patients had clinical characteristics similar to those entered into the MADIT trials. Congestive heart failure (NYHA class II or III) was present in 73% of patients. The ICD had no impact on survival with a 2-year actuarial mortality of 18%. The effect of the ICD on mortality in patients with recent myocardial infarction was studied in the Defibrillator in Acute Myocardial Infarction Trial (DINAMIT) [24]. Patients ($n = 674$) with a recent acute myocardial infarction (6–40 days) and an LVEF < 35% were randomly assigned to an ICD or standard medical therapy. There was no difference in overall survival during the follow-up period (30 ± 13 mo) although the ICD was associated with a reduction in arrhythmic death. Although the reasons for the failure of the ICD to improve survival in these two trials is unclear, the data suggest that the risk factors for sudden death are quite complex and that there may be factors other than poor left ventricular function, such as ischemia or recent myocardial infarction, which have a major impact on outcome.

Summary of primary prevention ICD trials

The seven major randomized clinical trials of the ICD for primary prevention randomized 5840 patients. The entry criteria varied but focused on an EF < 30–35% as a marker of left ventricular dysfunction. These studies demonstrate that the ICD is associated with a 28% relative risk reduction in overall mortality [25]. The average 2-year mortality was 17.3% in the standard medical therapy group and 14.3% in the ICD group, which translates to a 3% absolute reduction in mortality. These data indicate that the ICD provides a significant reduction in mortality in patients with left ventricular dysfunction, regardless of whether they present with ischemic or nonischemic cardiomyopathy.

The ICD for primary prevention: some unanswered questions

While the ICD reduces mortality in patients with heart failure, a number of questions remain.

Is LVEF the sole risk factor for SCD? The major randomized clinical trials of the ICD for primary prevention utilized LVEF as the major criterion for study entry. It is well known that the 1-year mortality following myocardial infarction markedly rises as the EF falls below 40% [26]. But is EF the sole risk factor for SCD? In a prospective analysis of cardiac arrest, more than half of the deaths in patients with coronary artery disease occurred in those with an EF > 30% [27]. In 20% of patients the EF was normal. In MUSTT, mortality was greater in patients with an EF < 30% as compared to those with an EF between 30 and 40%. However, the percentage of death due to arrhythmia was equally common in both groups. Furthermore, patients with an EF > 30% who had inducible sustained VT had a similar risk of SCD as those with an EF < 30%. Therefore, a low EF was not solely responsible for an increased risk of arrhythmic death. Low EF alone does not predict a high event rate. In the two largest ICD primary prevention clinical trials, the major entry criterion was EF. In MADIT II, an EF < 30% identified a control group with a 20-month mortality rate of 19.8% (annual mortality rate = 12%), while in SCD-HeFT an EF < 35% identified a control group with a 5-year mortality of 36.1% (annual mortality = 7.2%). In MUSTT, the finding of low EF alone predicted a 2-year total mortality of 6.2% and a 2-year event rate for cardiac arrest or arrhythmic death of only 3.5%. Therefore, EF alone is not an ideal predictor of sudden death.

Can other risk factors for cardiac arrest besides low EF help identify a higher risk group? In MADIT I, the annual mortality rate in the control group was 16%, while SCD-HeFT observed a much lower annual mortality rate of 7.2%. What accounts for these differences? The differing observed event rates among the control groups suggest that there must be important clinical risk factors in addition to EF. It is well recognized that cardiac arrest arises from the complex interaction of myocardial substrate, triggers in the form of premature ventricular contractions, and transient modulating factors such as ischemia [28]. EF is one measurement of an abnormal myocardial substrate. Triggers can be analyzed from ambient electrocardiographic recordings. There are data to suggest that complex ventricular ectopy is associated with poor outcome in patients with prior myocardial infarction [13]. Finally, transient modulating factors may include such factors as ischemia, electrolytes, and catecholamines. Predicting cardiac arrest is exceedingly difficult and complex as myocardial substrate, triggers, and modulating factors change over time. The MUSTT investigators identified clinical predictors of a poor outcome [29]. These factors included digitalis therapy, EF < 30%,

left bundle branch block or other intraventricular conduction delay, age > 65 years, and nonsustained VT while hospitalized. Other clinical factors such as cigarette smoking, hypertension, left ventricular hypertrophy, intraventricular conduction delay, and age have been associated with a higher risk for sudden death [28]. Clinical heart failure seems to place patients at particular risk [5,30]. These data suggest that we may be able to develop a clinical algorithm to more accurately assess the risk for sudden death. EF would be one but not the only element.

Are there clinical tests to assess the risk for sudden death? In MUSTT, inducibility to sustained VT predicted a poor outcome. A variety of noninvasive tests have also been evaluated to assess arrhythmic risk [31]. These include the signal-averaged electrocardiogram to detect late potentials, T-wave alternans, and heart rate variability. It remains to be determined whether a single or group of tests will improve patient selection for ICD implantation.

Is the ICD cost-effective? ICD implantation is associated with a low rate of complications ranging from 2 to 5% [18,20]. Inappropriate shocks due to lead complications or transient atrial tachyarrhythmias may also occur. Nonetheless, ICD implantation is associated with an improved quality of life [32]. In addition, cost analyses from the major clinical trials suggest that the ICD compares favorably with other acceptable therapies. Investigators from MADIT II reported that during the 3.5-year study the ICD resulted in a cost of $235,000 per year of life saved. When projected to 12 years, the cost fell to a range of $78,600–114,000 [33]. In SCD-HeFT, cost analysis also concluded that the ICD compared favorably with a cost of $38,389 per year of life saved [34]. Further efforts to improve risk stratification should improve this number.

Secondary prevention ICD trials

Patients who have suffered a cardiac arrest due to VT or VF are at particularly high risk for a recurrent event [8]. Evaluation of the patient having suffered a malignant ventricular arrhythmia involves identifying and treating reversible triggers, understanding the underlying cardiac substrate including ventricular function, and, if possible, securing electrocardiographic documentation of the arrhythmia. Triggers of ventricular arrhythmias

Table 2.2 Summary of secondary prevention ICD trials.

ICD Trial	# of patients and Rx arms	Inclusion criteria	Ejection fraction	% CAD	Medications	Follow-up and results
CASH	n = 230 ICD Rx: 59 (26%) Drug Rx: 171 (74%) Amiodarone: 56 Metoprolol: 59 Propafenone: 56	SCD survivors	ICD Rx: 42% Drug Rx Amiodarone: 38% Metoprolol: 44% Propafenone: 43%	ICD Rx: 41% Drug Rx Amiodarone: 45% Metoprolol: 50% Propafenone: 46%	Amiodarone 400–600 mg/day Metoprolol ≤ 200 mg/day Propafenone ≤ 900 mg/day	Mean f/u 11 mo: No mortality difference among ICD, amiodarone, and metoprolol). Propafenone associated with increased risk of death
AVID	n = 1016 ICD Rx: 507 (50%) Drug Rx 509 (50%)	Resuscitated VF Unstable VT	ICD Rx: 32% Drug Rx: 31%	ICD Rx: 81% Drug Rx: 81%	Drug Rx Amiodarone: 95.8% Sotalol: 2.8%	3 yr f/u:Overall survival of ICD Rx: 75.4% Drug Rx: 64.1% (p < 0.02)
CIDS	n = 659 ICD Rx: 328 (50%) Amiodarone Rx: 331 (50%)	SCD survivors Unstable VT Unmonitored syncope likely due to VT	ICD Rx: 34% Amiodarone Rx: 33%	ICD Rx: 83% Amiodarone Rx: 82%	Amiodarone Rx: 1200 mg/day for ≥1 wk ≥400 mg/day for ≥10 wk ≥300 mg/day for remainder of the study	Mean f/u of 3 yr: ICD Rx: 19.7% Relative risk reduction in death by ICD (p = 0.142)

CAD, coronary artery disease; f/u, follow-up; SCD, sudden cardiac death; VF, ventricular fibrillation; VT, ventricular tachycardia.

include ischemia, electrolyte imbalances, and drug proarrhythmia. Patients with ischemia-induced VT should be evaluated for potential revascularization. Electrolyte abnormalities should be corrected and offending drugs removed. Despite identifying transient or correctable risk factors, such patients remain at high risk for death [35]. Three trials enrolling separately in Europe, the United States, and Canada were performed to evaluate the effectiveness of ICD compared to antiarrhythmic drug therapy in reducing mortality in sudden death survivors (Table 2.2).

The Cardiac Arrest Study Hamburg (CASH) trial compared ICD therapy to antiarrhythmic drug therapy with amiodarone, metoprolol, or propafenone in reducing mortality of SCD survivors [36]. After baseline clinical testing, enrolled patients were randomized to one of the four regimens. Nearly half the patients had coronary artery disease. After a mean follow-up of 11 months in 230 patients, no significant difference in mortality was observed among patients randomized to ICD, amiodarone, and metoprolol. Propafenone was associated with an increase in mortality resulting in early termination of this arm of the trial.

The larger Antiarrhythmics Versus Implantable Defibrillator (AVID) study was published in 1997 and compared ICD implantation to antiarrhythmic drug therapy in patients with either resuscitated VF or hemodynamically intolerable VT [37]. Enrolled patients were randomized to either ICD implantation or a type III antiarrhythmic drug (96% amiodarone, 3% sotalol). Eighty-one percent of patients had coronary artery disease. After a follow-up of 3 years in 1016 patients, ICD therapy was superior to antiarrhythmic drug therapy in improving survival (75.4% vs 64.1%, $p < 0.02$).

The Canadian Implantable Defibrillator Survival (CIDS) trial published in 2000 hypothesized that ICD therapy improves survival compared to amiodarone in SCD survivors and patients suffering unmonitored syncope likely due to VT [38]. Enrolled patients were randomized either to ICD therapy or to amiodarone, and after a mean follow-up of approximately 3 years in 659 patients, a nonsignificant reduction in the risk of death (19.7% relative risk reduction, $p = 0.142$) and arrhythmic death (32.8% relative risk reduction, $p = 0.094$) was observed with ICD therapy.

Summary of secondary prevention ICD trials

A meta-analysis of the three major secondary prevention trials showed the superiority of ICD therapy over amiodarone in improving survival of patients having suffered VF or hemodynamically unstable VT [39]. The relative risk of death was reduced by 28% with ICD implantation due almost entirely to a 50% reduction in arrhythmic death. Patients with an EF $\leq$ 35% derived more benefit than patients with preserved left ventricular function. Based on these data, implantation of an ICD has a class I indication for survivors of cardiac arrest due to VF or sustained VT after exclusion of completely reversible causes [40].

Future directions

As our understanding of the mechanisms underlying VT and VF improve so will our ability to stratify high-risk patients and better identify those requiring an ICD. Advances in technology will lead to newer defibrillator designs, such as a leadless ICD, as well as smaller and longer lasting devices. Such improvements will lead to more cost-effective therapy.

References

1. Myerburg R, Kessler KM, Castellanos A. Sudden cardiac death: epidemiology, transient risk, and intervention assessment. Ann Intern Med 1993;119:1187–1197.

2. DiMarco JP, Haines, DE. Sudden cardiac death. Curr Probl Cardiol 1990;15:187–232.

3. Robertson ME. Sudden death from cardiac arrest—improving the odds. N Engl J Med 2000;343:1259–1260.

4. Moss AJ. Sudden cardiac death and national health. PACE 1993;16:2190–2191.

5. Josephson M, Wellens HJJ. Implantable defibrillators and sudden cardiac death. Circulation 2004;109:2685–2691.

6. Mirowski M. The automatic implantable cardioverter-defibrillator: an overview. J Am Coll Cardiol 1985;6:461–466.

7. Josephson ME, Callans DJ, Buxton AE. The role of the implantable cardioverter-defibrillator for prevention of sudden cardiac death. Ann Intern Med 2000;133:901–910.

8. Myerburg RJ, Mitrani R, Interian A, Castellanos A. Interpretation of outcomes of antiarrhythmic clinical trials: design features and population impact. Circulation 1998;97:1514–1521.

9. Kannel WB, Plehn JF, Cupples A. Cardiac failure and sudden death in the Framingham study. Am Heart J 1988;115:869–875.

10. Tamburro P, Wilber D. Sudden death in idiopathic dilated cardiomyopathy. Am Heart J 1992;124:1035–1045.

11. Cohn JN, Archibald DG, Zieche S, et al. Effect of vasodilator therapy on mortality in chronic heart failure: results of a Veterans Administration Cooperative Study. N Engl J Med 1986;314:1547–1552.

12. SOLVD Investigators. Effect of enalapril on mortality and the development of heart failure in asymptomatic patients with reduced left ventricular ejection fractions. N Engl J Med 1992;327:685–691.

13. Sweeney MO. Sudden death in heart failure associated with reduced left ventricular function: substrates, mechanisms, and evidence-based management (Part I). PACE 2001;24:871–888.

14. Greene H, Richardson D, Barker A, et al. Classification of deaths after myocardial infarction as arrhythmic or nonarrhythmic (the Cardiac Arrhythmia Pilot Study). Am J Cardiol 1989;63;1–6.

15. Davis H, DeCamilla J, Bayer L, Moss A. Survivorship patterns in the posthospital phase of myocardial infarction. Circulation 1979;60:1252–1258.

16. Moss AJ, Hall WJ, Cannom DS, et al. Improved survival with an implanted defibrillator in patients with coronary disease at high risk for ventricular arrhythmia. N Engl J Med 1996;335:1933–1940.

17. Buxton AE, Lee KL, Fisher JD, Josephson ME, Prystowsky EN, Hafley G; Multicenter Unsustained Tachycardia Trial Investigators. A randomized study of the prevention of sudden death in patients with coronary artery disease. N Engl J Med 1999;341:1882–1890.

18. Moss AJ, Fadl Y, Zareba W, Cannom DS, Hall WJ; Multicenter Automatic Defibrillator Implantation Trial Research Group. Survival benefit with an implanted defibrillator in relation to mortality risk in chronic coronary heart disease. Am J Cardiol 2001;88:516–520.

19. Moss AJ, Zareba W, Hall WJ, et al. Prophylactic implantation of a defibrillator in patients with myocardial infarction and reduced ejection fraction. N Engl J Med 2002;346:877–883.

20. Bardy GH, Lee KL, Mark DB, et al. Amiodarone or an implanted cardioverter-defibrillator for congestive heart failure. N Engl J Med 2005;352:225–237.

21. Kadish A, Dyer A, Daubert JP, et al. Prophylactic defibrillator implantation in patients with nonischemic dilated cardiomyopathy. N Engl J Med 2004;350:2151–2158.

22. Desai AS, Fang JC, Maisel WH, Baughman KL. Implantable defibrillators for the prevention of mortality in patients with nonischemic cardiomyopathy: a meta-analysis of randomized controlled trials. JAMA 2004;292:2874–2879.

23. Bigger JT; Coronary Artery Bypass Graft (CABG) Patch Trial Investigators. Prophylactic use of implanted cardiac defibrillators in patients at high risk for ventricular arrhythmias after coronary-artery bypass graft surgery. N Engl J Med 1997;337:1569–1575.

24. Hohnloser SH, Kuck KH, Dorian P, et al. Prophylactic use of an implantable cardioverter-defibrillator after acute myocardial infarction. N Engl J Med 2004;351:2481–2488.

25. Moss AJ. Everyone with an ejection fraction less than or equal to 30% should receive an implantable defibrillator. Circulation 2005;111:2542–2548.

26. The Multicenter Postinfarction Research Group. Risk stratification and survival after myocardial infarction. N Engl J Med 1983;309:331–336.

27. deVreede-Swagemakers JJ, Gorgels AP, Dubois-Arbouw WI, et al. Out-of-hospital cardiac arrest in the 1990s: a population-based study in the Maastricht area on incidence, characteristics, and survival. J Am Coll Cardiol 1997;30:1500–1505.

28. Zipes DP, Wellens HJJ. Sudden cardiac death. Circulation 1998;98:2334–2351.

29. Buxton AE, Lee KL, Hafley GE, et al. A simple model using the MUSTT database can stratify total mortality and sudden death risk of coronary disease patients. J Am Coll Cardiol 2004;43:425A.

30. Singh JP, Hall WJ, McNitt S, et al. Factors influencing appropriate firing of the implanted defibrillator for ventricular tachycardia/fibrillation. J Am Coll Cardiol 2005;46:1712–1720.

31. Passman R, Kadish A. Sudden death prevention with implantable devices. Circulation 2007;116:561–571.

32. Burke J, Hallas C, Clark-Carter D, White D, Connelly D. The psycho-social impact of the implantable cardioverter-defibrillator: a meta-analytic review. Br J Health Psychol 2003;8:165–178.

33. Zwanziger J, Hall W, Dick A, et al. The cost effectiveness of implantable cardioverter-defibrillators: results from the Multicenter Automatic Defibrillator Implantation Trial (MADIT)-II. J Am Coll Cardiol 2006;47:2310–2318.

34. Mark D, Nelson C, Anstrom K, et al. Sudden cardiac death in Heart Failure Trial Investigators. Cost-effectiveness of defibrillator therapy or amiodarone in chronic stable heart failure: results from the sudden cardiac death in Heart Failure Trial (SCD-HeFT). Circulation 2006;114:135–142.

35. Wyse DG, Friedman PL, Brodsky MA, et al. Life-threatening ventricular arrhythmias due to transient or correctable causes: high risk for death in follow-up. J Am Coll Cardiol 2001;38:1718–1724.

36. Siebels J, Cappato R, Ruppel R, et al. for the Cardiac Arrest Study Hamburg (CASH) Investigators. Preliminary

results of the Cardiac Arrest Study Hamburg (CASH). Am J Cardiol 1993;72:109F–113F.

37. The Antiarrhythmics Versus Implantable Defibrillators (AVID) Investigators. A comparison of antiarrhythmic-drug therapy with implantable defibrillators in patients resuscitated from near-fatal ventricular arrhythmias. N Engl J Med 1997;337:1576–1583.

38. Connolly SJ, Gent M, Roberts RS, *et al.* for the CIDS Investigators. Canadian Implantable Defibrillator Study (CIDS): a randomized trial of the implantable cardioverter defibrillator against amiodarone. Circulation 2000;101:1297–1302.

39. Connolly SJ, Hallstrom AP, Cappato R, *et al.* Meta-analysis of the implantable cardioverter defibrillator secondary prevention trials. Eur Heart J 2000;21:2071–2078.

40. Epstein AE, DiMarco JP, Ellenbogen KA, *et al.* ACC/AHA/HRS 2008 guidelines for device-based therapy of cardiac rhythm abnormalities. J Am Coll Cardiol 2008;51:e1–e62.

CHAPTER 3

Chronic Implantable Monitoring

Nisha Aggarwal, & David J. Whellan
Jefferson Medical College, Philadelphia, PA, USA

Heart failure (HF) is a growing problem that is associated with high mortality, frequent hospitalizations, and poor quality of life. According to the American Heart Association, 5 million people in the United States suffer from HF, with over 500,000 new cases a year [1]. Moreover, HF accounts for over 1 million hospital discharges annually and for almost $30 billion in expenditures for care and management of patients with HF, based on American Heart Association statistics from 2006 [1].

As a chronic disease, HF is characterized by remissions and exacerbations and thus demands frequent follow-up and acute visits with physicians. The rehospitalization rate in these patients is high. Most patients hospitalized for acute decompensated HF have a previous diagnosis of HF. In a 3-year retrospective study of Medicare patients in the state of Connecticut ($n = 17,448$) who survived an HF-related hospitalization, the 6-month rehospitalization rate was as high as 44% [2].

Addressing this high rehospitalization rate through preventive efforts is clearly warranted. However, signs and symptoms of HF are not reliable indicators of cardiopulmonary status and are therefore poor predictors of whether a patient needs medication readjustment or is likely to decompensate. Stevenson and Perloff [3] reported in 1989 that rales, edema, and elevated mean jugular venous pressure were absent in 18 of 43 patients with pulmonary capillary wedge pressures (PCWP) greater than or equal to 22 mmHg, yielding a sensitivity of only 58%. In another study, 39% of patients with high PCWPs did not show signs of pulmonary congestion on chest radiography [4].

Given the unreliability of physical signs and symptoms, researchers have tried to identify more direct methods for assessing HF status, such as pulmonary catheterization. Reductions in HF symptoms, jugular venous pressure, mortality, and length of hospital stay were shown after inpatient catheterization in the ESCAPE study (Evaluation Study of Congestive Heart Failure and Pulmonary Artery Catheterization Effectiveness) [5]. However, catheterization is an invasive procedure that must be done on an inpatient basis and is associated with such risks as arrhythmias, rupture of the pulmonary artery, pneumothorax, infection, and internal bleeding.

Implantable monitors provide a noninvasive means to monitor HF events outside the hospital setting and have the potential to reduce hospital readmissions and decrease associated health care costs related to inpatient care. Unlike pulmonary artery catheters, which must be inserted after the patient's presentation with decompensated HF, implantable devices can be used to monitor patients during relative stability and can detect early signs of decompensation. Detection of hemodynamic congestion prior to clinical symptoms could then allow time to change the natural history of acute HF.

Extensive efforts to monitor hemodynamic variables on an outpatient basis have been evaluated in a number of studies. Investigators in the Trans-European Network Homecare Monitoring Study (TEN-HMS), a large-scale randomized prospective clinical trial, compared usual care, telephone support, and home telemonitoring (twice-daily home measurements of blood pressure, echocardiography [ECG], and weight) and found consistent improvement in the primary endpoint of number of days lost to hospitalization or death with increased intensity of care. However, this benefit did not extend to the percentage of patient-days lost as a result of hospitalization in patients who received home telemonitoring [6]. Results from other studies indicate that patient education, home monitoring, and early physician notification can reduce resource use and hospitalizations [7,8]. Systematic reviews suggest that disease management programs decrease hospitalizations and costs, but whether they affect HF mortality is unclear [9,10].

Results from other large-scale trials of more intensive monitoring have been equivocal. The European InSync Sentry Observational Study was conducted in patients who had received an impedance monitoring device. In 373 subjects, 53 alerts and 53 clinical events were reported during a median of 4.2 months, with 60% sensitivity (95% CI 46–73) and, likewise, a positive predictive value of 60% (95% CI 46–73) [11]. Higher New York Heart Association (NYHA) class at baseline accurately predicted alert events in follow-up ($P < 0.05$). The COMPASS Chronicle trial (Chronicle Offers Management with Advanced Signs and Symptoms of Heart Failure), a randomized, single-blind, parallel-controlled study, investigated the safety and efficacy of implantable cardioverter-defibrillators (ICDs) developed by Medtronic (Minneapolis, MN). In 2/4 NYHA class III or IV patients, an 8% rate of system-related complications was established. However, the efficacy endpoint was not met, with only a nonsignificant 21% lower rate of HF-related events in the treatment group versus the control group ($P = 0.03$) and a 36% reduction in hospital admissions ($P = 0.03$) [12]. A subsequent trial of the implantable hemodynamic monitor (IHM) concept combined with an ICD is currently underway [13].

Implantable device parameters

Although use of implanted devices has been based on their efficacy in reducing clinical events, decreasing mortality, and decreasing hospitalizations, another strength of ICDs and cardiac resynchronization therapy (CRT) systems is that they provide monitoring for a number of patient parameters. These parameters include heart rate variability (HRV), physical activity, intrathoracic impedance, right ventricular pressure, maximum positive and maximum negative rate of change of right ventric-

ular pressure (dP/dt_{max}), and estimated pulmonary arterial diastolic pressure (ePADP). Table 3.1 provides a summary of changes in these parameters and their relationship to monitoring.

Heart rate variability

Over the past several years, our understanding of the pathophysiology of HF has shifted from pump failure mechanisms to a neurohormonal hypothesis [14]. We now believe that patients with HF have an imbalance in cardiac autonomic control, with decreased parasympathetic control and increased sympathetic activity. The Task Force of the European Society of Cardiology and the North American Society of Pacing and Electrophysiology reported in 1996, based on results from several studies, that sympathetic tone is increased in HF and that mortality decreases with neurohormonal influence through autonomic drug therapy [15].

HRV is an indirect, noninvasive measurement of cardiac autonomic tone. Traditionally measured via continuous ECG recordings from short-term Holter monitoring, HRV is defined as the standard deviation of the normal-to-normal (SDNN) RR intervals. Several prospective studies have investigated the predictive value of SDNN in HF mortality and sudden death. Researchers in a retrospective analysis of 127 patient ECGs from the Veterans Affairs' Survival Trial of Antiarrhythmic Therapy in Congestive Heart Failure (CHF-STAT) found that HRV was associated with sudden death and mortality in patients with moderate-to-severe ischemic HF [16]. Patients in the lowest quartile (SDNN < 65.3 ms) were at significantly increased risk for all-cause mortality ($P = 0.0001$). In fact, each 10-millisecond increase in the SDNN led to a 20% decrease in mortality risk. These results were confirmed in a study reported in 2003, in which a decrease in short-term HRV measured by a decrease in the low-versus-high-frequency power component of the HRV spectrum was an independent predictor of sudden cardiac death in chronic HF patients (relative risk 3.7). In a subset of these patients, plasma catecholamines were assessed, and peripheral noradrenaline was significantly higher in patients who had markedly reduced HRV [17].

The prognostic value of deriving HRV for continuous Holter monitoring has also been shown

Table 3.1 Monitored parameters in implantable devices.

Parameter↑	Effect on disease state	Theoretical use
Heart rate variability (HRV)	HF → ↓ Vagal tone → tachycardia and ↓ HRV	↓ HRV → intensified monitoring and therapy
	Tachycardia secondary to unregulated sympathetic tone worsens heart function	• Neurohormonal blocking agents (β-blockers, ACE-I) decrease sympathetic tone and reduce morbidity and mortality
	↓ HRV → poorer prognosis	• AV nodal blocking agents (low-dose digoxin) for atrial and ventricular tachycardia, especially in patients with concomitant atrial fibrillation
Intrathoracic impedance	HF → pulmonary congestion → ↓ intrathoracic impedance	↓ Intrathoracic impedance precedes symptom onset
	↓ Intrathoracic impedance associated with acute decompensation	Diuretics initiated prior to acute decompensation
Ventricular pressure	HF → volume overload and ventricular failure → ↑ cardiac filling pressures	↑ Ventricular pressure precedes symptom onset
• RVSP, RVDP, dP/dt_{max}, ePADP	↑ Ventricular pressures associated with acute decompensation	Diuretics initiated prior to acute decompensation
		Reduction in need for invasive methods of measuring ventricular pressures
Cardiac output (CO)	HF → ventricular failure → ↓ CO → decreased perfusion of vital organs	Detection of ↓ CO → use of positive inotropic therapy—however not always recommended due to potential increase in oxygen demand and arrhythmias
		Reduction in need for invasive methods of measuring CO and oxygenation

ACE-I, angiotensin-converting enzyme inhibitor; AV, arteriovenous; dP/dt_{max}, maximum positive rate of pressure development; ePADP, estimated pulmonary arterial diastolic pressure; HF, heart failure; HRV, heart rate variability; RVSP, right ventricular systolic pressure.

for HRV derived from implantable devices. In the InSync III trial, HRV was derived using the standard deviation of 5-minute median atrial–atrial intervals (SDAAM) [18,19]. This study was based on three hypotheses: (1) that longer term, device-based SDAAM values are associated with risk for mortality or hospitalizations; (2) that SDAAM is different between groups at high and low risk for subsequent clinical decompensation; and (3) that SDAAM changes as HF patients decline clinically. As predicted, all-cause mortality was higher in the low-SDAAM group (SDAAM < 50 ms), with a hazard ratio of 3.20 ($P = 0.02$). The hazard ratio for cardiovascular deaths specifically was 4.43 ($P = 0.01$). Absolute SDAAM values were significantly lower in patients who were hospitalized or who died. SDAAM also declined significantly over the 9–12 weeks before hospitalization. Using a SDAAM detection algorithm created for a threshold of 200 millisecond-days, a sensitivity of 70% was associated with a 2.4 false-positive rate per patient-year of follow-up. The median time between crossing of the threshold and hospital admission was 16 days. Also, night heart rate increased and patient activity declined as patients neared hospital admission [18,19].

Intrathoracic impedance

Pulmonary congestion is a common sign of decompensation in patients with HF. Detection of accumulating pulmonary fluid before acute symptoms develop can enable appropriate therapeutic interventions and therefore potentially prevent decompensation and hospital admission. One method of detecting pulmonary fluid is through intrathoracic impedance measurement. *Impedance* is defined as the sum of forces that oppose conductance and is equivalent to resistance in a circuit that obeys Ohm's law (voltage = current × resistance). Accumulation of intrathoracic fluid allows better conductance, resulting in decreased resistance and thus decreased impedance.

Impedance monitoring was first accomplished externally. Early studies investigated the use of impedance monitoring in surgical and trauma patients, with changes in impedance reflecting alterations in intrathoracic fluid volume [20]. Investigators also measured hemodynamic parameters such as stroke volume and cardiac output using continuous whole-body bioimpedance monitoring with wrist and ankle electrodes. They calculated cardiac output from increases in measurable conductance in the periphery that were proportional to stroke volume and thermodilution. In 1979, Fein et al. [21] sought to determine the role of transthoracic electrical impedance monitoring for clinical use. Using a tetrapolar impedance plethysmograph, they found that patients who were continuously monitored and had a greater than 5% decrease from initial impedance values also had physical and roentgenographic findings consistent with pulmonary edema. However, the authors reported that isolated measurements of transthoracic impedance were not helpful in detecting pulmonary congestion.

Limitations to external impedance monitoring include lack of reproducibility due to inaccuracy of skin electrode placement, inability to continuously monitor patients in an ambulatory setting, and need for frequent physician visits. Also, placement of electrodes on the neck can lead to interference from carotid artery blood flow. In a recent study, internal transthoracic impedance was monitored noninvasively using the Edema Guard Monitor model RS-207 (RS Medical Monitoring, Jerusalem, Israel). Differences between the Edema Guard Monitor and other noninvasive plethysmographs include movement of electrodes to the lung area (thorax) rather than near large arteries and separation of skin to electrode impedance from internal thoracic impedance (ITI), so that the calculated ITI truly reflects only internal impedance [22]. ITI correlated well with cardiogenic pulmonary edema, with ITI falling before onset of physical signs and symptoms.

Researchers are now exploring internal methods of calculating thoracic impedance. Wang et al. [23] first attempted intrathoracic impedance monitoring via a modified pacemaker in a canine HF model. They found an inverse relationship between left ventricular end-diastolic pressure and impedance [23]. Yu et al. [24] were the first to assess the feasibility and clinical usefulness of intrathoracic impedance monitoring. In their study, the Medtronic Impedance Diagnostics in Heart Failure Patients Trial (MIDHeFT), these investigators followed 33 NYHA class III and IV patients during chronic and acute phases of their disease. An ICD lead was implanted in the right ventricular apex, and a pacemaker with two sensors for activity and minute ventilation was placed in the left pectoral region. The device measured impedance between the coil electrode of the ICD lead and the device case, and provided ventricular rate support when indicated. After implantation of the monitoring device, the intrathoracic impedance first decreased for about 30 days due to wound healing and subsequently stabilized. A patient's reference impedance value was calculated using days 31–34 after implant, and this value was then compared with daily impedance measurements. In 24 HF hospitalizations, the daily intrathoracic impedance was below the reference value for an average of 18.3 days leading up to hospital admission. Impedance decreased by an average of 12.3% ($P < 0.001$) from baseline to the day before hospitalization, reflecting the gradual accumulation of pulmonary fluid. The decrease in impedance preceded symptom onset by an average of 15 days, suggesting that impedance monitoring could warn clinicians of a patient's status and provide an opportunity for early intervention. The researchers also found a good inverse correlation between intrathoracic impedance and PCWP. Seventeen patients were intravenously diuresed in the critical care unit during the MIDHeFT study. As their fluid load decreased, impedance increased significantly (17.1%), and PCWP, as measured by Swan-Ganz catheter, decreased by 45.1%. After MIDHeFT showed the value of intrathoracic impedance monitoring in humans, investigators in the Fluid Accumulation Status Trial (FAST) used the InSync Marquis CRT-D to prospectively evaluate if impedance monitoring could predict HF-related health care use events. They found that decreases in daily impedance and increases in the cumulative difference between impedance measurements and the patient's reference impedance were consistent with pulmonary congestion-related HF decompensation events [25].

Data from the MIDHeFT study were used to develop an algorithm for fluid status monitoring for which they used the OptiVol system (Medtronic, Inc.; see the following text for detailed discussion of OptiVol and other IHM systems). Using this algorithm, impedance is measured every 20 minutes from noon to 5 p.m. These values are then averaged to obtain a daily impedance value. The OptiVol fluid index is the final variable. It contains two pieces of information: the magnitude of the reduction in impedance from reference impedance (measured in ohms) and the sustainability of the reduction (measured in days). The index thus has a measurement unit of ohm-days. The threshold can then be set on an individual basis. A threshold of 60 ohm-days was set for the MIDHeFT data and yielded a sensitivity of 76.9% and 1.5 false-positive detections per patient-year of monitoring. The authors attributed many of these false-positive results to patients whose medications were adjusted by their physicians so that the patients did not require hospitalization. Another study using the InSync Sentry biventricular ICD with the OptiVol alert system confirmed the inverse correlation between intrathoracic impedance and both PCWP and fluid balance; however, the researchers proposed an alarm sensor threshold of 120 ohm-days to optimize sensitivity and specificity [26].

Additional findings on impedance monitoring with the OptiVol system were presented by investigators from the PARTNERS trial (Program to Access and Review Trending INformation and Evaluate CoRrelation to Symptoms in Patients with Heart Failure) at the 2008 meeting of the Heart Failure Society of America. The 12-month study of 797 subjects was designed to test the hypothesis that changes in intrathoracic impedance monitored by implantable devices can predict subsequent HF-related adverse events. Impedance data recorded at 3-month intervals indicated that patients with a fluid index that crossed the device threshold were twice as likely to experience subsequent HF events after adjustment for other clinical variables.

Given the results of studies to date, intrathoracic impedance monitoring seems to be a promising method of predicting future decompensation in patients with HF. However, this method has limitations. When the device is implanted, the tissue in the area becomes edematous and undergoes soft-tissue changes, and thus impedance measurements are unreliable during the first 30 days after implantation. Thoracic impedance may also vary considerably with body position changes, especially upright to supine changes. Also, secondary thoracic phenomena can elevate or decrease impedance. Such disease processes as ipsilateral pneumonia or pleural effusion may decrease impedance for reasons that are not related to the cardiovascular system. Air, on the other hand, is an insulator and increases impedance. Research is needed to assess the use of this method for monitoring patients with chronic obstructive pulmonary disease in which lung air volumes may change over time.

Right ventricular pressure

Seventy-five percent of acute HF hospitalizations are for volume overload leading to elevated cardiac filling pressures. While hospitalized, these patients often require invasive procedures to assess their cardiopulmonary status and adjust therapy. Right heart catheterizations are done to measure pulmonary artery and right ventricular pressures, putting patients at increased risk of bleeding and infection as well as requiring additional costs.

These acute HF exacerbations may be preceded by increases in right ventricular pressure due to pulmonary congestion and ventricular failure [27]. Therefore, as is the case with measuring intrathoracic impedance, monitoring cardiac pressures could facilitate early identification of patients at risk for decompensation. However, current invasive methods are not feasible for this purpose because they cannot be done in the outpatient setting and only give values for a single point in time. Thus, continuous hemodynamic monitoring with an innovative implantable device is an excellent alternative. Hemodynamic monitors (IHMs) have the capability to measure right ventricular systolic pressure (RVSP), right ventricular diastolic pressure (RVDP), dP/dt_{max}, and ePADP, as described below.

ePADP is calculated at the point when right ventricular pressure equals pulmonary artery pressure, and this point in the cardiac cycle is associated with dP/dt_{max} in the ventricle. The IHM can detect dP/dt_{max} and record the simultaneous right ventricular pressure through its lead. ePADP can then be measured, and this finding reflects left ventricular end-diastolic pressure (LVEDP) in patients without valvular insufficiency, mitral stenosis, or pulmonary vascular disease.

In an early study, Chuang et al. [28] assessed the correlation between actual pulmonary artery diastolic pressure measured using a high-fidelity Millar catheter (Millar Instruments, Houston, TX) and right ventricular transducer-sensed ePADP. Ten NYHA class III and IV patients with varying degrees of disease severity were assessed at rest and during several provocative maneuvers. The overall correlation was 0.92 ($r^2 = 0.878$), and no significant difference was observed between the two measure-

ments during Valsalva maneuver ($r = 0.96$, $r^2 = 0.943$), submaximal bicycle exercise ($r = 0.87$, $r^2 = 0.756$), or infusions of dobutamine and nitroglycerin ($r = 0.82$, $r^2 = 0.73$). ePADP is therefore a valid approximation of the actual pulmonary artery diastolic pressure in HF patients with abnormal hemodynamics, reduced systolic function, and variable degrees of mitral valve and tricuspid regurgitation. Ohlsson et al. [29] and Reynolds et al. [30] made similar observations.

Magalski et al. [31] investigated the feasibility and accuracy of IHMs in measuring cardiac pressures in a small series of patients. They used IHM recordings of heart rate, patient activity levels, RVSP, RVDP, and ePADP measured with a balloon-tipped catheter, and their results were comparable with standard reference values (Figure 3.1). Thirty-two patients were monitored with an IHM and right heart catheterization at implantation and at 3, 6, and 12 months during supine rest, peak response of Valsalva maneuver, sitting, peak of a two-stage upright bicycle stress test, and final rest period. The pressure transducer was accurate over the study period.

More recently, Zile et al. [32,33] observed relationships between changes in right ventricular pressure and ePADP pressures based on additional findings from the COMPASS-HF study. They reported progressive rises in filling pressures occurring over days to weeks preceding symptomatic decompensation based on 163 HF events in 90 of the 274 enrolled patients. They also extended the potential

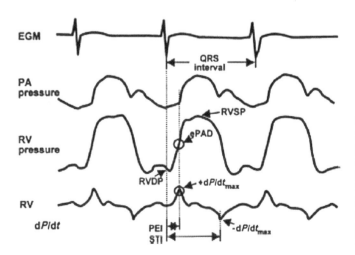

Figure 3.1 Electrocardiogram showing right ventricular (RV) pressure, pulmonary artery (PA) pressure, and right ventricular diastolic maximum positive ($+dP/dt$) and maximum negative diastolic pressure. EGM, Edema Guard Monitor; ePAD, estimated pulmonary artery diastolic pressure; PEI, preejection interval; STI, systolic time interval. (From [31], with permission.)

application of hemodynamic monitoring by describing the similarity of the hemodynamic patterns in patients with preserved LVEF (>50%) to those with reduced LVEF. In addition, they reported on the impact of hemodynamic monitoring in reducing HF events in patients with preserved LVEF [33]. Although the study was not powered to detect statistical significance in this subgroup analysis, the potential for a clinical management tool for use in patients with preserved LVEF is intriguing because no other devices or drug therapies have proved useful for these patients.

Cardiac output

Cardiac output is another hemodynamic variable that can be measured in HF patients with the use of an IHM. Originally, cardiac output was determined according to the Fick principle, which requires invasive catheterization of both pulmonary and systemic arteries. Later, dye dilution and thermodilution methods were developed, but these, too, required right heart catheterization. With an IHM, oxygen saturation can be measured through biosensor technology. A strong correlation has been observed between IHM-sensed oxygen saturation and pulmonary artery blood samples at the time of IHM implantation and after 2, 6, and 11 months. Cardiac output calculated from biosensor values also correlated to values obtained with an invasive technique [34,35].

Preliminary reports indicate that it may be possible to track and derive cardiac output by processing of the right ventricular pressure waveform—a pulse contour cardiac output (PCCO) method adapted to the right ventricular signal. Karamanoglu and coworkers [36,37] have reported promising pilot observations in canine and clinical studies. In their canine study, the investigators evaluated the PCCO method over a wide range of cardiovascular stresses while comparing the derived PCCO signals to actual pulmonary arterial flow using ultrasonic flow probes on the pulmonary artery [36]. Subsequently, in 8 patients with pulmonary arterial hypertension, the investigators compared PCCO measures to Fick cardiac outputs while patients were undergoing vasodilator infusions. They found that the breath-by-breath cardiac index correlated with the right ventricular pressure waveform estimates ($r^2 =$ 0.95) [37]. Further validation of this concept could lead to continuous, even ambulatory cardiac output measurements.

IHM summary

Implantable hemodynamic monitors have advanced considerably over the past decade. These advances are documented in Table 3.2. Ease of use has improved considerably over the past few years. Patients who are implanted carry the external pressure reference with them and make adjustments for changes in barometric pressure. Data can now be transmitted using radiofrequency-linked telemetry from the clinic or from the patient's home (Figure 3.2). Data transmitted to a central server, like the Chronicle Information Network online, make it possible for health care workers to access the data remotely. In a retrospective study, 93% of patients rated the Chronicle system "very easy to use" and said the training material was user-friendly, informative, and thorough. The success rate for data transmission was 86%, with the most common reasons for failed data transfer being interrupted telephone connections and errors related to external pressure reference. The overall success rate was acceptable, and no differences were observed in age, gender, or severity of illness [40].

The OptiVol system

The OptiVol system, discussed previously in the text, was the first IHM manufactured by Medtronic, Inc. (referred to as IHM-0). It consisted of a right ventricular lead that contained a *relative* pressure sensor for measurement of right ventricular pulse pressure and dP/dt_{max} as well as an oxygen saturation sensor. Five patients—four with HF and one with chronic obstructive pulmonary disease—were studied with this IHM, and long-term ambulatory monitoring of ePADP and SvO$_2$ was found to be feasible and potentially useful in HF management. The parameters showed adequate and significant response to various hemodynamic situations, including rest, 6-minute hall walk, supine or sitting maximal bicycle exercise testing, and activities of daily living [34].

The next IHM, the CHF-Pacer (IHM-1), measured *absolute* pressure from a lead implanted in the pulmonary artery, but this device did not have data storage capabilities. However, it contained a

Table 3.2 Evolution of implantable hemodynamic monitoring devices.

Device	Company	Parameters measured	Sensor	Data storage/gathering	Studies
IHM-O	Medtronic, Inc. (Minneapolis, MN)	RV pulse pressure, dP/dt_{max}, HR, activity levels	SvO_2 and dynamic pressure sensors	RAM, radiofrequency device	Ohlsson et al. [34,35]
CHF-Pacer		SvO_2, ECG, absolute PA pressure	SvO_2 and absolute and actual PA pressure sensors	No memory, radiofrequency device	Ohlsson et al. [34]
IHM-1	Medtronic, Inc.	SvO_2, absolute RV pressure, ePADP	SvO_2 and dynamic and absolute pressure sensors	Memory capacity, radiofrequency device	Ohlsson et al. [34,35]
Chronicle (IHM-2)	Medtronic, Inc.	RV pressures, ePADP	Dynamic and absolute pressure sensors	Memory capacity, radiofrequency device	Bourge et al. [12] COMPASS-HF
EndoSure	CardioMEMS (Atlanta, GA	Pressure waveforms	Wireless, MEMS technology		Ongoing prospective trial
ImPressure	Remon Medical	Diastolic PA pressure	Wireless, acoustic energy	No storage capability as of now	Prospective trial planned [38]
HeartPod	St. Jude Medical/Savacor	LA pressure, intracardiac ECG, core body temperature	Implanted through transseptal approach, sits flush against LA septum; connected to antenna implanted in abdomen	Handheld pocket PC-type device (Patient Advisory Module)	Ritzema et al. [39]
LVP-1000 LV Pressure Monitoring System	Transoma Medical	Intraventricular pressure	LV apical sensor placed via subxiphoid puncture		Two ongoing prospective trials

dP/dt_{max}, maximum positive rate of pressure development; ECG, echocardiography; ePADP, estimated pulmonary arterial diastolic pressure; HR, heart rate; LA, left arterial; LV, left ventricular; PA, pulmonary artery; RV, right ventricular; SvO_2, saturated venous oxygen.

pressure sensor in the right ventricular lead and was capable of continuous recording of absolute pressure as well as data storage. The device was found to be stable, reproducible, and accurate when compared with standard reference right heart catheterizations over 1 year [35].

Adamson et al. [27] studied the newest IHM (the Chronicle, IHM-2 from Medtronic) in 32 patients with HF. They found that hospitalizations were decreased with the use of this device. They measured RVSP, RVDP, heart rate, and pressure derivatives. Data were collected for 9 months without changes in clinical management and then for follow-up until 17 months, with data available to clinicians. During 36 volume overload events, RVSP increased by an average of 25%, RVDP by 265%, ePADP by 26%, and heart rate by 11%. Pressure increased an average of 4 days before acute decompensation in 9 of the 12 events requiring hospitalization, but early pressure increases occurred in only 9 of 24 events with minor exacerbations. In all exacerbations, pressure increased 24 hours before clinical intervention. Also, during 8 volume depletion episodes, all pressure measurements decreased significantly. All parameters returned to baseline with successful therapy. Guiding management with the IHM resulted in

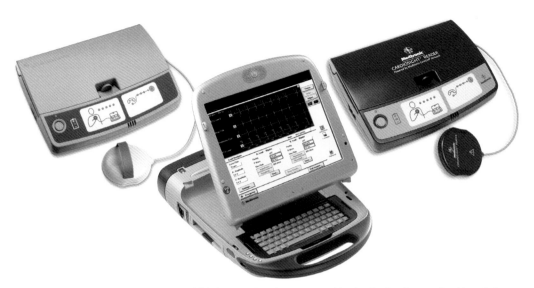

Figure 3.2 Three different systems are available for accessing data generated by the Cardiac Compass in a Heart Failure Management Report: Medtronic CareLink Network, CardioSight, and Medtronic CareLink Programmer. (Courtesy of Medtronic, Inc.)

fewer hospitalizations, decreasing the rate from 1.08 per patient-year when data were not available to clinicians to 0.47 per patient-year when clinicians had access to IHM data.

The OptiVol alert systems now available for clinical use are the ICD (Virtuoso and Secura, Medtronic, Inc.) and the CRT-D devices (InSync Sentry, Concerto, and Consulta). Prospective randomized trials are needed to establish an appropriate alarm threshold and to confirm the clinical utility of impedance monitoring. Figure 3.3 is a report generated for a patient using one of these devices. The report documents a possible fluid accumulation that exceeded the expected threshold of the system. The three panels in Figure 3.4 demonstrate the device's capacity to monitor fluid status continuously over time. The graph in Figure 3.5 depicts an upward trend, indicating the possible beginning of an HF event.

Left atrial pressure systems

Left arterial pressure is one of the characteristic manifestations of HF, but the pressure increase is gradual and usually begins before symptoms arise. The ability to monitor the increase before the patient becomes symptomatic would be helpful to the physician in determining a treatment plan. A left arterial pressure system suitable for ambulatory

monitoring is in development from St. Jude Medical/Savacor (St. Paul, MN). Results from an initial experience with 8 patients at 12-week follow-up showed that 87% of measurements were within ± 5 mmHg of PCWP readings over a wide range of pressures (1.6–71 mmHg). The investigators reported no complications or deaths and no unplanned clinic visits or hospital admissions for HF (Figure 3.6) [39]. A larger phase I/II trial (NCT00547729; $n = 40$) initiated in 2005 is now nearing completion.

Also under study is a left ventricular pressure system by Transoma (St. Paul, MN). Enrollment in two multicenter, randomized, controlled clinical studies of this device (the VALAD study and the LVP-HF Study for Open Chest Patients) is ongoing. More information is available at the Transoma Web site, accessible at http://www.transomamedical.com.

Other new developments

Wireless monitors

Another notable technologic advancement is the development of wireless monitoring devices, such as the CardioMEMS (Atlanta, GA) EndoSure Wireless Pressure Measurement System. The CardioMEMS consists of an implanted sensor and external electronics module. The sensor is placed in the pulmonary artery and held there using wire

Heart Failure Management Report

Device: **Concerto C154DWK**	Serial Number:	Date of Visit: **01-Mar-2006 13:39:07**
Patient:	ID:	Physician:

Date of Birth	EF, on	20% Jun 1, 2005	Hospital
History	Implant	01-Jun-2005	

Clinical Status (01-Oct-2005 to 01-Mar-2006)

Treated VT/VF	0 episodes	V. Pacing	99.8%	Lower Rate	50 ppm
AT/AF	22 episodes	Atrial Pacing	17.2%	Upper Rate	130 ppm
Time in AT/AF	< 0.1% hr/day (0.2%)			Battery	OK

Observations (1) (01-Oct-2005 to 01-Mar-2006)

Possible fluid accumulation: exceeded OptiVol Threshold, 28-Feb-2006 – ongoing.

OptiVol Fluid Trends (Jun 2005 to Mar 2006)

OptiVol fluid index is an accumulation of the difference between the daily and reference impedance.

P = Program
I = Interrogate
_ = Remote

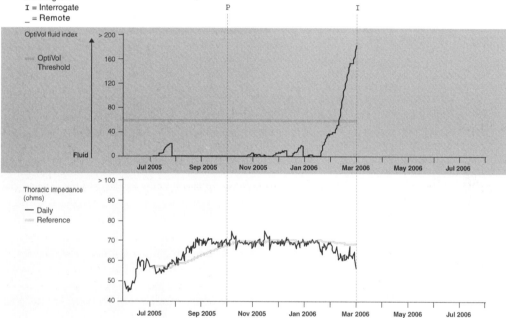

Figure 3.3 Sample of a Heart Failure Management Report generated from the Concerto C154dWK OptiVol system. (Courtesy of Medtronic, Inc.)

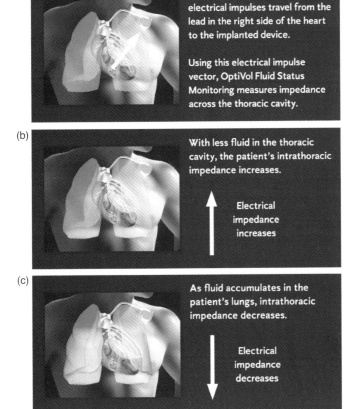

(a) Many times during the day, electrical impulses travel from the lead in the right side of the heart to the implanted device.

Using this electrical impulse vector, OptiVol Fluid Status Monitoring measures impedance across the thoracic cavity.

(b) With less fluid in the thoracic cavity, the patient's intrathoracic impedance increases.

Electrical impedance increases

(c) As fluid accumulates in the patient's lungs, intrathoracic impedance decreases.

Electrical impedance decreases

Figure 3.4 Fluid changes are tracked by electrical impulses with the use of a hemodynamic monitoring system, such as OptiVol. Panel (a) shows the path of the electrical impulses from the thoracic cavity to the monitor; Panel (b) shows the relationship between decreased fluid and increased impedance; and Panel (c) shows the relationship between fluid accumulation and decreased impedance. (Courtesy of Medtronic, Inc.)

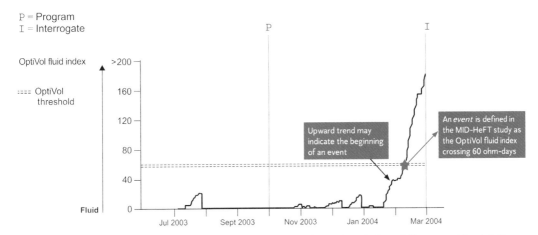

Figure 3.5 The upward trend on the fluid index indicates the possible beginning of a heart failure event. The definition of a heart failure event is taken from the results of the MID-HeFT study. (Data from [25]; courtesy of Medtronic, Inc.)

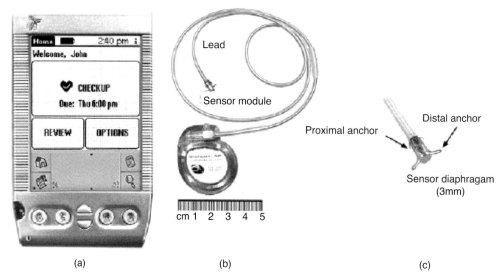

Figure 3.6 This left atrial pressure sensing device, called the HeartPOD, is now in development from St. Jude Medical/Savacor. Panel (a) shows the patient advisory module; Panel (b) shows the sensing device; and Panel (c) is a close-up image of the sensor tip. (From [30]; with permission).

loops made from nickel–titanium alloy (nitinol). The sensor uses passive resonance instead of batteries to absorb radiofrequency energy transmitted from an external electronics module and resonates at a frequency proportional to the pressure detected by the sensor. The data are then processed and displayed as a pressure waveform on the external electronics module, which consists of the internal signal processing electronics (main unit), an antenna to wirelessly communicate with the sensor, and a graphic user interface [41]. CardioMEMS hopes to apply its EndoSure technology to HF care and began its feasibility study in the United States in 2006. Their primary endpoint is avoidance of hospitalizations [42]. A prospective randomized, multicenter study of 450 NYHA class III patients is also planned, with a primary endpoint of HF hospitalizations and secondary endpoints of number of patients hospitalized, time to first hospitalization, and number of days patients remain alive out of hospital.

A wireless device developed by Remon Medical Technologies (Caesaria Industrial Park, Israel) measures pulmonary artery pressure using acoustic energy, which penetrates deep into the body. This type of energy differs from electromagnetic energy, which requires a large antenna and is therefore unsuitable for deep body implants [38]. In a pilot trial the wireless device was implanted in 8 pigs and 10

human patients via right heart catheterization. In both animals and human patients, results with the wireless device were comparable to those with a Millar catheter (Millar Instruments, Houston, TX). At 6 months, a macroscopic and histopathologic examination of the animals showed no device-related complications. The addition of a miniature battery, now in development, would make the device suitable for home monitoring.

Carotid monitoring and stimulation

Due to the decreased vagal tone in patients with HF, HRV decreases as well. Carotid stimulation of the vagus nerve, a treatment that has been used for epilepsy and other neurologic conditions, was recently described for use in patients with HF [43,44]. As described in a case report by Mohaupt et al. [44], electrodes were placed around the carotid adventitial surface, and leads were connected to the implantable stimulation device, which was placed subcutaneously in the subclavian artery. The investigators found that device stimulation caused a decrease in blood pressure (systolic more than diastolic) and heart rate. The newest implantable carotid stimulating device is the Rheos, by CVRx, Inc. (Minneapolis, MN) [43,44]. These devices may have the capacity to work as monitors in patients with HF and to deliver carotid stimulation based on detection of such changes as decreased HRV due to loss of autonomic control. This technology could take implantable monitoring to the next level, delivering immediate therapy just as an ICD does [45].

Conclusion: applications in disease management

HF is a growing epidemic and economic burden. With the advent of implantable monitoring, clinicians have a more reliable source for information on their patients' hemodynamic status and can anticipate the need for therapeutic interventions prior to acute decompensation. This capacity may decrease the number of costly hospitalizations and invasive procedures and expand our understanding of the natural history and pathophysiology of HF.

Diagnostic monitoring with implantable hemodynamic devices has shown feasibility and favorable outcomes in HF patients. Other potential uses for IHMs are in patients with chronic obstructive pulmonary disease [29], in hemodialysis patients with other indications for device management [46], in pulmonary arterial hypertension patients [47], and in patients during exercise stress testing [48]. Another possibility to be explored is for continuous monitoring of biomarker levels, such as B-type natriuretic peptide.

Device management has the potential to bring patients and clinicians closer together but will also require cooperation among cardiology subspecialty practitioners. Until now, electrophysiologists have had the primary responsibility for controlling patient heart rate and heart rhythm with such devices as pacemakers and ICDs, whereas HF specialists have managed their patients' cardiopulmonary status with medication adjustments and transplant assessment. As indications for device management expand to include hemodynamic monitoring, electrophysiologists and HF specialists will need to join forces to enhance disease management. Further data from prospective randomized trials are needed to establish clinical outcomes, risks versus benefits, and indications for use.

References

1. Thom T, Haase N, Rosamond W, *et al*. Heart disease and stroke statistics—2006 update: a report from the American Heart Association Statistics Committee and Stroke Statistics Subcommittee. Circulation 2006;113:e85–e151; Erratum appears in Circulation 113, e696.

2. Krumholz HM, Parent EM, Tu N, *et al*. Readmission after hospitalization for congestive heart failure among Medicare beneficiaries. Arch Intern Med 1997;157:99–104.

3. Stevenson LW, Perloff JK. The limited reliability of physical signs for estimating hemodynamics in chronic heart failure. JAMA 1989;261:884–888.

4. Chakko S, Woska D, Martinez H, *et al*. Clinical, radiographic, and hemodynamic correlations in chronic congestive heart failure: conflicting results may lead to inappropriate care. Am J Med 1991;90:353–359.

5. Binanay C, Califf RM, Hasselblad V, *et al*. Evaluation study of congestive heart failure and pulmonary artery catheterization effectiveness: the ESCAPE trial [comment]. JAMA 2005;294:1625–1633.

6. Cleland JG, Louis AA, Rigby AS, *et al*. Noninvasive home telemonitoring for patients with heart failure at high risk of recurrent admission and death: the Trans-European Network-Home-Care Management System (TEN-HMS) Study. J Am Coll Cardiol 2005;45:1654–1664.

7. Whellan DJ. Heart failure disease management: implementation and outcomes. Cardiol Rev 2005;13:231–239.

8. Heidenreich PA, Ruggerio CM, Massie BM. Effect of a home monitoring system on hospitalization and resource use for patients with heart failure. Am Heart J 1999;138:633–640.

9. Gonseth J, Guallar-Castillon P, Banegas JR, Rodriguez-Artalejo F. The effectiveness of disease management programmes in reducing hospital re-admission in older patients with heart failure: a systematic review and meta-analysis of published reports [review]. Eur Heart J 2004;25:1570–1595.

10. McAlister FA, Lawson FM, Teo KK, Armstrong PW. A systematic review of randomized trials of disease management programs in heart failure. Am J Med 2001;110:378–384.

11. Vollmann D, Nagele H, Schauerte P, *et al*. Clinical utility of intrathoracic impedance monitoring to alert patients with an implanted device of deteriorating chronic heart failure. Eur Heart J 2007;28:1835–1840.

12. Bourge RC, Abraham WT, Adamson PB, *et al*. Randomized controlled trial of an implantable continuous hemodynamic monitor in patients with advanced heart failure: the COMPASS-HF Study. J Am Coll Cardiol 2008;51:1073–1079.

13. Adamson PB, Conti JB, Smith AL, *et al*. Reducing events in patients with chronic heart failure

(REDUCEhf) Study Design: continuous hemodynamic monitoring with an implantable defibrillator. Clin Cardiol 2007;30:567–575.

14. Francis GS. Pathophysiology of chronic heart failure. Am J Med 2001;110:37S–46S.

15. Task Force of the European Society of Cardiology and the North American Society of Pacing and Electrophysiology. Heart rate variability: standards of measurement, physiological interpretation and clinical use. Circulation 1996;93:1043–1065.

16. Bilchick KC, Fetics B, Djoukeng R. Prognostic value of heart rate variability in chronic congestive heart failure (Veterans Affairs Survival Trial of Antiarrhythmic Therapy in Congestive Heart Failure). Am J Cardiol 2002;90:24–28.

17. La Rovere MT, Pinna GD, Maestri R, et al. Short-term heart rate variability strongly predicts sudden cardiac death in chronic heart failure patients. Circulation 2003;107:565–570.

18. Adamson PB, Kleckner KJ, VanHout WL. Cardiac resynchronization therapy improves heart rate variability in patients with symptomatic heart failure. Circulation 2003;110:266–269.

19. Adamson PB, Smith AL, Abraham WT, et al. Continuous autonomic assessment in patients with symptomatic heart failure: prognostic value of heart rate variability measured by an implanted cardiac resynchronization device. Circulation 2004;110:2389–2394.

20. Pomerantz M, Baumgartner R, Lauridson J, Eiseman B. Transthoracic electrical impedance for the early detection of pulmonary edema. Surgery 1969;66:260–268.

21. Fein A, Grossman RF, Jones JG, et al. Evaluation of transthoracic electrical impedance in the diagnosis of pulmonary edema. Circulation 1979;60:1156–1160.

22. Shochat M, Charach G, Meyler S. Prediction of cardiogenic pulmonary edema onset by monitoring right lung impedance. Intensive Care Med 2006;32:1214–1221.

23. Wang L, Lahtinen S, Lentz L, et al. Feasibility of using an implantable system to measure thoracic congestion in an ambulatory chronic heart failure canine model. Pacing Clin Electrophysiol 2005;28:404–411.

24. Yu CM, Wang L, Chau E, et al. Intrathoracic impedance monitoring in patients with heart failure: correlation with fluid status and feasibility of early warning preceding hospitalization. Circulation 2005;112:841–848.

25. Abraham WT, Foreman B, Fishel R, et al. Fluid accumulation status trial (FAST). Heart Rhythm 2005;2:S65–S66.

26. Maines M, Catanzariti D, Cemin C, et al. Usefulness of intrathoracic fluids accumulation monitoring with an implantable biventricular defibrillator in reducing hospitalizations in patients with heart failure: a case-control study. J Interv Card Electrophysiol 2007;19:201–207.

27. Adamson PB, Magalski A, Braunschweig F, et al. Ongoing right ventricular hemodynamics in heart failure: clinical value of measurements derived from an implantable monitoring system. J Am Coll Cardiol 2003;41:565–571.

28. Chuang PP, Wilson RF, Homas DC. Measurement of pulmonary artery diastolic pressure from a right ventricular pressure transducer in patients with heart failure. J Card Fail 1996;2:41–46.

29. Ohlsson A, Bennett T, Nordlander R, et al. Monitoring of pulmonary arterial diastolic pressure through a right ventricular pressure transducer. J Card Fail 1995;1:161–168.

30. Reynolds DW, Bartelt N, Taepke R, Bennett TD. Measurement of pulmonary artery diastolic pressure from the right ventricle. J Am Coll Cardiol 1995;25:1176–1182.

31. Magalski A, Adamson P, Gadler F, et al. Continuous ambulatory right heart pressure measurements with an implantable hemodynamic monitor: a multicenter, 12-month follow-up study of patients with chronic heart failure. J Card Fail 2002;8:63–70.

32. Zile MR, Bemmett TD, Sutton MSJ, et al. Transition from chronic compensated to acute decompensated heart failure: pathophysiological insights obtained from continuous monitoring of intercardiac pressures. Circulation 2008;118:1433–1441.

33. Zile MR, Bourge RC, Bennett TD, et al. Application of implantable hemodynamic monitoring in the management of patients with diastolic heart failure: a sub-study of the COMPASS-HF trial. J Card Fail 2008;14:816–823.

34. Ohlsson A, Bennett T Ottenhoff F, et al. Long-term recording of cardiac output via an implantable haemodynamic monitoring device. Eur Heart J 1996;17:1902–1910.

35. Ohlsson A, Kubo SH, Steinhaus D. Continuous ambulatory monitoring of absolute right ventricular pressure and mixed venous oxygen saturation in patients with heart failure using an implantable haemodynamic monitor: results of a 1 year multicentre feasibility study. Eur Heart J 2001;22:942–954.

36. Karamanoglu M, Bennett TD. A right ventricular pressure waveform based pulse contour cardiac output algorithm in canines. Cardiovasc Eng 2006;6:83–92.

37. Karamanoglu M, McGoon M, Frantz RP, et al. Right ventricular pressure waveform and wave reflection analysis in patients with pulmonary arterial hypertension. Chest 2007;132:37–43.

38. Rozenman Y, Schwartz RS, Shah H, Parikh KH. Wireless acoustic communication with a miniature pressure sensor in the pulmonary artery for disease surveillance and therapy of patients with congestive heart failure. J Am Coll Cardiol 2007;49:784–789.

39. Ritzema J, Melton IC, Richards AM, *et al.* Direct left atrial pressure monitoring in ambulatory heart failure patients: initial experience with a new permanent implantable device. Circulation 2007;116:2952–2959.

40. Kjellstrom B, Igel D, Abraham J, *et al.* Trans-telephonic monitoring of continuous haemodynamic measurements in heart failure patients. J Telemed Telecare 2005;11:240–244.

41. Ohki T, Ouriel K, Silveira PG, *et al.* Initial results of wireless pressure sensing for endovascular aneurysm repair: the APEX Trial—Acute Pressure Measurement to Confirm Aneurysm Sac EXclusion. J Vasc Surg 2007;45:236–242.

42. Verdejo HE, Castro PF, Concepcion R, *et al.* Comparison of a radiofrequency-based wireless pressure sensor to Swan-Ganz catheter and echocardiography for ambulatory assessment of pulmonary artery pressure in heart failure. J Am Coll Cardiol 2007;50:2375–2382.

43. Filippone JD, Bisognano JD. Baroreflex stimulation in the treatment of hypertension. Curr Opin Nephrol Hypertens 2007;16:403–408.

44. Mohaupt M, Schhmidli G, Luft J, *et al.* Management of uncontrollable hypertension with a carotid sinus stimulation device. Hypertension 2007;50: 825–828.

45. Krapohl BD, Deutinger M, Komurcu F. Vagus nerve stimulation: treatment modality for epilepsy. Medsurg Nurs 2007;16:39–44.

46. Braunschweig F, Kjellstrom B, Soderhall M, *et al.* Dynamic changes in right ventricular pressures during haemodialysis recorded with an implantable haemodynamic monitor. Nephrol Dial Transplant 2006;21:176–183.

47. Frantz RP, Benza RL, Kjellstrom B, *et al.* Continuous hemodynamic monitoring in patients with pulmonary arterial hypertension. J Heart Lung Transplant 2008;27:780–788.

48. Ohlsson A, Steinhaus D, Kjellstrom B, *et al.* Central hemodynamic responses during serial exercise tests in heart failure patients using implantable hemodynamic monitors. Eur J Heart Fail 2003;5:253–259.

CHAPTER 4

Cardiac Contractility Modulation by Electrical Signals Applied during the Absolute Refractory Period as a Treatment for Chronic Heart Failure

Daniel Burkhoff[1,2], Hani N. Sabbah[3], Christian Butter[4], Yuval Mika[2], & Martin Borggrefe[5]

[1]Columbia University, New York, NY, USA
[2]IMPULSE Dynamics USA, Orangeburg, NY, USA
[3]Henry Ford Health System, Detroit, MI, USA
[4]Heart Center Brandenburg Bernau/Berlin, Bernau, Germany
[5]Fakultät für klinische, Medizin der Universität Heidelberg, Mannheim, Germany

Clinical studies have shown that cardiac resynchronization therapy (CRT) improves patient symptoms, quality of life, exercise tolerance and reduces hospitalizations in patients with advanced heart failure and prolonged electrical activation (i.e., increased QRS duration) [1,2]. The results of a recent study showed that patients with mechanical dyssynchrony by tissue Doppler imaging but a normal QRS duration did not benefit from CRT [3]. Thus, QRS duration remains paramount in patient selection for CRT. In view of the fact that greater than 70% of patients with heart failure have a normal QRS duration [4], development of a device-based treatment for such patients with persistent symptoms despite optimal medical therapy would have an important impact.

Cardiac contractility modulating (CCM) signals are nonexcitatory signals applied during the absolute refractory period that have been shown to enhance the strength of left ventricular (LV) contraction in studies carried out in animals and humans with heart failure. Since the signals impact cell function without any impact on activation sequence, the effects are independent of QRS duration and additive to those of CRT in patients with prolonged QRS. We review here the concept and available basic and clinical results concerning the evaluation of CCM as a treatment for heart failure. Reviews of early findings have appeared previously [5,6].

CCM concept and underlying mechanisms

One cellular defect that underlies myocardial contractile dysfunction in heart failure is reduction in the peak and broadening of the time course of the intracellular calcium transient [7]. Such abnormalities reflect heart failure-associated changes

Heart Failure: Device Management. Edited by Arthur Feldman. © 2010 Blackwell Publishing.

in expression of genes encoding calcium handling proteins and posttranslational modification of their associated proteins. Several of the commonly discussed abnormalities include downregulation of genes encoding for the sarcoplasmic reticular ATPase-dependent calcium pump (SERCA2a) [8–11], changes in expression and hypophosphorylation of phospholamban (PLB) [10–15], altered regulation of the sodium–calcium exchanger [11,16,17], and hyperphosphorylation of the ryanodine release channel [18–20]. Accordingly, it has been proposed that treatments aimed at improving the calcium transient in heart failure could be therapeutic [21].

Early studies of isolated cardiac muscle showed that use of voltage clamping techniques to modulate the amplitude and duration of membrane depolarization could modulate calcium entry and contractility in isolated papillary muscles [22–25]. Increases in the duration and amplitude of depolar-

ization have each been associated with increases in the strength of cardiac muscle contraction, which have been linked with increased calcium influx, increased calcium loading of the sarcoplasmic reticulum, and increased calcium release to the myofilaments. However, because voltage clamping is not applicable to the intact heart, this approach was never considered as a treatment option for heart failure. A conceptual breakthrough occurred with recognition and experimental demonstration in isolated superfused muscle strips that similar effects could be achieved when extracellular fields with relatively high current densities are applied over relatively long durations during the absolute refractory period (Figure 4.1) [26,27]. These so-called *CCM signals* contain ∼100 times the amount of energy delivered in standard pacemaker impulse. These signals do not initiate the contraction; they do not recruit additional contractile elements; and there is no additional action potential (as would be

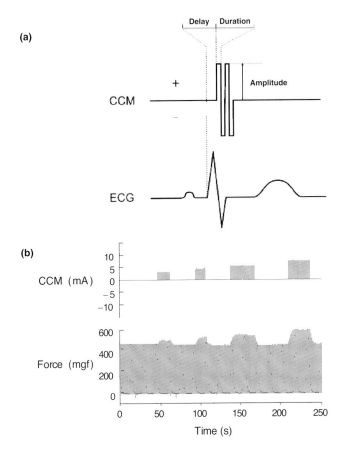

Figure 4.1 (a) Cardiac contractility modulating (CCM) signals employed in clinical study are biphasic pulses delivered after a defined delay from detection of local electrical activation. (b) Effects of CCM signals on isometric force measured from trabecular muscle of an end-stage failing heart obtained at heart transplant [27].

observed with paired pacing or post-extra systolic potentiation). CCM signals are thus referred to as nonexcitatory.

Borrowing from the earlier literature on voltage clamping [22–25], several studies were undertaken to investigate contributing mechanisms of the effects of CCM signals in isolated superfused muscles. Initial evidence suggested that CCM signals influence calcium entry, thus enhancing the strength of the heartbeat [26–28]. Whether this mechanism is in effect during intermediate (hours) or long-term (days and beyond) signal application is still not known, largely because methods to measure calcium transients in intact animals are not available.

Nevertheless, the next series of experiments were aimed at studies in large animal models, including animal models of heart failure. In vivo field stimulation of entire hearts of larger mammals is not feasible because of practical considerations related to power availability and nonspecific stimulation of other tissues (e.g., nerves and skeletal muscles). Studies were therefore undertaken to understand the impact of regional CCM signal delivery on regional contractile function and to test the degree to which such signals could impact on global contractility (Figure 4.2) [29]. The results indeed showed that CCM signals impact on myocardial function in the region where they are applied (assessed by regional pressure-segment length loops), that these

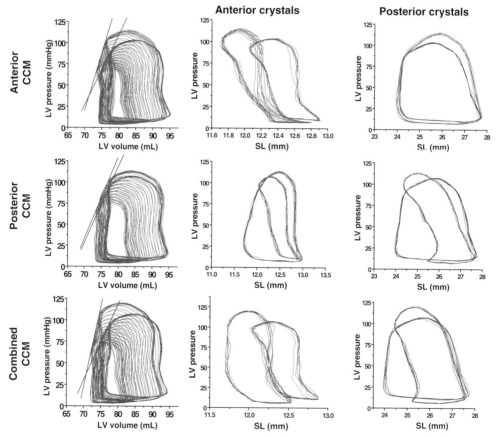

Figure 4.2 Effects of cardiac contractility modulating (CCM) signals on global function assessed by pressure–volume relations (first column) and on regional function in the anterior wall (second column) and posterior wall (third column) assessed by pressure-segment length loops when signals are applied to the anterior wall (first row), posterior wall (second row), and simultaneously to both walls (third row) [29]. Baseline shown in blue; measurements during CCM signal application shown in red. LV, left ventricular; SL, segment length. (Reproduced with permission from the American Physiological Society).

Table 4.1 Comparison between Sham-operated untreated and CCM-treated heart failure dogs for changes (Δ) between pre- and posttreatment (3-mo period) measurements.

	Sham group	CCM-treated group	p value
ΔHeart rate (beats/min)	12 ± 8	8 ± 4	NS
ΔSystolic aortic pressure (mmHg)	6 ± 6	1 ± 7	NS
ΔLV EDP (mmHg)	1 ± 2	−6 ± 2	0.029
ΔLV EDV (mL)	10 ± 1	−4 ± 2	0.0001
ΔLV ESV (mL)	11 ± 1	−7 ± 2	0.0001
ΔLV EF (%)	−4 ± 1	6 ± 1	0.0001
ΔStroke volume (mL)	−1 ± 0.5	3 ± 0.4	0.0001

CCM, cardiac contractility modulating signals; EDP, end-diastolic pressure; EDV, end-diastolic volume; EF, ejection fraction; ESV, end-systolic volume; LV, left ventricle; NS, nont significant.

effects are significant enough to exert an influence on the strength of global contractility (as assessed by global pressure–volume relationships), and that the effects are additive when applied simultaneously to different regions of the heart.

More important, these signals have been shown to have a similar effect in animals with heart failure. In one series of experiments, heart failure was induced by multiple sequential intracoronary microembolizations until ejection fraction (EF) was ≤40% [30,31]. Hemodynamic parameters and myocardial oxygen consumption were measured in an open chest, anesthetized state, with epicardial electrodes used to administer CCM signals. The results showed that while heart rate and peak LV pressure were not significantly influenced, acute CCM therapy decreased LV end-diastolic pressure and end-systolic volume. Consequently, LVEF and cardiac output increased significantly. The improvement in LV systolic function seen in this study was accompanied by unchanged total LV coronary blood flow and unchanged myocardial oxygen consumption.

To further explore the mechanisms underlying the chronic effects, dogs with heart failure induced by repeated coronary microembolization were implanted with a device to deliver CCM signals. Following implantation, dogs were randomized either to receive active CCM treatment for 5 h/day or for the device to remain off; both groups were followed for 3 months. At the end of the follow-up period, CCM-treated dogs had a significantly lower LV end-diastolic pressure, end-diastolic volume, and end-systolic volume, and significantly higher LV EF and stroke volume (Table 4.1). It should be emphasized

that these hemodynamic measurements were made at a time when CCM signals were turned off. That means that the noted improvements in hemodynamic measurements reflect changes in intrinsic muscle properties, not just acute effects of CCM signals.

Therefore, in view of prior literature showing that electromagnetic fields can impact on protein–protein interaction and gene expression [26], we hypothesized that CCM signals may have a direct impact on cellular physiology beyond acute effects on calcium handling. To explore this hypothesis, myocardial samples were taken for molecular and biochemical analysis. Tissue samples were available from the animals from both the acute and chronic studies discussed above [32,33]; samples were also available from normal animals. In all cases, samples were taken from the interventricular septum (near the site of CCM signal delivery) and in a remote area on the LV free wall. Findings related to SERCA2a gene expression are illustrated by the Northern blots of Figure 4.3. For both acute and chronic experiments, glyceraldehyde 3-phosphate dehydrogenase (GAPDH) band intensities show relatively equal loading in each lane. Compared to normals, SERCA2a expression was decreased in all untreated heart failure animals in both the interventricular septum ("near") and remote from the LV free wall ("remote"). For tissue obtained from animals with acute (4 h) CCM treatment, SERCA2a expression increased in the region near the site of CCM signal administration, but not in the remote region. In the chronic setting, however, SERCA2a expression was improved in both near and remote

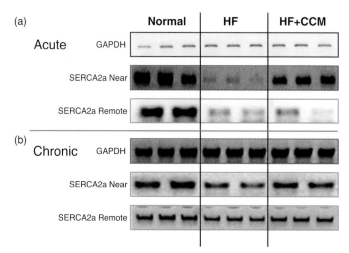

Figure 4.3 Northern blots showing impact of (a) acute (6 h) and (b) chronic (3 mo) cardiac contractility modulating (CCM) signal application on myocardial SERCA2a gene expression, both near and remote from the site of signal delivery. Tissue obtained from normal dogs, dogs with heart failure induced by repeated coronary microembolization, and similar heart failure dogs exposed to CCM treatment. As shown, acute CCM improve gene expression only in the region near where signals are delivered. However, in the chronic setting, gene expression is improved both near and remote from the site of signal delivery. (Reproduced with permission from [33]).

regions. These findings are representative of findings obtained with PLB. B-type natriuretic peptide (BNP) expression was also examined, but in this case, BNP was overexpressed in untreated heart failure, decreased acutely only in the region near the CCM pacing site, and decreased in both the near and remote sites with chronic CCM treatment. The fact that gene expression is improved in the short term only near the area of treatment implies that the effects of CCM treatment are local and direct. However, in the long run, where expression is improved in both near and remote sites, two possible factors may contribute. First, changes in gene expression in remote areas may be secondary to the global hemodynamic benefits provided by chronic regional CCM treatment. Alternatively, there may be some direct effect that is transmitted to remote sites via gap junctions. Which, if either, of these is contributory or dominant remains to be elucidated.

In the chronic study, mRNA expression of a larger array of genes was examined [33]. These included the housekeeping genes GAPDH and calsequestrin (CSQ), the fetal program genes consisting of β_1-adrenergic receptor (β_1-AR), α-myosin heavy chain (α-MHC), and A-type (ANP) and B-type (BNP) natriuretic peptides and the cardiac SR genes SERCA-2a, PLB, and RYR. Expression of GAPDH and CSQ was unchanged among the study groups (i.e., normal dogs, sham-operated heart failure dogs, and heart failure CCM-treated dogs). mRNA expression of β_1-AR, α-MHC, SERCA-2a, PLB, and RYR (ryanodine receptor) decreased and expression of ANP and BNP increased significantly in sham-operated heart failure dogs compared to normals. CCM therapy restored the expression of all genes to near-normal levels.

In addition to looking at mRNA expression, myocardial protein expression was examined in the myocardium from sites both near and remote from the site of CCM signal application. Protein levels of CSQ (a housekeeping gene product) were unchanged among the three study groups. Protein levels of β_1-AR, SERCA-2a, PLB, and RYR decreased and that of ANP and BNP increased significantly in sham-operated controls compared to normals. CCM therapy restored the expression of all measured proteins except for total PLB. The restoration of genes and proteins after 3 months of CCM therapy was the same in LV tissue obtained from

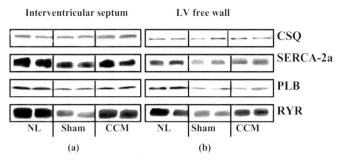

Figure 4.4 (a) Western blots of sarcoplasmic reticulum proteins in tissue obtained from the *interventricular septum* of 2 normal dogs (NL), 2 sham-operated heart failure dogs (Sham), and 2 cardiac contractility modulation (CCM) treated dogs [33]. (b) Western blots of the same proteins in tissue obtained from the *left ventricular (LV) free wall* of the same dogs as in (a) [33]. CSQ, calsequestrin; PLB, phospholamban; RYR, ryanodine receptor; SERCA-2a, calcium ATPase. (Reproduced with permission from [33]).

the interventricular septum, the site nearest to the CCM signal delivery leads, and the LV free wall, a site remote from the CCM leads (Figure 4.4).

Although protein levels of total PLB did not change with CCM, levels of PLB that was phosphorylated (P-PLB) at serine-16 and threonine-17 in tissue obtained from both the interventricular septum and the LV free wall were significantly lower in sham-operated heart failure dogs compared to normal dogs and returned to near-normal levels after 3 months of CCM therapy (Figure 4.5, Table 4.2). In both the interventricular septum and LV free wall, the ratio of P-PLB at serine-16 to total PLB and the ratio of P-PLB at threonine-17 were also significantly lower in sham-operated heart failure dogs compared to normal dogs. Thus, the long-term CCM therapy resulted in a significant increase

of both ratios in both the interventricular septum and the LV free wall (Table 4.2).

In summary, in the chronic setting, CCM signals have hemodynamic effects that persist even when the signals are turned off, at least for short (hours) periods of time. The longevity of those effects is not yet established. CCM signals applied to myocardium of dogs with chronic heart failure have relatively rapid impact on gene expression, but only in the region where they are applied. In the chronic setting, however, improved gene expression is present both local to and remote from the region of signal delivery. These findings potentially imply both direct and indirect effects of the signals on gene expression. Furthermore, similar improvements are seen at the protein level. Interestingly, as was the case for PLB for which total

(a)   **Interventricular septum**

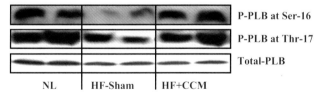

(b)   **LV free wall**

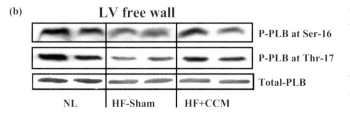

Figure 4.5 (a) Western blots of phospholamban (PLB) in tissue obtained from the interventricular septum of 2 normal dogs (NL), 2 sham-operated heart failure dogs (HF-Sham), and 2 cardiac contractility modulation treated heart failure dogs (HF + CCM). (b) Western blots of the same protein in tissue obtained from the left ventricular (LV) free wall of the same dogs as in (a). P-PLB at Ser-16, phosphorylated phospholamban at serine-16; P-PLB at Thr-17, phosphorylated phospholamban at threonine-17. (Reproduced with permission from [33]).

Table 4.2 Protein expression of total PLB and phosphorylated PLB at serine-16 and threonine-17 in the interventricular septum and left ventricle free wall of normal dogs (NL) ($n = 6$), Sham-operated untreated heart failure dogs (Sham; $n = 7$), and CCM-treated heart failure dogs (CCM; $n = 7$).

	Interventricular septum			LV free wall		
	NL	Sham	CCM	NL	Sham	CCM
Total PLB (du)	445 ± 7	$305 \pm 23^*$	$299 \pm 16^*$	446 ± 19	$305 \pm 19^*$	$299 \pm 9^*$
P-PLB Ser-16 (du)	85 ± 6	$47 \pm 5^*$	$79 \pm 6^\dagger$	128 ± 11	$50 \pm 12^*$	$87 \pm 11^{*\dagger}$
P-PLB Thr-17 (du)	146 ± 6	$62 \pm 10^*$	$129 \pm 12^\dagger$	137 ± 4	$56 \pm 7^*$	$109 \pm 18^\dagger$
P-PLB Ser-16/Total PLB	0.19 ± 0.01	$0.15 \pm 0.01^*$	$0.27 \pm 0.02^\dagger$	0.29 ± 0.03	$0.16 \pm 0.03^*$	$0.29 \pm 0.04^\dagger$
P-PLB Thr-17/Total PLB	0.33 ± 0.01	$0.21 \pm 0.04^*$	$0.44 \pm 0.05^\dagger$	0.31 ± 0.02	$0.19 \pm 0.03^*$	$0.36 \pm 0.05^\dagger$

$p < 0.05$ vs NL.

$p < 0.05$ vs Sham.

CCM, cardiac contractility modulating signals; du, densitometric units; PLB, phospholamban; P-PLB, phosphorylated phospholamban; Ser-16, serine-16; Thr-17, theonine-17.

protein expression was not changed significantly, the ratio of total-to-phosphorylated PLB improved in a manner that would result in improved SR calcium handling. Thus, the mechanisms by which CCM signal impact myocardial properties appear to go far beyond the original hypotheses related to acute augmentation of calcium handling.

Initial clinical study of acute CCM signals

The initial clinical study of CCM signals involved short-term (10–30 min) CCM signal application using a desktop signal generator and temporarily placed electrodes in patients with heart failure who had a clinical indication for an electrophysiology procedure (such as a CRT and/or ICD implantation or a study for evaluation of ventricular or supraventricular arrhythmias) [34,35]. This study involved patients with an average ($\pm$SD) age of 60 ± 11 years with EF $28 \pm 6\%$, having either ischemic or idiopathic cardiomyopathy. The findings showed the feasibility of delivering CCM treatment in humans and demonstrated that contractile performance could be enhanced. The signals were applied to patients with normal and prolonged QRS complexes and similar acute effects were identified in both groups (Figure 4.6). The data from all patients studied showed an average $\sim$10% increase in dP/dt_{max}, which was independent of baseline QRS duration (Figure 4.6a). In a subgroup of the patients with long QRS, CCM signals were also applied simultaneously with biventricular pacing (which is

equivalent to CRT); the effects on acute contractile performance as quantified by dP/dt_{max} of CRT and CCM were shown to be additive in most patients (Figure 4.6b) [34].

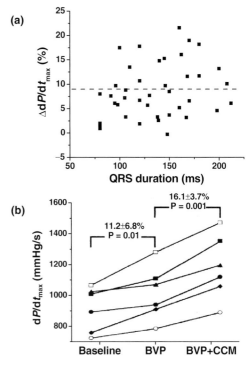

Figure 4.6 (a) Acute effects of cardiac contractility modulating (CCM) signals on dP/dt_{max} in patients with heart failure. Average CCM effect (dashed line) was independent of QRS duration. (b) In patients with prolonged QRS duration, CCM effects were additive to those of biventricular pacing (BVP). (Reproduced with permission from [34]).

Another study examined the impact of acute CCM signal application on myocardial oxygen consumption [36]. Patients were instrumented to measure coronary flow velocity in the left main artery; quantitative angiography was performed to measure left main diameter at the site of velocity measurement (for calculation of cross-sectional area). Coronary flow was therefore estimated as the product of velocity and cross-sectional area. Myocardial oxygen extraction was estimated from measurements of arterial and coronary venous blood pO_2 and hemoglobin content. Myocardial oxygen consumption, in turn, was estimated as the product of oxygen extraction and coronary flow. This study was performed in a group of 11 patients, 6 having idiopathic cardiomyopathy and 5 having ischemic cardiomyopathy in whom EF averaged $26 \pm 4\%$ and peak VO_2 averaged 13.9 ± 2.3 mL O_2/kg/min. The results showed that myocardial oxygen consumption was 13.6 ± 9.7 mL O_2/kg/min at baseline versus 12.5 ± 7.2 mL O_2/kg/min during CCM ap-

plication ($p = NS$). This was in the setting of an average $8.8 \pm 4.8\%$ increase in dP/dt_{max}.

Device description and implantation procedure in humans

In the clinical setting, CCM signals are delivered to the heart by an implantable pulse generator that looks like a pacemaker and connects to the heart via standard commercially available pacing leads (Figure 4.7). The device, called the OPTIMIZER System [37], does not have pacing or antitachycardia therapy capabilities but is designed to work in concert with pacemakers (including CRT devices) and internal defibrillators. The implantable pulse generator has a rechargeable battery that the patients recharge at home once per week via a transcutaneous energy transfer charging unit. In addition, the system includes an acute monitoring system used to measure hemodynamic responses during the system implant and the system programmer.

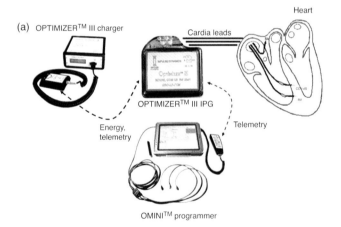

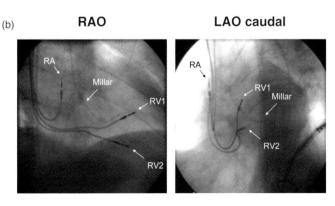

Figure 4.7 (a) System overview with the implantable pulse generator, the leads connecting to the heart, the charger and charging wand, the acute hemodynamic monitoring system used to measure hemodynamic responses during the system implant, and the programmer. (b) Right anterior oblique (RAO) and left lateral oblique (LAO) fluoroscopic images of electrode placement during OPTIMIZER System implant. One lead is placed in the right atrium (RA) and two leads are placed on the right ventricular septum (RV1, RV2) approximately midway between the base and apex, one near the anterior and one near the posterior interventricular groove. The LAO caudal view shows the electrode tips point toward the patient's left, into the septum. A micromanometer (Millar) is placed temporarily to measure physiologic response to acute CCM signal application.

The implant procedure is also similar to that of a standard dual chamber pacemaker and has been described in detail previously, along with a detailed description of the system [5]. In brief, a pocket is made in the right subclavian region (a pacemaker/ICD usually residing on the left subclavian region) and three electrodes are introduced into the subclavian vein in a standard manner. One electrode is positioned in the right atrium and is used only for sensing atrial activity as part of an arrhythmia detection algorithm that inhibits CCM signal delivery during arrhythmias. The other two electrodes are positioned on the right ventricular (RV) septum. The electrodes are positioned under fluoroscopic guidance approximately halfway between the base and the apex; one ideally placed near the anterior interventricular groove and the other in the posterior groove (Figure 4.7).

Chronic signal application in heart failure patients

The initial experiences with chronic CCM signal applications were reported in two papers describing results obtained in patients with New York Heart Association (NYHA) class III symptoms and QRS duration $\leq$ 120 milliseconds [37,38]. The study described in these reports (the FIX-HF-3 study) were multicenter, unblinded, uncontrolled, treatment only, feasibility studies designed mainly to test the functionality of an implanted device that automatically delivers CCM signals [37,38]. The OPTIMIZER System was implanted in 23 patients with an average age of 62 ± 9 years who were primarily male (92%) and were split between idiopathic and ischemic cardiomyopathy (41 and 59%, respectively). Baseline EF averaged 22 ± 7% and Minnesota Living with Heart Failure Questionnaire (MLWHFQ) score averaged 43 ± 22. Patients were well medicated with diuretics (88%), β-blockers (88%), and angiotensin-converting enzyme inhibitors (100%). The study revealed that the device operated as intended; there was no change in ambient ectopy observed between baseline and 8 weeks of treatment; and no overt safety concerns were revealed. In addition, improvements were reported in patient symptoms (assessed by NYHA class), quality of life (assessed by MLWHFQ), and EF.

This was followed by a second feasibility study carried out in the United States (the FIX-HF-5 Phase I study) [39]. Forty-nine subjects with EF $\leq$ 35%, normal QRS duration (105 ± 15 ms), and NYHA class III or IV despite medical therapy received a CCM pulse generator. Two weeks after implantation, patients were randomized to a treatment group in which their devices were programmed to deliver CCM signals for 5 h/day ($n = 25$) or to a control group in which the device remained off ($n = 24$). All patients were followed for 6 months; both patients and investigators were blinded to the treatment group. Evaluations included NYHA, 6-minute walk, cardiopulmonary stress test, MLWHFQ, and Holter. Although most baseline features were balanced between groups, EF (31.4 ± 7.4 vs 24.9 ± 6.5%, $p = 0.003$), end-diastolic dimension (52.1 ± 21.4 vs 62.5 ± 6.2 mm, $p = 0.01$), peak VO$_2$ (16.0 ± 2.9 vs 14.3 ± 2.8 mL O$_2$/kg/min, $p = 0.02$), and anaerobic threshold (12.3 ± 2.5 vs 10.6 ± 2.4 mL O$_2$/kg/min, $p = 0.01$) were all worse in the treatment group as compared to the control group. Nevertheless, there was 1 death in the control group and more treatment group patients were free of hospitalization for any cause at 6 months (84% vs 62%; Figure 4.8b). Compared to baseline, changes in 6-minute walk (13.4 m), peak VO$_2$ (0.2 mL O$_2$/kg/min), and anaerobic threshold ($\sim$0.8 mL O$_2$/kg/min, Figure 4.8a) were more positive in the treatment group than in the control group. None of these differences was statistically significant because of the small sample size. Nevertheless, despite a distinctly sicker population in the treatment group, no safety concerns emerged with chronic CCM signal administration and there were trends toward better outcomes and improved symptoms in response to CCM treatment.

These feasibility studies were followed by a multicenter randomized, double blind, double crossover study of CCM in heart failure patients with NYHA class II or III symptoms despite optimal medical therapy (the FIX-HF-4 study) [40]. One hundred sixty-four subjects with EF < 35% and NYHA class II (24%) or III (76%) symptoms received a CCM pulse generator. Patients were randomly assigned to Group 1 ($n = 80$, CCM treatment 3 mo, sham treatment second 3 mo) or Group 2 ($n = 84$, sham treatment 3 mo, CCM treatment second 3 mo). The coprimary endpoints were changes in peak oxygen

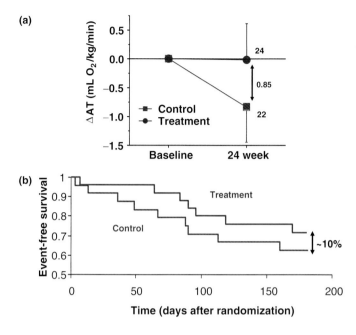

Figure 4.8 Key findings from the US feasibility study (called the FIX-HF-5 Phase I study) of cardiac contractility modulating (CCM). (a) In this prospective, double blind study in which all 49 patients were implanted with an OPTIMIZER System, average anaerobic threshold (measured on cardiopulmonary stress testing) decreased by 0.85 mL O_2/kg/min in the Sham control group and remained constant in the active treatment group. (b) The event-free survival (i.e., the proportion of patients alive without being hospitalized) also trended better in the treatment group. With the small number of patients, the differences were not statistically different. (Reproduced with permission from [39]).

consumption ($VO_{2,peak}$) and MLWHFQ. Baseline EF (29.3±6.69% vs 29.8 ± 7.8%), $VO_{2,peak}$ (14.1 ± 3.0 vs 13.6 ± 2.7 mL O_2/kg/min), and ML-WHFQ (38.9 ± 27.4 vs 36.5 ± 27.1) were similar between groups. $VO_{2,peak}$ increased similarly in both groups during the first 3 months (0.40 ± 3.0 vs 0.37 ± 3.3 mL O_2/kg/min) (Figure 4.9a). This was interpreted as evidence of a prominent placebo effect. During the next 3 months, however, $VO_{2,peak}$ decreased in the group switched to sham (−0.86 ± 3.06 mL O_2/kg/min) and increased in patients switched to active treatment (0.16 ± 2.50 mL O_2/kg/min). At the end of the second phase of the study, the difference in peak VO_2 between groups was approximately 1 mL O_2/kg/min. MLWHFQ behaved similarly, trending only slightly better with treatment (−12.06 ± 15.33 vs −9.70 ± 16.71) during the first 3 months (again consistent with a large placebo effect) (Figure 4.9b). During the second 3 months, MLWHFQ increased in the group switched to sham (+4.70 ± 16.57) and decreased further in patients switched to active treatment (−0.70 ± 15.13). Serious cardiovascular adverse events were tracked carefully in both groups. The most frequently reported events were episodes of decompensated heart failure, atrial fibrillation, bleeding

at the OPTIMIZER System implant site, and pneumonia. Importantly, there were no significant differences between ON and OFF phases in the number or types of adverse events.

Hospitalizations and mortality were compared for the first period of the study (since these will be difficult to interpret following crossover). In all, there were 14 hospitalizations in Group 1 patients (CCM ON phase) compared to 20 hospitalizations in Group 2 patients (CCM OFF phase). In addition, there was 1 death in a Group 2 patient versus no deaths in Group 1 patients. With the relatively small sample size, the overall event-free survival (Figure 4.9c) did not reach statistical significance ($p = 0.31$), but showed trends of magnitude that were similar to those reported for CRT [1].

In aggregate, the data from the feasibility and larger randomized FIX-HF-4 study show that in patients with heart failure and LV dysfunction, CCM signals appear to be safe and improve exercise tolerance and quality of life.

Currently, a randomized, 12-month, parallel group study that enrolled 428 patients with NYHA class III or IV despite optimal medical therapy is underway at 50 centers in the United States (the FIX-HF-5 Phase II study).

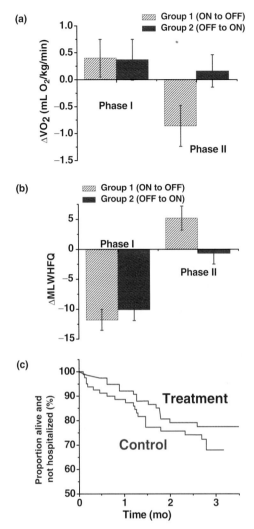

Figure 4.9 Key results of the FIX-HF-4 study [40]. (a) Changes in peak VO$_2$ between baseline and end of Phase I (labeled "Phase I") and changes between end of Phase I and end of Phase II (labeled "Phase II"). (b) Changes in MLWHFQ with the same format as in (a). For both, parameters were significant but similar during the study Phase I, which was attributed to a placebo effect. Clinically and statistically significant differences emerged between the groups during the second phase of the study, which revealed treatment benefits. (c) Kaplan–Meier analysis of the proportion of patients surviving without being hospitalized during the first phase of the study between baseline and end of Phase I (labeled "Phase I") and changes between end of Phase I and end of Phase II (labeled "Phase II"). Bar graphs of VO$_2$, MLWHFQ, and event-free survival. With the relatively small number of patients, the differences were not statistically significant.

Evidence of molecular remodeling in patients with heart failure

To explore mechanisms of CCM effects in patients with heart failure, the effects of CCM therapy on myocardial gene expression were investigated in a substudy of 11 patients of the FIX-HF-4 study described above [41]. Endomyocardial biopsies were obtained at baseline (prior to CCM therapy) and 3 and 6 months thereafter. As detailed above, patients were randomized either to get CCM therapy for the first 3 months followed by sham treatment (Group 1) or to receive sham treatment first followed by active treatment (Group2). mRNA expression was analyzed in core laboratory blinded to treatment sequence. Expression of ANP, BNP, MHC, the SR genes SERCA-2a, PLB, RYR, and the stretch response genes p38 mitogen-activated protein kinase (MAPK) and p21ras was measured using reverse transcription polymerase chain reaction and bands quantified in densitometric units (du). The 3 months' OFF therapy phase was associated with increased expression of ANP, BNP, p38-MAPK, and p21ras and decreased expression of α-MHC, SERCA-2a, PLB, and RYR. In contrast, the 3 months' ON therapy phase resulted in decreased expression of ANP, BNP, p38-MAPK, and p21ras and increased expression of α-MHC, SERCA-2a, PLB, and RYR.

A detailed analysis of the findings pertaining to α-MHC is shown in Figure 4.10. Band intensities were normalized to their respective values obtained in the baseline heart failure state. Data from patients with ischemic and idiopathic cardiomyopathy are shown with dashed and solid lines, respectively. At the end of Phase 1, α-MHC expression increased in Group 1 patients (device ON, Figure 4.10a) and stayed the same or decreased in Group 2 patients (device OFF, Figure 4.10b). After crossover, expression decreased in Group 1 patients when the device was switched off and increased in Group 2 patients when the device was switched on. The overall comparisons are summarized in Figure 4.10c, where results from ON periods and OFF periods are pooled. As shown, there was a statistically significant ~62.7 ± 45.3% increase in α-MHC expression above the heart failure baseline state in response to CCM treatment. As shown in this typical example,

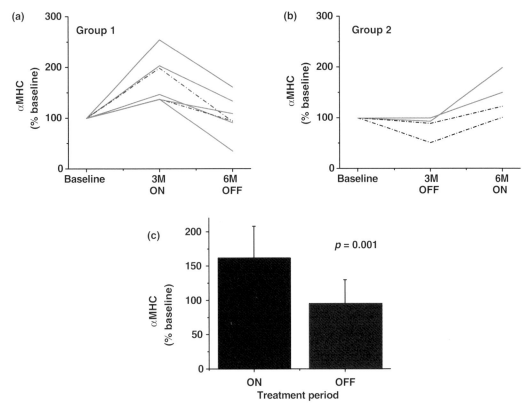

Figure 4.10 Changes in α-MHC (α-myosin heavy chain) expression (quantified as percentage of baseline) at the end of study periods in Group 1 (a) and Group 2 (b) patients. Data summarized by pooling of the end of "ON" periods from the two groups and end of "OFF" periods from the two groups (c). Solid lines show data from patients with idiopathic cardiomyopathy whereas dashed lines are from patient with ischemic cardiomyopathy [41].

there was no substantive difference in the response identified in hearts with idiopathic and ischemic cardiomyopathies. These findings were representative of those obtained with the other genes examined except, as detailed above, expression of ANP, BNP, p38-MAPK, and p21ras were decreased during CCM therapy.

Most interestingly, there were significant correlations between improvements in gene expression correlated with improvements in peak VO_2 and MLWHFQ [41]. As one example, the correlations between changes in these parameters of functional status and changes in SERCA2a expression are summarized in Figure 4.11. As shown, these correlations were present for both ischemic and idiopathic cardiomyopathy.

These findings indicated that CCM treatment reversed cardiac maladaptive fetal gene program and normalized expression of key SR Ca^{2+} cycling and stretch response genes. These findings, which are confirmatory of those identified in response to CCM treatment in animals with heart failure discussed above, support a novel mechanism of action by which CCM improves LV function in patients with heart failure.

Combining CCM with CRT

As discussed above, CCM signals applied in the acute setting to heart failure patients simultaneously receiving CRT provide additive effects on LV contractility indexed by dP/dt_{max}. Because symptoms persist in more than ∼30% patients with prolonged QRS duration receiving CRT, we have postulated that addition of CCM treatment may provide an option for these patients. We have previously reported on the initial experience of combining CCM in CRT nonresponders [42]. It was

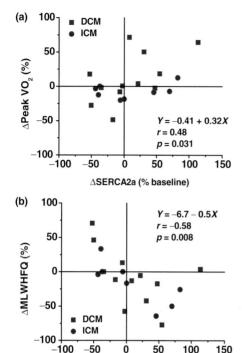

Figure 4.11 Changes in (a) peak VO$_2$ and (b) MLWHFQ score versus changes in expression of SERCA2a from the subset of 11 patients of the FIX-HF-4 study [41]. DCM, dilated cardiomyopathy; ICM, ischemic cardiomyopathy.

demonstrated that the implantation procedure is technically feasible, that the OPTIMIZER System and CRT-D devices can coexist without interference, and that acute hemodynamic and clinical improvements can be observed. These preliminary results have provided the impetus for initiation of a prospective study that is now planned to systematically investigate the effects of CCM in CRT nonresponders.

Summary and conclusions

Studies of CCM signals performed in isolated muscle strips and in intact hearts of animals with congestive heart failure have suggested that these signals can enhance myocardial contractile strength. CCM signal delivery with a pacemaker-like device connected to the heart with standard pacing leads has been shown to be straightforward to implement clinically. More recent basic research has demon-

strated that CCM signals effect significant changes in myocardial gene expression (including a reversal of several aspects of the fetal gene program expressed in heart failure), improved expression and phosphorylation of the sodium–calcium exchanger and connexin 43, and improved ratio of total PLB to phosphorylated PLB [33,41]. These findings point toward novel mechanisms of action of this electrical form of treatment.

Results obtained in patients with symptomatic heart failure with reduced EF have been encouraging and support both safety and efficacy. A large, randomized, controlled clinical trial is underway in the United States. Future studies could also evaluate whether CCM is effective in patients with wide QRS who declare themselves nonresponsive to CRT [42] or if combining CRT with CCM is more effective than CRT alone. Testing of these hypotheses would be facilitated by development of a single device that incorporates pacing, anti-tachycardia therapies, and CCM.

Acknowledgment

The research presented in this study was supported by grants from IMPULSE Dynamics, Inc.

References

1. Abraham WT, Fisher WG, Smith AL, *et al.* Cardiac resynchronization in chronic heart failure. N Engl J Med 2002;346:1845–1853.
2. Bristow MR, Saxon LA, Boehmer J, *et al.* Cardiac-resynchronization therapy with or without an implantable defibrillator in advanced chronic heart failure. N Engl J Med 2004;350:2140–2150.
3. Beshai JF, Grimm RA, Nagueh SF, *et al.* Cardiac-resynchronization therapy in heart failure with narrow QRS complexes. N Engl J Med 2007;357:2461–2471.
4. Shenkman HJ, Pampati V, Khandelwal AK, *et al.* Congestive heart failure and QRS duration: establishing prognosis study. Chest 2002;122:528–534.
5. Lawo T, Borggrefe M, Butter C, *et al.* Electrical signals applied during the absolute refractory period: an investigational treatment for advanced heart failure in patients with normal QRS duration. J Am Coll Cardiol 2005;46:2229–2236.
6. Burkhoff D, Ben Haim SA. Nonexcitatory electrical signals for enhancing ventricular contractility: rationale and initial investigations of an experimental treat-

ment for heart failure. Am J Physiol Heart Circ Physiol 2005;288:H2550–H2556.

7. Gomez AM, Valdivia HH, Cheng H, *et al.* Defective excitation–contraction coupling in experimental heart failure. Science 1997;276:800–806.

8. Hasenfuss G, Reinecke H, Studer R, *et al.* Relation between myocardial function and expression of sarcoplasmic reticulum Ca^{2+}-ATPase in failing and nonfailing human myocardium. Circ Res 1994;75:434–442.

9. Frank KF, Bolck B, Brixius K, Kranias EG, Schwinger RH. Modulation of SERCA: implications for the failing human heart. Basic Res Cardiol 2002;97(Suppl 1):I72–I78.

10. Mishra S, Gupta RC, Tiwari N, Sharov VG, Sabbah HN. Molecular mechanisms of reduced sarcoplasmic reticulum Ca(2+) uptake in human failing left ventricular myocardium. J Heart Lung Transplant 2002;21:366–373.

11. O'rourke B, Kass DA, Tomaselli GF, *et al.* Mechanisms of altered excitation–contraction coupling in canine tachycardia-induced heart failure: I. Experimental studies. Circ Res 1999;84:562–570.

12. Haghighi K, Gregory KN, Kranias EG. Sarcoplasmic reticulum Ca-ATPase–phospholamban interactions and dilated cardiomyopathy. Biochem Biophys Res Commun 2004;322:1214–1222.

13. Frank K, Kranias EG. Phospholamban and cardiac contractility. Ann Med 2000;32:572–578.

14. Schmidt U, Hajjar RJ, Kim CS, *et al.* Human heart failure: cAMP stimulation of SR Ca(2+)-ATPase activity and phosphorylation level of phospholamban. Am J Physiol 1999;277:H474–H480.

15. Schwinger RH, Munch G, Bolck B, *et al.* Reduced Ca(2+)-sensitivity of SERCA 2a in failing human myocardium due to reduced serin-16 phospholamban phosphorylation. J Mol Cell Cardiol 1999;31:479–491.

16. Studer R, Reinecke H, Bilger J, *et al.* Gene expression of the cardiac Na^+–Ca^{2+} exchanger in end-stage human heart failure. Circ Res 1994;75:443–453.

17. Heerdt PM, Holmes JW, Cai B, *et al.* Chronic unloading by left ventricular assist device reverses contractile dysfunction and alters gene expression in end-stage heart failure. Circulation 2000;102:2713–2719.

18. Marx SO, Reiken S, Hisamatsu Y, *et al.* PKA phosphorylation dissociates FKBP12.6 from the calcium release channel (ryanodine receptor): defective regulation in failing hearts. Cell 2000;101:365–376.

19. Wehrens XH, Lehnart SE, Marks AR. Intracellular calcium release channels and cardiac disease. Annu Rev Physiol 2005;67:69–98.

20. Li Y, Kranias EG, Mignery GA, Bers DM. Protein kinase A phosphorylation of the ryanodine receptor does not affect calcium sparks in mouse ventricular myocytes. Circ Res 2002;90:309–316.

21. Dorn GW, Molkentin JD. Manipulating cardiac contractility in heart failure: data from mice and men. Circulation 2004;109:150–158.

22. Wood EH, Heppner RL, Weidmann S. Inotropic effects of electric currents: 1. Positive and negative effects of constant electric currents or current pulses applied during cardiac action potential. Circ Res 1969;24:409–445.

23. Wood EH, Heppner RL, Weidmann S. Inotropic effects of electric currents: 2. Hypotheses: calcium movements, excitation–contraction coupling and inotropic effects. Circ Res 1969;24:409–445.

24. Antoni H, Jacob R, Kaufmann R. Mechanical response of the frog and mammalian myocardium to changes in the action potential duration by constant current pulses. Pflugers Arch 1969;306:33–57.

25. Kaufmann RL, Antoni H, Hennekes R, *et al.* Mechanical response of the mammalian myocardium to modifications of the action potential. Cardiovasc Res 1971;1(Suppl 70):64–70.

26. Blank M, Goodman R. Initial interactions in electromagnetic field-induced biosynthesis. J Cell Physiol 2004;199:359–363.

27. Burkhoff D, Shemer I, Felzen B, *et al.* Electric currents applied during the refractory period can modulate cardiac contractility in vitro and in vivo. Heart Fail Rev 2001;6:27–34.

28. Mohri S, Shimizu J, Mika Y, *et al.* Electric currents applied during the refractory period enhance contractility and systolic calcium in Ferret. Am J Physiol Heart Circ Physiol 2002;284:1119–1123.

29. Mohri S, He KL, Dickstein M, *et al.* Cardiac contractility modulation by electric currents applied during the refractory period. Am J Physiol Heart Circ Physiol 2002;282:H1642–H1647.

30. Sabbah HN, Stein PD, Kono T, *et al.* A canine model of chronic heart failure produced by multiple sequential coronary microembolizations. Am J Physiol 1991;260:H1379–H1384.

31. Sabbah HN, Shimoyama H, Kono T, *et al.* Effects of long-term monotherapy with enalapril, metoprolol, and digoxin on the progression of left ventricular dysfunction and dilation in dogs with reduced ejection fraction. Circulation 1994;89:2852–2859.

32. Morita H, Suzuki G, Haddad W, *et al.* Cardiac contractility modulation with nonexcitatory electric signals improves left ventricular function in dogs with chronic heart failure. J Card Fail 2003;9:69–75.

33. Imai M, Rastogi S, Gupta RC, *et al.* Therapy with cardiac contractility modulation electrical signals improves left ventricular function and remodeling in dogs with chronic heart failure. J Am Coll Cardiol 2007;49:2120–2128.

34. Pappone C, Rosanio S, Burkhoff D, *et al.* Cardiac contractility modulation by electric currents applied during the refractory period in patients with heart failure secondary to ischemic or idiopathic dilated cardiomyopathy. Am J Cardiol 2002;90:1307–1313.

35. Pappone C, Vicedomini G, Salvati A, *et al.* Electrical modulation of cardiac contractility: clinical aspects in congestive heart failure. Heart Fail Rev 2001;6:55–60.

36. Butter C, Wellnhofer E, Schlegl M, *et al.* Enhanced inotropic state of the failing left ventricle by cardiac contractility modulation electrical signals is not associated with increased myocardial oxygen consumption. J Card Fail 2007;13:137–142.

37. Stix G, Borggrefe M, Wolpert C, *et al.* Chronic electrical stimulation during the absolute refractory period of the myocardium improves severe heart failure. Eur Heart J 2004;25:650–655.

38. Pappone C, Augello G, Rosanio S, *et al.* First human chronic experience with cardiac contractility modulation by nonexcitatory electrical currents for treating systolic heart failure: mid-term safety and efficacy results from a multicenter study. J Cardiovasc Electrophysiol 2004;15:418–427.

39. Neelagaru SB, Sanchez JE, Lau SK, *et al.* Nonexcitatory, cardiac contractility modulation electrical impulses: feasibility study for advanced heart failure in patients with normal QRS duration. Heart Rhythm 2006;3:1140–1147.

40. Borggrefe M, Lawo T, Butter C, *et al.* Randomized, double blind study of non-excitatory, cardiac contractility modulation (CCM) electrical impulses for symptomatic heart failure. Eur Heart J 2008;29:1019–1028.

41. Butter C, Rastogi S, Minden HH, *et al.* Cardiac contractility modulation electrical signals improve myocardial gene expression in patients with heart failure. J Am Coll Cardiol, 2008;51:1784–1789.

42. Butter C, Meyhofer J, Seifert M, Neuss M, Minden HH. First use of cardiac contractility modulation (CCM) in a patient failing CRT therapy: clinical and technical aspects of combined therapies. Eur J Heart Fail 2007; 9:955–958.

CHAPTER 5

The Role of Cardiac Restraint Devices in the Treatment of Patients with Dilated Cardiomyopathy

Douglas L. Mann

Baylor College of Medicine, Houston, TX, USA

Introduction

Heart failure is currently viewed as a syndrome that develops and progresses as a result of the overexpression of biologically active molecules that are capable of exerting deleterious effects on the heart and circulation [1]. The evidence in support of this point of view is derived from experimental models that have shown that pathophysiologically relevant concentrations of neurohormones are sufficient to mimic some aspects of the heart failure phenotype (reviewed in [1]). Clinical studies have likewise shown that antagonizing "neurohormones" with angiotensin-converting enzyme inhibitors and β-blockers lead to clinical improvement for patients with heart failure [2–5]. Nonetheless, despite the many strengths of the neurohormonal model in terms of explaining disease progression, it is becoming increasingly clear that heart failure continues to progress despite optimal medical therapy with neurohormonal antagonists.

Left ventricular remodeling as a mechanism for disease progression in heart failure

Natural history studies have shown that progressive left ventricular (LV) remodeling is directly related to future deterioration in LV performance and a less favorable clinical course in patients with heart failure [6–8]. Although some investigators currently view LV remodeling simply as the end-organ response that occurs following years of exposure to the deleterious effects of long-term neurohormonal stimulation, others have suggested that LV remodeling may contribute independently to the progression of heart failure. Although a complete discussion of the complex changes that occur in the heart during LV remodeling is well beyond the intended scope of this brief review, it is worth emphasizing that the process of LV remodeling extends to and impacts importantly on the biology of the cardiac myocyte, the volume of myocyte and nonmyocyte components (reviewed in [1]) of the myocardium, as well as on the geometry and architecture of the LV chamber (Table 5.1). Although each of these various components of the remodeling process may contribute importantly to the overall development and progression of heart failure, what determines the reversibility of heart failure is whether or not the changes that occur at the level of the myocyte, the myocardium, or the LV chamber are reversible. In this regard, it is interesting to note that the changes that occur at the level of the myocyte and the LV chamber appear to be at least partially reversible in some experimental and/or clinical models [9–12].

A number of changes that occur during the process of LV remodeling may contribute to worsening heart failure. Principal among these changes is the increase in LV wall stress that occurs during LV remodeling. Indeed, one of the first observations with

Heart Failure: Device Management. Edited by Arthur Feldman.
© 2010 Blackwell Publishing.

Table 5.1 Mechanical disadvantages created by left ventricular remodeling.

Increased wall stress (afterload)
Afterload mismatch
Episodic subendocardial hypoperfusion
Increased oxygen utilization
Functional mitral regurgitation
Worsening hemodynamic overloading
Worsening activation of compensatory mechanisms
Activation of maladaptive gene expression
Activation of maladaptive signal transduction pathways

respect to the abnormal geometry of remodeled ventricle was the consistent finding that the remodeled heart was not only larger, but was also more spherical in shape [13]. As depicted in Table 5.1, the increase in LV size and resultant change in LV geometry from the normal prolate ellipse to a more spherical shape creates a number of de novo mechanical burdens for the failing heart, most notably an increase in LV end-diastolic wall stress. Insofar as the load on the ventricle at end diastole contributes importantly to the afterload that the ventricle faces at the onset of systole, it follows that LV dilation itself will increase the work of the ventricle, and hence the oxygen utilization as well. In addition to the increase in LV end-diastolic volume, LV wall thinning occurs as the ventricle begins to remodel. The increase in wall thinning along with the increase in afterload created by LV dilation leads to a functional "afterload mismatch" that may further contribute to a decrease in forward cardiac output [14,15–17]. Moreover, the high end-diastolic wall stress might be expected to lead to episodic hypoperfusion of the subendocardium with resultant worsening of LV function [18–20], as well as increased oxidative stress, with the resultant activation of families of genes that are sensitive to free radical generation (e.g., tumor necrosis factor and interleukin-1 ∃). Finally, increased LV wall stress may lead to sustained expression of stretch-activated genes (angiotensin II, endothelin, and tumor necrosis factor [21–23]) and/or stretch activation of hypertrophic signaling pathways.

The suggestion that LV remodeling contributes to the progression of heart failure raises the inter-esting possibility that therapeutic strategies that are specifically designed to prevent and/or antagonize LV remodeling may also be beneficial in heart failure. Thus far, several innovative approaches have been evaluated to address LV remodeling, including cardiomyoplasty, partial left ventriculectomy ("Batista procedure"), and the endoventricular circular patch plasty (the "Dor procedure") [24–26]. Although cardiomyoplasty has largely been abandoned, one of the important observations that arose from these studies was that the beneficial effects of the cardiomyoplasty on LV remodeling were largely dependent on the external girdling provided by the skeletal muscle wrap, as opposed to the systolic assistance provided by the skeletal muscle contraction [26]. In the section that follows, we will review the role of cardiac support devices in preventing and/or inhibiting LV remodeling in patients with moderate to advanced heart failure.

Cardiac support devices

As noted above, the current generation of passive cardiac support devices arose out of original observations with dynamic cardiomyoplasty, which was originally intended to act as an auxiliary pump for the failing heart (reviewed in [27]). Subsequent hemodynamic assessments in animals and humans suggested that much of the observed benefit of dynamic cardiomyoplasty appeared to be derived from the passive girdling effect of the muscle wrap, which limited ventricular dilatation, reduced LV wall stress, and prevented LV remodeling [27]. These early experiences with dynamic cardiomyoplasty and the insights into its biological effects have led to the ongoing development of cardiac support devices that were specifically aimed at inhibiting LV remodeling. At the time of this writing, there are two different passive cardiac support devices that have been developed: the CorCap™ Cardiac Support Device (CSD; Acorn Cardiovascular, Inc., St. Paul, MN, USA) and the Paracor® device (Paracor Medical Inc., Sunnyvale, CA, USA).

CorCap™ Cardiac Support Device

The CorCap™ Cardiac Support Device (CSD; Acorn Cardiovascular, Inc., St. Paul, MN, USA) is a fabric mesh device that is surgically implanted around the heart (Figure 5.1). The general

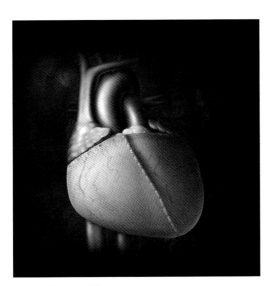

Figure 5.1 CorCap™ cardiac support device.

surgical procedure, which requires a median sternotomy and general anesthesia, takes approximately 2 hours if there is no concomitant (e.g., mitral) surgery. Although the procedure can be performed without going on cardiopulmonary bypass, it is often necessary to use cardiopulmonary bypass for the more unstable patients. The CSD is designed to provide circumferential diastolic support and reduce LV wall stress, thereby leading to reverse cardiac remodeling. Mechanistic preclinical studies in a canine model of heart failure have shown that treatment with the CSD leads to beneficial changes in the biology of the failing cardiac myocyte, including reversal of the fetal gene program and increased adrenergic sensitivity [12,28], changes in the extracellular matrix including decreased fibrosis and increased capillary density [29], as well as energetically favorable changes in the size and shape of the ventricle, with a return of the LV to a smaller and more elliptically shaped left ventricle that has improved pump performance [29]. Moreover, early nonrandomized safety studies with the CSD, implanted either alone or in conjunction with mitral valve repair, mitral valve replacement, or coronary artery bypass grafting, have shown that the CSD was safe and was associated with improvements in ventricular structure and function that were maintained after more than 4 years of follow-up [30]. Based on these early preclinical and clinical stud-

ies, a randomized, prospective, controlled trial was conducted to evaluate the safety and efficacy of the CorCap CSD in patients with dilated cardiomyopathy [31].

The Acorn trial [31]

The primary objective of the Acorn trial was to determine the safety and efficacy of the CorCap CSD in patients with New York Heart Association (NYHA) class III or IV heart failure of nonischemic etiology who were receiving optimal medical therapy. Patients had a LV ejection fraction (EF) < 0.35%, LV dilation (defined as an LV end-diastolic dimension [EDD] > 60 mm, or an LVEDD index > 30 mm/m^2 as determined by transthoracic echocardiography), a 6-minute walk distance < 450 m (1476 ft), and acceptable laboratory and pulmonary function tests. Patients were excluded from the trial if they had a planned cardiac surgical procedure other than mitral valve repair and/or replacement (MVR) with or without tricuspid valve repair or an ablation for atrial fibrillation, hypertrophic obstructive cardiomyopathy, significant cardiomegaly which was estimated to exceed the largest available size of the CSD, expectation of existing cardiothoracic adhesions that would limit circumferential access to the heart, any condition considered a contraindication for extracorporeal circulation, an existing patent coronary artery bypass grafts, a need for surgical revascularization as determined by an angiogram, a need for an intra-aortic balloon pump or intravenous inotropic or vasoactive agents, with a current or anticipated need for LV assist device or cardiac replacement device, or were on an active cardiac transplant list or had an anticipated need for heart transplant within the next 2 years.

Patients were enrolled into one of two strata, depending on whether they required MVR (Figure 5.2). Patients who had significant mitral regurgitation and a clinical indication for MVR were enrolled in the MVR stratum (193 patients) and were then randomized to either treatment (MVR surgery plus the CSD) or control (MVR surgery alone). Patients without a clinical indication for mitral surgery were enrolled in the no-MVR stratum, and were randomized to either treatment (CSD implant) plus optimal medical therapy or control (optimal medical therapy alone). The primary analysis of the data was prespecified to include all patients from

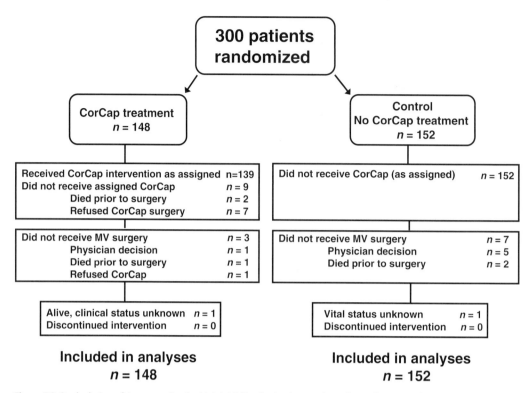

Figure 5.2 Study design of Acorn randomized trial. MVR, mitral valve repair and/or replacement. (Reproduced with permission from [31].)

both strata. The primary endpoint of the Acorn trial was a composite ordinal endpoint based on three outcomes: vital status, occurrence of a major cardiac procedure for progression of heart failure, and change in NYHA classification. The proportion of patients who improved, remained unchanged, and/or worsened was analyzed.

A total of 300 patients at 29 centers were enrolled in the Acorn trial. As specified in the treatment protocol, the trial was stopped on a common closing day after the last patient enrolled in the study had been followed for 1 year. The median duration of follow-up was 22.9 months, with a range of 12–48 months. Ninety-two percent of the patients had at least 12 months of follow-up. The Acorn trial showed that the use of a CSD resulted in salutary changes in LV structure (decreased LV volumes and decreased LV sphericity) that were accompanied by significant improvements in patient's functional status and quality of life. In patients who were receiving optimal medical care with angiotensin-converting enzyme inhibitors/angiotensin receptor

blockers (97%), β-blockers (84%), aldosterone antagonists (76%), and diuretics (98%), more CSD-treated patients were considered improved and fewer were worsened when compared to patients in the control group. The proportional odds ratio for the clinical composite score, the primary endpoint of the trial, showed that CSD-treated patients had a 73% likelihood of having a better clinical outcome relative to patients in the control arm (1.73 [(95% CI 1.07–2.79, $p = 0.02$]). When the individual components of the clinical composite score were examined, there was a significant ($p < 0.01$) reduction in the need for major cardiac procedures in the CSD treatment arm when compared to the control arm. The Kaplan–Meier curves depicting the percentage of patients who did not receive a major cardiac procedure because of worsening heart failure began to diverge early, and continued to diverge over the course of the trial (Figure 5.3), reflecting the greater need for invasive cardiac interventions in the control group. Indeed, the CSD treatment group received fewer cardiac transplantations, LV assist

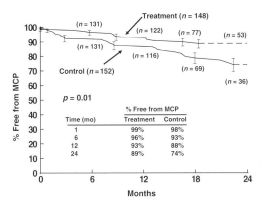

Figure 5.3 Kaplan–Meier curves for freedom from major cardiac procedures (MCP) in both the Cardiac Support Device treatment and control groups. (Reproduced with permission from [31].)

devices, repeat mitral and tricuspid valve surgeries, and biventricular pacemakers. Treatment with the CSD led to a significant decrease in LV end-diastolic ($p < 0.009$) and end-systolic volumes ($p < 0.017$), and a significant increase in the LV sphericity in-

dex ($p = 0.026$), as shown in Figure 5.4. Although LVEF increased significantly in the CSD treatment arm at 12 months ($p < 0.0009$), there was no significant difference in LVEF between groups ($p = 0.45$). These changes in LV structure were accompanied by significant improvement in patient's quality of life, as shown by the significant decrease in the Minnesota Living with Heart Failure score ($p = 0.04$) as well as by a significant improvement ($p < 0.015$) in the Short Form-36 scores. Overall, 81% of patients in the control group and 85% of patients in the treatment group had an adverse event, reflecting the surgical nature of the trial. The number of patients and the type of adverse events were not statistically different ($p = 0.27$) between the treatment and control groups. There were no adverse events related to sizing or fitting of the CorCap CSD. Special attention was given to the hypothetical concern with respect to the development of constrictive physiology following placement of the CSD. There were no acute constrictive physiology events during the postoperative period when patients were

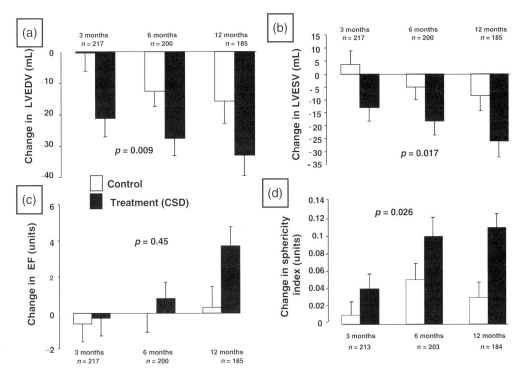

Figure 5.4 Change in left ventricular (LV) structure in the Cardiac Support Device (CSD) treatment and control groups. (a) Change in LV end-diastolic volume (LVEDV; mL) from baseline; (b) change in LV end-systolic volume (LVESV; mL) from baseline; (c) change in LV ejection fraction (EF; units) from baseline; (d) change in LV sphericity index (ratio of LV long axis/LV short axis; units) at 3, 6, and 12 months. (Reproduced with permission from [31].)

monitored in the intensive care unit. There were no adverse events related to constrictive physiology in either the control or treatment groups. The total number of all-cause rehospitalizations occurring during the 22-month median follow-up period was similar in the treatment and control groups (305 vs 307, $p = 0.44$).

Because of the invasive nature of device implantation, it has been suggested that patient selection criteria should be individualized and optimized so that devices are implanted in those patients who are the most likely to receive a maximal benefit from the device when compared to subjects who do not receive a device. To this end the Acorn trial utilized a cumulative trends analysis to identify a "focused cohort of patients" who had the largest and most consistent treatment effect. This analysis showed that patients with an LVEDD that was $\exists$ 30 mm/m^2 and 40 mm/m^2 were the most likely to

benefit from the CSD treatment, based on analysis of the primary composite endpoint (OR 2.45, $p = 0.011$), freedom from major cardiac procedures ($p = 0.013$), and mortality (34% decrease, $p = 0.17$). Moreover, the treatment effects were consistent in the no-MVR and MVR strata, with the largest benefit in the no-MVR stratum. These more selective patient criteria may prove useful in selecting those patients who will be most likely to benefit from CSD implantation.

The results of the long-term follow-up of the Acorn trial have been published [32]. Over the entire duration of follow-up, there were 41 deaths among 152 patients in the control group (crude mortality rate 27.0%) and 38 deaths among 148 patients in the treatment group (crude mortality rate 25.7%) (Figure 5.5). This resulted in a relative risk reduction of 4.8%, favoring the treatment group. Although this small difference was not

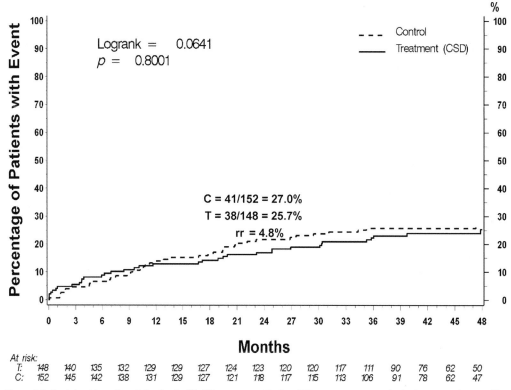

Figure 5.5 Sustained benefits of the CorCap™ CSD. Kaplan–Meier mortality curves for the CorCap CSD treatment group (T; solid line) and the control group (C; dotted line) for patients followed up to 4 years. The CorCap CSD treatment group had a lower crude mortality rate (25.7%) when compared to the control group (27.0%, risk reduction 4.8%), but this difference was not significant. (Reproduced with permission from [32].)

statistically significant, there was no late adverse effect on mortality associated with implantation of the CorCap CSD. It bears emphasis that the Acorn study was not powered to detect a mortality benefit. Patients treated with the CorCap CSD had sustained long-term reductions in LV end-diastolic volume (average difference 18.8 mL, $p = 0.005$) and LV end-systolic volume (average difference 15.6 mL, $p = 0.013$) compared to the control group when followed over 3 years. Moreover, the LV sphericity index was also significantly increased in the treatment group (average difference 0.045 units, $p = 0.018$). Importantly, the improvements in LV size and shape were observed when the CorCap CSD was implanted concomitantly with mitral value surgery (MVR stratum) or by itself (no-MVR stratum). In this regard, it is worth noting that in the control group the standard mitral valve surgery with either a mitral valve ring or mitral valve replacement (control group) also led to a progressive improvement in LV size and shape. Adding the CorCap CSD with mitral valve surgery resulted in an additional improvement in LV size and shape. Thus the CSD appears to provide a sustained beneficial effect on remodeling when used independently, as well as incremental benefit when used with concomitant therapies such as mitral valve surgery.

Paracor® Cardiac HeartNet ventricular support system

The Paracor® HeartNet device (Paracor Medical Inc., Sunnyvale, CA, USA) is a nitinol mesh weave that is surgically implanted around the ventricle. The mesh is flexible over a wide range of sizes, which allows it to be collapsed into a delivery system that conforms to the ventricle upon deployment (Figure 5.6). A suction device contained with the delivery system allows for ventricular stabilization and placement of bypass through a small minimally invasive anterior thoracotomy that is performed under general anesthesia. The theoretical and therapeutic concept of the Paracor device is similar to the Acorn CSD, but the device has not been as extensively studied as the Acorn CSD.

Recently the results of a feasibility pilot trial with the Paracor HeartNet device have been reported [33]. In this study, 51 patients (mean age 52 yr, range 30–73 yr) with an EF $\leq 35\%$ and a NYHA class II or III heart failure who were receiving optimal medi-

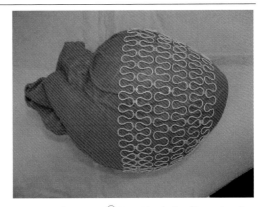

Figure 5.6 The Paracor® HeartNet device. (Reproduced with permission from [33].)

cal therapy for at least 3 months were enrolled at 15 sites (3 in Europe, 12 in the United States) to undergo implantation of the HeartNet device. Patients were evaluated at baseline and at 6-month follow-up by echocardiography, a 6-minute walk test, cardiopulmonary exercise testing (partial oxygen pressure in mixed venous blood), NYHA class, and the Minnesota Living with Heart Failure questionnaire. Implantation of the HeartNet was accomplished in 50 of 51 patients (98%). After 6 months of follow-up there was a significant improvement in the 6-minute walk test ($p < 0.002$) and Minnesota Living with Heart Failure scores ($p < 0.002$). Echocardiographic parameters also demonstrated significant improvement at 6 months, with improvements in LVEDD (mean decrease 3 mm, $p < 0.038$), end-diastolic volume (mean decrease 25.7 cm^3, $p < 0.025$), end-systolic volume (mean decrease 23.5 cm^3, $p < 0.037$), and LV mass (mean decrease 23.1 g, $p < 0.046$). There was a trend toward improvement in the NYHA class at 3, 6, and 12 months, as well as a trend toward improvement in the maximal oxygen consumption by treadmill testing. Thus, the overall results with the Parcor HeartNet device are consistent with those observed in the Acorn trial. The adverse events with the implantation of the HeartNet included 2 in-hospital deaths secondary to pulmonary complications (4%), additional pulmonary complications in 7 patients (14%), arrhythmia in 14 patients (27%), epicardial laceration in 2 patients (4%), and empyema in 1 patient (2%). Interestingly, as with the findings in the Acorn trial, major complications occurred with the patients with the largest ventricles.

Currently the HeartNet Ventricular Support System is being evaluated in the Prospective Evaluation of Elastic Restraint to LESSen the Effects of Heart Failure (PEERLESS-HF) trial, which will determine whether the device will benefit symptomatic Stage C heart failure patients with an EF $\leq$ 30% who are being treated with optimal medical therapy including angiotensin-converting enzyme inhibitors or angiotensin receptor blockers. The use of β-blockers, diuretics, and aldosterone inhibitors is at the discretion of the investigator. The primary outcome measures are peak VO_2 and 6-minute walk at 6 months, quality of life at 6 months, and all-cause mortality at 12 months. The trial is expected to enroll 272 patients, with an anticipated completion date of June 2010.

Summary and conclusions

In the present chapter review we have described the role of LV remodeling in the pathogenesis of heart failure, with a focus on how the current generation of cardiac support devices therapies change LV size and shape in the failing ventricle. Thus far, the results of the completed Acorn trial with the CorCap CSD and the early results with the HeartNet device appear remarkably consistent in terms of their effects of cardiac remodeling. Moreover, the effects of these devices on clinical outcomes also appear encouraging, in terms of stabilizing the progression of heart failure as well as improving patient's quality of life. Insofar as there are no therapies that are specifically designed to address the problem of cardiac remodeling and many patients will have progressive heart failure in spite of intensive medical regimens and biventricular pacemakers, the use of cardiac support devices fits an unmet clinical need for patients with advanced heart failure and LV dilation. Improvements in the technique of implanting the device using less invasive means, optimizing patient selection, as well as combining this technology with other technologies (e.g., cell-based therapy) may allow for even greater clinical benefits than have already been observed thus far. Accordingly, the use of cardiac support devices may prove to be a novel adjunctive therapy for stabilizing the progression of heart failure in patients who remain symptomatic despite optimal medical therapy.

Acknowledgement

This work was supported, in part, by research funds from the NIH (P50 HL-O6H and RO1 HL58081-01, RO1 HL61543-01, HL-42250-10/10).

References

1. Mann DL. Mechanisms and models in heart failure: a combinatorial approach. Circulation 1999;100: 999–1088.
2. Cohn JN, Johnson G, Ziesche S, *et al.* A comparison of enalapril with hydralazine-isosorbide dinitrate in the treatment of chronic congestive heart failure. N Engl J Med 1991;325:303–310.
3. The SOLVD Investigators. Effect of enalapril on mortality and the development of heart failure in asymptomatic patients with reduced left ventricular ejection fraction. N Engl J Med 1992;327:685–691.
4. Bristow MR, Gilbert EM, Abraham WT, *et al.* Carvedilol produces dose-related improvements in left ventricular function and survival in subjects with chronic heart failure. Circulation 1996;94:2807–2816.
5. Packer M, Bristow MR, Cohn JN, et al; U.S. Carvedilol Heart Failure Study Group. The effect of carvedilol on morbidity and mortality in patients with chronic heart failure. N Engl J Med 1996;334:1350–1355.
6. Cohn JN. Structural basis for heart failure: ventricular remodeling and its pharmacological inhibition. Circulation 1995;91:2504–2507.
7. Douglas PS, Morrow R, Ioli A, Reicheck N. Left ventricular shape, afterload, and survival in idiopathic dilated cardiomyopathy. J Am Coll Cardiol 1989;13:311–315.
8. Vasan RS, Larson MG, Benjamin EJ, Evans JC, Levy D. Left ventricular dilation and the risk of congestive heart failure in people without myocardial infarction. N Engl J Med 1997;336:1350–1355.
9. Tsutsui H, Spinale FG, Nagatsu M, *et al.* Effects of chronic β-adrenergic blockade on the left ventricular and cardiocyte abnormalities of chronic canine mitral regurgitation. J Clin Invest 1994;93:2639–2648.
10. Hall SA, Cigarroa CG, Marcoux L, Risser RC, Grayburn PA, Eichhorn EJ. Time course of improvement in left ventricular function, mass and geometry in patients with congestive heart failure treated with beta-adrenergic blockade. J Am Coll Cardiol 1995;25:1154–1161.
11. Doughty RN, Whalley GA, Gamble G, MacMahon S, Sharpe N. Left ventricular remodeling with carvedilol in patients with congestive heart failure due to ischemic heart disease. J Am Coll Cardiol 1998;29:1060–1066.
12. Sabbah HN, Sharov VG, Gupta RC, *et al.* Reversal of chronic molecular and cellular abnormalities due to

heart failure by passive mechanical ventricular containment. Circ Res 2003;93(11):1095–1101.

13. Linzbach AJ. Heart failure from the point of view of quantitative anatomy. Am J Cardiol 1960;5:370–382.

14. Ross J Jr. Afterload mismatch in aortic and mitral valve disease: implications for surgical therapy. J Am Coll Cardiol 1985;5:811–826.

15. Ross JJ. Mechanisms of cardiac contraction. What roles for preload, afterload and inotropic state in heart failure? Eur Heart J 1983;4(Suppl A):19–28.

16. Hirota Y, Saito T, Kita Y, Shimizu G, Kino M, Kawamura K. The natural history of dilated cardiomyopathy and pathophysiology of congestive heart failure. J Cardiogr Suppl 1986;(9):67–76.

17. Pouleur H, Rousseau MF, van Eyll C, Melin J, Youngblood M, Yusuf S; SOLVD Investigators. Cardiac mechanics during development of heart failure. Circulation 1993;87(5 Suppl):IV14–IV20.

18. Vatner SF. Reduced subendocardial myocardial perfusion as one mechanism for congestive heart failure. Am J Cardiol 1988;62(8):94E–98E.

19. Shannon RP, Komamura K, Shen YT, Bishop SP, Vatner SF. Impaired regional subendocardial coronary flow reserve in conscious dogs with pacing-induced heart failure. Am J Physiol 1993;265(3 Pt 2):H801–H809.

20. LeGrice IJ, Takayama Y, Holmes JW, Covell JW. Impaired subendocardial function in tachycardia-induced cardiac failure. Am J Physiol 1995;268(5 Pt 2):H1788–H1794.

21. Kapadia S, Oral H, Lee J, Nakano M, Taffet GE, Mann DL. Hemodynamic regulation of tumor necrosis factor-α gene and protein expression in adult feline myocardium. Circ Res 1997;81:187–195.

22. Sadoshima JI, Xu Y, Slayter HS, Izumo S. Autocrine release of angiotensin II mediates stretch-induced hypertrophy of cardiac myocytes in vitro. Cell 1993;75:977–984.

23. Ruwhof C, Van Der LA. Mechanical stress-induced cardiac hypertrophy: mechanisms and signal transduction pathways. Cardiovasc Res 2000;47(1):23–37.

24. Batista R. Partial left ventriculectomy—the Batista procedure. Euro J Cardiothor Surg 1999;15(Suppl I):S12–S19.

25. Dor V, Saab M, Coste P, Kornaszewska M, Montiglio F. Left ventricular aneurysm: a new surgical approach. Thorac Cardiovasc Surg 1989;37(1):11–19.

26. Kass DA, Baughman KL, Pak PH, et al. Reverse remodeling from cardiomyoplasty in human heart failure: external constraint versus active assist. Circulation 1995;91(9):2314–2318.

27. Starling RC, McCarthy PM, Yamini MH. Surgical treatment of chronic congestive heart failure. In: Mann DL, editor. Heart Failure: A Companion to Braunwald's Heart Disease. Philadelphia: Saunders; 2003:717–736.

28. Saavedra WF, Tunin RS, Paolocci N, et al. Reverse remodeling and enhanced adrenergic reserve from passive external support in experimental dilated heart failure. J Am Coll Cardiol 2002;39:2069–2076.

29. Chaudhry PA, Mishima T, Sharov VG, et al. Passive epicardial containment prevents ventricular remodeling in heart failure. Ann Thorac Surg 2000;70(4):1275–1280.

30. Oz MC, Konertz WF, Kleber FX, et al. Global surgical experience with the Acorn cardiac support device. J Thorac Cardiovasc Surg 2003;126(4):983–991.

31. Mann DL, Acker MA, Jessup M, et al. Clinical evaluation of the CorCap Cardiac Support Device in patients with dilated cardiomyopathy. Ann Thorac Surg 2007;84(4):1226–1235.

32. Starling RC, Jessup M, Oh JK, et al. Sustained benefits of the CorCap Cardiac Support Device on left ventricular remodeling: three year follow-up results from the Acorn clinical trial. Ann Thorac Surg 2007;84(4):1236–1242.

33. Klodell CT Jr, Aranda JM Jr, McGiffin DC, et al. Worldwide surgical experience with the Paracor HeartNet cardiac restraint device. J Thorac Cardiovasc Surg 2008;135(1):188–195.

CHAPTER 6

The Role of Right Heart Catheterization in the Management of Patients with Heart Failure

Sandeep A. Kamath, & Mark H. Drazner
University of Texas, Southwestern Medical Center, Dallas, TX, USA

Introduction

The pulmonary artery catheter (PAC), also referred to as a right heart catheter or Swan-Ganz catheter, is frequently used in patients with heart failure (HF) to measure ventricular filling pressures and cardiac output. Whether routine insertion of a PAC in these patients provides any meaningful benefit has been called into question over the last decade [1–6]. This chapter will outline the historical basis for measurement of hemodynamics with PAC in patients with HF, review large clinical trials assessing the utility of the PAC in the critically ill, with a focus on the recently published Evaluation Study of Congestive Heart Failure and Pulmonary Artery Catheterization Effectiveness (ESCAPE) trial [1], and discuss clinical surrogates for PAC measurements. Finally, we will conclude with our recommendations regarding the use of PAC in HF.

Rationale for PA catheter use: therapy tailored to specific hemodynamic goals

In the mid-1970s, Kovick [7] studied the effects of chronic oral vasodilator therapy in a group of 15 patients with HF that was refractory to standard therapy with digoxin and furosemide. Prior to acute therapy with sodium nitroprusside infusion,

mean right atrial pressure (RAP), pulmonary artery pressure (PAP), and pulmonary capillary wedge pressure (PCWP) were 14, 43, and 30 mmHg, respectively. With nitroprusside infusion, these values were all significantly decreased. A fall in systemic vascular resistance and a corresponding rise in cardiac index were observed with no change in mean systemic artery pressure or heart rate. Patients were also given oral isosorbide dinitrate and responses to acute administration were similar to nitroprusside in terms of a rise in cardiac index and a fall in PCWP. Patients were then given a combination of oral isosorbide dinitrate and phenoxybenzamine. At a mean follow-up period of 6 months, 12 of 15 patients were alive but only 9 underwent repeat PA catheterization. In these 9 patients, the benefits of acute vasodilator therapy were maintained with chronic oral vasodilator therapy. Clinical improvement was seen in all 12 survivors with concomitant reduction in diuretic dose. These findings supported the prevailing hypothesis that hemodynamic derangements were responsible for the clinical sequelae of the HF syndrome and the additional hypothesis that treatment of these hemodynamic derangements with vasodilator therapy would result in reduced HF symptoms and perhaps alter the natural history of the disease.

Subsequently, a series of studies by Stevenson and coworkers reported benefits of tailoring therapy to specific hemodynamic goals as measured by PAC in patients with advanced HF [8]. Target hemodynamic goals included achieving a PCWP

Heart Failure: Device Management. Edited by Arthur Feldman.
© 2010 Blackwell Publishing.

< 16 mmHg, RAP < 8 mmHg, and SVR (systemic vascular resistance) between 1000 and 1200 (dyn s)/cm^5 while maintaining an SBP (systolic blood pressure) > 80 mmHg. Important observations that came from these studies included that cardiac output could be maintained at normal filling pressures in individuals with dilated cardiomyopathy and that therapy tailored to reduce filling pressures (initially with intravenous nitroprusside and diuretics, followed by an oral regimen consisting of angiotensin-converting enzyme (ACE) inhibitors, nitrates, and occasionally hydralazine) in acutely decompensated patients could be maintained long term, resulting in sustained improvement in symptoms [9] and a decreased need for urgent cardiac transplantation [10]. Stevenson further demonstrated in a study of 152 patients referred for cardiac transplantation with high initial filling pressures (mean PCWP 28 mmHg) that patients achieving PCWP ≤ 16 mmHg had 1-year survival of 83% vs 38% for those patients not able to achieve PCWP ≤ 16 mmHg [11]. Other investigators found improvement in exercise tolerance in HF patients who underwent PAC-guided diuresis when there was evidence of elevated RAP and PCWP but no clinical evidence of volume overload [12], suggesting that PAC insertion was of benefit in these individuals.

These studies demonstrated the benefits of defining hemodynamics in advanced HF patients, particularly those listed for cardiac transplantation [13], and using this information to determine prognosis and guide therapy. However, although patients who responded to such therapy had a better prognosis than those who did not achieve target goals [11] it remained unclear whether this strategy altered the natural history of the disease process or whether this strategy merely identified survivors (i.e., those individuals who met hemodynamic goals were less ill than those who did not meet the specific hemodynamic goals, and therefore would have had a better outcome irrespective of whether or not they underwent PAC-guided therapy).

Large trials of PAC use in the critically ill

From a historical perspective, bedside pulmonary artery catheterization was introduced in the early 1970s, which resulted in widespread use of the PAC; this was prior to the Food and Drug Administration (FDA) gaining oversight of device therapy [14] and so the PAC was granted grandfather status and was not subject to FDA regulation. Thus, no study demonstrating the safety and efficacy of the PAC was needed before its widespread adoption in clinical practice.

The first large prospective study examining the use of the PAC in critically ill patients was reported in 1996. In this nonrandomized cohort study of 5735 critically ill patients at five participating centers, PAC use was associated with longer length of stay in the ICU, higher cost, and increased mortality at 30 days. Logistic regression was used to determine variables associated with a propensity toward PAC use, and these variables were subsequently matched in cases (PAC use) vs controls (no PAC), minimizing selection bias in this analysis. Subgroup analysis revealed no patient group, diagnosis, or site in which PAC use was associated with improved outcomes [2]. An accompanying editorial to this publication suggested that a moratorium on PAC use should occur until further studies were completed showing its safety and effectiveness [15].

Subsequently, a randomized study on the PAC was conducted in the United Kingdom. In the Assessment of the Clinical Effectiveness of Pulmonary Artery Catheters in Management of Patients in Intensive Care (PAC-man) trial [4], 1041 patients from 65 UK intensive care units (ICUs) were enrolled, with randomization stratified by age and presumptive clinical syndrome at the time of randomization. There was a 5% crossover rate from the control arm to the PAC arm. In addition, 7% of patients randomized to the PAC arm did not have the PAC inserted, owing to difficulties with insertion, clinical improvement of the patient so as not to warrant PAC insertion, and safety concerns in individuals with coagulopathy. There were no differences between groups with regard to in-hospital mortality, ICU length of stay, and overall length of stay. Subgroups stratified by Acute Physiology and Chronic Health Evaluation II (APACHE II) score and major presumptive clinical syndrome also showed no differences with regard to the primary outcome variable. There was a 10% complication rate with PAC insertion, the most frequent being hematomas at the insertion site, arterial punctures, and arrhythmias needing treatment within 1 hour of insertion. Eighty percent of the patients in the PAC arm had one or more changes in clinical management made within 2 hours of PAC insertion as a direct result of PAC-derived data: infusion of fluid >200 mL above maintenance levels in 1 hour (42%), a greater than 25% change in the dose of vasoactive drug (43%), and introduction of vasoactive drugs (32%) [4]; these changes had no effect on the primary outcome. Despite showing a lack of benefit of PAC use, this study appeared to refute the findings of Connors [2], which demonstrated that PAC use was associated with harm.

In 2003, Sandham et al. [3] reported results of a randomized trial of PAC use in 1994 high-risk surgical patients who were scheduled for urgent or elective major surgery followed by a stay in an ICU. There were no differences in either group with respect to 10-day mortality, total hospital length of stay, and 6-month mortality. Patients in the PAC arm were more likely to suffer pulmonary thromboembolism compared to those not managed with PAC [3]. Patients in the PAC arm were also more likely to receive therapy with intravenous inotropes.

Recently, a randomized trial of CVC (central venous catheter) vs PAC use in 1000 patients with established acute lung injury was reported. In this trial there were also no significant differences between groups in lung or kidney function, rates of hypotension, ventilator settings, or use of dialysis or vasopressors. Approximately 90% of protocol instructions were followed in both groups, with a 1% crossover rate from CVC- to PAC-guided therapy. Fluid balance was similar in the two groups, as was the proportion of instructions given for fluid and diuretics. There was an increased incidence of both atrial and ventricular arrhythmias in the PAC group, particularly during PAC insertion, but this may have been secondary to underreporting of CVC-insertion related events [6].

ESCAPE: a randomized trial of PAC in advanced HF

The ESCAPE trial [1] was an NHLBI-sponsored randomized trial designed to determine whether PAC use was safe and improved clinical outcomes in patients hospitalized with severe symptomatic and recurrent HF. A total of 433 patients were randomized at 26 experienced HF centers in the United States and Canada during the years 2000–2003. In order to be eligible for the study the patient had to have been hospitalized for HF within the past year, had an emergency department visit within the past month, or required more than 160 mg of furosemide (or equivalent) daily for the past month. In addition, patients required 3 months of symptoms despite therapy with ACE inhibitors and diuretics, LVEF (left ventricular ejection fraction) $\leq$ 30%, SBP $\leq$ 125 mmHg, and at least one symptom and one sign of congestion. Exclusion criteria designed to minimize confounding and the likelihood of urgent crossover included creatinine >3.5 mg/dL, prior use of dopamine or dobutamine >3 mcg/kg/min, or any prior use of milrinone during the current hospitalization. A concurrent PAC registry was established to characterize hospitalized patients receiving PACs considered by their physician to be required during HF management. Patients were randomized to two groups: therapy guided by clinical assessment alone and therapy guided by clinical assessment and PAC.

The goal of therapy in the clinical arm was resolution of the clinical signs and symptoms of congestion, particularly jugular venous pressure (JVP) elevation, edema, and orthopnea. Treatment goals in the PAC group were the same, with the additional hemodynamic goals of PCWP of 15 mmHg and RAP of 8 mmHg. Therapy was adjusted in both groups to avoid progressive renal dysfunction or symptomatic systemic hypotension. Investigators were encouraged to follow national guidelines for the treatment of HF and to primarily use intravenous diuretics and vasodilators. The use of inotropic agents was consistently and explicitly discouraged. The primary outcome variable was the number of days alive outside of the hospital at 6 months. There were several secondary outcome variables, including B-type natriuretic peptide (BNP), 6-minute walk distance, and quality of life indices.

The clinical and PAC groups were well-matched with regard to baseline characteristics. Mean age was 56 years, almost 75% were male, and about 60% were white. Ischemic etiology of HF comprised about half the group in each arm, mean LVEF was 20%, mean creatinine was 1.5 mg/dL, mean sodium was 137 mEq/L, and mean BNP was around

1000 pg/mL. Those assigned to the PAC registry were older, more often white, and had lower sodium and higher creatinine than the randomized group. The enrollment goal was 500 patients, but the trial was stopped early by the data and safety monitoring board due to concerns of early adverse events and the unlikelihood of achieving a significant difference in the primary endpoint. At the time of trial stoppage, 433 patients had been enrolled ($n = 215$ PAC, $n = 218$ clinical). Due to withdrawal of permission and loss to follow-up, a total of 206 patients in the PAC arm and 207 patients in the clinical arm were analyzed for the primary endpoint. Within the PAC-guided arm, mean RAP was reduced from 14 to 10 mmHg, mean PCWP was decreased from 25 to 17 mmHg, and mean cardiac index was increased from 1.9 to 2.4 L/min/m^2. Despite these hemodynamic improvements, there was no difference between the two groups with regard to number of days alive outside the hospital, time to death or hospitalization, number of deaths, or days hospitalized at 6 months (Figure 6.1). Further, there were no patient characteristics that identified subgroups in which PA catheter use was either beneficial or

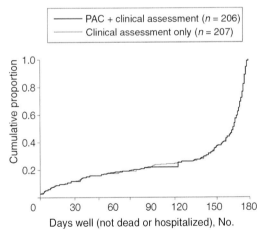

Figure 6.1 ESCAPE trial, cumulative primary endpoint (days alive and out of hospital). Cumulative proportion of patients contributing each possible numeric outcome for the number of days neither dead nor hospitalized during the 180 possible days of follow-up. Patients at the far left side of the curve represent early deaths, while those counted as 180 days survived for 6 months without rehospitalization. There was no significant difference in the primary endpoint whether subjects were randomized to pulmonary artery catheterization or not. (From [1], with permission.)

harmful. Importantly, individuals stratified by use of intravenous vasoactive therapy (inotropes, vasodilators, neither) did similarly well whether they did or did not receive PA-catheter guided therapy. In a subsequent analysis, it was found that PAC-guided therapy was associated with smaller changes in creatinine from baseline to discharge versus clinical assessment. PAC use was also associated with lower discharge diuretic dose [16].

One explanation for the discrepancy between earlier studies (PAC beneficial) and the ESCAPE trial (no benefit of PAC) may lie in the evolution of both HF therapies and the HF population. Early experiences with tailored therapy, performed in the late 1980s and early 1990s, involved patients with very high baseline systemic vascular resistance. More recently, patients with severe HF had lower SVR than found in earlier studies, perhaps owing to longer duration of ACE-inhibitor therapy. Specifically, systemic vascular resistance was 300 (dyn s)/cm^5 lower in ESCAPE than in earlier, nonrandomized experiences with PAC use [1]. In addition to having lower SVR, patients in ESCAPE more often had renal dysfunction [17] and diuretic resistance [18] owing to very poor cardiac output. PAC-guided therapy may have offered little advantage in this type of patient, given the absence of safe and effective medical therapies to improve a low-output state without a dramatically elevated SVR or high filling pressures. Intravenous inotropes have been found in several experiences to be harmful in patients with chronic HF [19,20]. It is also likely that in the experienced HF centers participating in ESCAPE, physicians had more expertise in the use of clinical surrogates to estimate both right- and left-sided filling pressures (e.g, the JVP), negating the benefit of PAC use.

Meta-analysis and declining use of PAC

A meta-analysis of all randomized trials of PAC use in critically ill patients, which included the ESCAPE trial, was also recently conducted [5]. The meta-analysis included 13 trials and a total of 5051 randomized patients, including those undergoing surgery, in the ICU, admitted with advanced HF, or diagnosed with acute respiratory distress syndrome and/or sepsis. There was no benefit or harm associated with PAC use with regard to mortality or number of days spent in the hospital. PAC use was associated with a higher frequency of intravenous vasodilator and intravenous inotrope use. The above trials suggest that PAC should not be routinely used in critically ill patients, regardless of indication (postsurgical, acute respiratory distress syndrome/sepsis, HF, admitted to ICU). One caveat to this conclusion is that patients were enrolled into these trials only if clinical equipoise existed. Whether PAC use is beneficial in critically ill patients who are felt by their physician to have a need for a PAC to guide management is not known. Nonetheless, a recently published analysis of the National Inpatient Sample, a large multistate inpatient registry, found a 65% decline in the rate of PAC use in 2004 as compared to 1993, likely due to increasing evidence that routine use in the critically ill does not result in reduced mortality [21]. This reduction in routine use of the PAC may have implications with regard to the overall safety of the procedure in the future, as fewer physicians and ICU nurses acquire sufficient experience to use this tool safely and effectively, leading some to question whether PAC use should be abandoned entirely [22].

Clinical surrogates of PAC measurements

Another explanation for the lack of benefit of PAC in the ESCAPE trial is that physicians are adept at noninvasively assessing hemodynamics. If so, there would be no real advantage of the invasive PAC, and it would only serve to expose patients to risk. Given that PAC use is declining, as described above, it is worthwhile to review the available data regarding the clinical assessment of hemodynamics (cardiac output and ventricular filling pressures), for increasingly these clinical assessments will guide physician decision making in patients with HF.

Surrogates for cardiac index

In the late 1980s, Stevenson and Perloff reported the correlation of physical findings and hemodynamic measurements by PAC in 50 patients with known chronic HF and mean LVEF < 20% [23]. Proportional pulse pressure [(SBP − DBP)/SBP] was found to correlate highly with cardiac index ($r = 0.82$), with proportional pulse pressure < 25% carrying a 91% sensitivity and 83% specificity for

a cardiac index < 2.2 L/min/m^2. However, recent data from the larger, randomized ESCAPE trial did not find a significant correlation between proportional pulse pressure and cardiac index as assessed by PAC [24].

Surrogates for elevated filling pressures

In the study discussed above by Stevenson and Perloff [23], rales, edema, and elevated mean JVP were totally absent in 18 of 43 patients with PCWP ≥ 22 mmHg. Presence of all three signs was 58% sensitive and 100% specific for PCWP ≥ 22 mmHg. JVP was a better predictor than peripheral edema or pulmonary rales for detecting elevated left-sided filling pressures [23]. In another study conducted in 52 patients referred for heart transplantation, the presence of elevated JVP or HJR (hepatojugular reflex) had 81% sensitivity and 80% specificity for PCWP ≥ 18 mmHg [25]. In a study of 1000 patients with advanced HF referred for cardiac transplant evaluation, RAP obtained by PAC did correlate with PCWP [26]. Whether physicians can reliably estimate the JVP has been questioned, as some have shown a frequent underestimation of RAP [27,28]. However, in a recent analysis of the ESCAPE trial, the physician's estimate of the RAP was accurate more than 80% of times for categories of invasively measured RAP (e.g., <8 or >12 mmHg) [24]. Further, the physician's estimate of the PCWP was associated with invasively measured PCWP [24].

Opinions regarding PAC use

There is considerable evidence that the routine use of PAC in a critically ill patient has no meaningful benefit [1–6]. These emerging data have resulted in reduced overall use of the PAC [21], which may further increase risk of PAC as physicians and nursing staff become less experienced with inserting and caring for the PAC and interpreting its data. Within the subgroup of decompensated or end-stage HF patients, the PAC has been traditionally used to determine filling pressures and to determine cardiac index. Skilled clinicians can accurately assess filling pressures via JVP in most patients. Cardiac index is difficult to assess noninvasively, but the lack of safe and effective therapies to raise cardiac index in the absence of elevated filling pressures make determination of cardiac index unnecessary except in the patients with the most advanced disease in whom cardiac transplantation or destination therapy with left ventricular assist device (LVAD) is being considered. In addition to end-stage HF patients, pulmonary artery catheterization may be of benefit in other patients with HF in a few key clinical situations where it may provide critical diagnostic information.

We offer our following recommendations regarding PAC use in patients with known left ventricular systolic dysfunction (Table 6.1):

1 PAC use should be performed in centers with sufficient experience in their use. This includes ICU nurses properly trained in routine care of and acquisition of hemodynamic data from the device and physicians trained in proper insertion/placement of the PAC and the proper use of hemodynamic data.

2 Initial estimation of filling pressures in patients hospitalized with HF should be made with clinical assessment (JVP/HJR), and clinical assessment should be used to guide empiric diuresis. PAC should not be routinely inserted in all patients with severe HF.

3 PAC should be considered in patients with known advanced HF who become frankly hypotensive

($<$75 mmHg), especially those who do not respond to intravenous fluids or require pressor support, particularly when other etiologies of shock besides cardiogenic shock may be operative. In these individuals, PAC insertion may provide diagnostic data as to the etiology of shock and subsequently guide therapy.

4 PAC can be considered in patients with HF and severe dyspnea who appear compensated by physical examination. In these cases, measured hemodynamics may demonstrate that the patient does have elevated left-sided filling pressures and the RAP is either low (occurs in 15% of patients) [26] or high (suggesting the physical examination was inaccurate). (See Figure 6.2.) Alternatively, the left-sided filling pressures may be normal suggesting a noncardiac cause of dyspnea.

5 PAC should be considered in decompensated patients who develop significant azotemia with diuresis in the setting of clinical symptoms and/or signs of volume overload. Discordance between clinical signs of volume overload and appropriate response to diuretic therapy may signify several possibilities, including an inadequate cardiac output, primary renal dysfunction, or that the usual relationship of right- and left-sided filling pressures (RAP one-half of PCWP) [26] does not exist (e.g.,

Table 6.1 Appropriate situations for the use of a pulmonary artery catheter in patients with heart failure (HF).

Major Indication #1: Patients with decompensated HF who are not responding as expected when decision making is based on noninvasive modalities

Specific examples

1. Development of frank hypotension (systolic blood pressure $<$ 75 mmHg) in patients with known advanced HF who do not respond to intravenous fluids or require pressor support, particularly when other etiologies of shock other than cardiogenic shock may be operative
2. Severe dyspnea in a patient with HF who appears compensated by physical examination
3. Development of significant azotemia with diuresis in a decompensated patient in the setting of clinical symptoms and signs of volume overload

Major indication #2: When therapies with significant risks are being considered

Specific examples

1. During the workup for cardiac transplantation to determine pulmonary artery pressures and to determine reversibility of pulmonary hypertension if present
2. During the initiation of continuous inotropic infusion for end-stage HF to establish both a need for and a benefit from this therapy
3. Prior to consideration of destination left ventricular assist device therapy

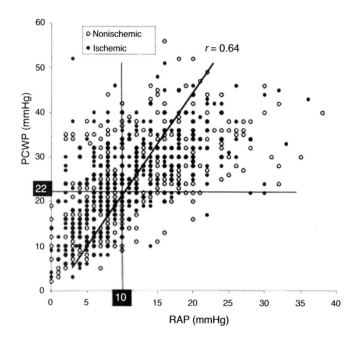

Figure 6.2 Scatterplot of the right atrial pressure (RAP) and pulmonary capillary wedge pressure (PCWP) in 1000 consecutive patients with advanced heart failure who were referred for cardiac transplantation at two major centers (from years 1986 to 1997). These values represent the initial hemodynamic measurement for each patient. Lines demarcate the PCWP (22 mmHg) and RAP (10 mmHg) arbitrarily defined as significantly elevated in this study. (From [26], with permission.)

a patient with right-sided filling pressures disproportionately elevated compared to the left-sided filling pressures, including those with restrictive physiology). In such cases, determination of cardiac index may be helpful in order to determine whether cardiac index is sufficient for adequate renal perfusion, and defining the right- and left-sided filling pressure relationships may avoid overdiuresis in attempts to drive the neck veins down when they do not reflect elevated left-sided filling pressures. Note that PA catheterization should not be considered as an initial intervention in patients who develop azotemia with diuresis in whom there is no clinical evidence of volume overload. In such patients, renal function should be reassessed after holding diuretics and/or administering fluids.

6 PA catheterization should be performed as part of a workup for cardiac transplantation to assess PAPs and to demonstrate reversibility of elevated PAPs if present.

7 PA catheterization should be performed to document that a patient will benefit from a continuous inotropic infusion as a palliative measure for end-stage HF.

8 PA catheterization should be performed prior to consideration of destination LVAD therapy.

Conclusions

Recently, the PAC has received much attention owing to several large randomized trials assessing its utility. Both in the critically ill patient and in those with advanced HF, the randomized trial data have not demonstrated benefit from the PAC. Fortunately, in patients with HF, much of the information gained from the PAC can often be obtained by a focused history and physical examination. Although routine use of PAC in patients with HF is no longer indicated, we believe there remain multiple situations in patients with HF where PAC is appropriate. These can be broadly grouped into two categories: (1) patients with decompensated HF who are not responding as expected when decision making is based on noninvasive (i.e., history and physical examination) modalities and remain either significantly hypotensive (<75 mmHg), have profound dyspnea, or develop renal failure; and (2) when therapies with significant risks are being considered (chronic inotropes, ventricular assist devices, or cardiac transplantation). In all cases, right heart catheterization should be performed in centers where physicians and nurses are adept at PAC insertion, maintenance, and interpretation to minimize its attendant risk. As PAC use declines nationwide, finding such expertise will become increasingly difficult.

Finally, the experience with the PAC in HF reminds us of the need to subject device therapy to rigorous, randomized clinical trials, in a manner analogous to pharmacological therapies, to improve patient outcomes. As device therapy is increasingly used in patients with HF [29–31], this is a lesson worth heeding.

References

1. Binanay C, Califf RM, Hasselblad V, *et al.* Evaluation study of congestive heart failure and pulmonary artery catheterization effectiveness: the ESCAPE trial. JAMA 2005;294:1625–1633.

2. Connors AF Jr, Speroff T, Dawson NV, *et al.* SUPPORT Investigators. The effectiveness of right heart catheterization in the initial care of critically ill patients JAMA 1996;276:889–897.

3. Sandham JD, Hull RD, Brant RF, *et al.* A randomized, controlled trial of the use of pulmonary-artery catheters in high-risk surgical patients. N Engl J Med 2003;348:5–14.

4. Harvey S, Harrison DA, Singer M, *et al.* Assessment of the clinical effectiveness of pulmonary artery catheters in management of patients in intensive care (PAC-Man): a randomised controlled trial. Lancet 2005;366:472–477.

5. Shah MR, Hasselblad V, Stevenson LW, *et al.* Impact of the pulmonary artery catheter in critically ill patients: meta-analysis of randomized clinical trials. JAMA 2005;294:1664–1670.

6. Wheeler AP, Bernard GR, Thompson BT, *et al.* Pulmonary-artery versus central venous catheter to guide treatment of acute lung injury. N Engl J Med 2006;354:2213–2224.

7. Kovick RB, Tillisch JH, Berens SC, *et al.* Vasodilator therapy for chronic left ventricular failure. Circulation 1976;53:322–328.

8. Stevenson LW, Tillisch JH. Maintenance of cardiac output with normal filling pressures in patients with dilated heart failure. Circulation 1986;74:1303–1308.

9. Steimle AE, Stevenson LW, Chelimsky-Fallick C, *et al.* Sustained hemodynamic efficacy of therapy tailored to reduce filling pressures in survivors with advanced heart failure. Circulation 1997;96:1165–1172.

10. Stevenson LW, Dracup KA, Tillisch JH. Efficacy of medical therapy tailored for severe congestive heart failure in patients transferred for urgent cardiac transplantation. Am J Cardiol 1989;63:461–464.

11. Stevenson LW, Tillisch JH, Hamilton M, *et al.* Importance of hemodynamic response to therapy in predicting survival with ejection fraction less than or equal to 20% secondary to ischemic or nonischemic dilated cardiomyopathy. Am J Cardiol 1990;66:1348–1354.

12. Chomsky DB, Lang CC, Rayos G, *et al.* Treatment of subclinical fluid retention in patients with symptomatic heart failure: effect on exercise performance. J Heart Lung Transplant 1997;16:846–853.

13. Campana C, Gavazzi A, Berzuini C, *et al.* Predictors of prognosis in patients awaiting heart transplantation. J Heart Lung Transplant 1993;12:756–765.

14. Parsons PE. Progress in research on pulmonary-artery catheters. N Engl J Med 2003;348:66–68.

15. Dalen JE, Bone RC. Is it time to pull the pulmonary artery catheter? JAMA 1996;276:916–918.

16. Nohria A, Hasselblad V, Stebbins A, *et al.* Cardiorenal interactions: insights from the ESCAPE trial. J Am Coll Cardiol 2008;51:1268–1274.

17. Weinfeld MS, Chertow GM, Stevenson LW. Aggravated renal dysfunction during intensive therapy for advanced chronic heart failure. Am Heart J 1999;138:285–290.

18. Butler J, Forman DE, Abraham WT, *et al.* Relationship between heart failure treatment and development of worsening renal function among hospitalized patients. Am Heart J 2004;147:331–338.

19. Cuffe MS, Califf RM, Adams KF Jr, *et al.* Short-term intravenous milrinone for acute exacerbation of chronic heart failure: a randomized controlled trial. JAMA 2002;287:1541–1547.

20. Thackray S, Easthaugh J, Freemantle N, *et al.* The effectiveness and relative effectiveness of intravenous inotropic drugs acting through the adrenergic pathway in patients with heart failure—a meta-regression analysis. Eur J Heart Fail 2002;4:515–529.

21. Wiener RS, Welch HG. Trends in the use of the pulmonary artery catheter in the United States, 1993–2004. JAMA 2007;298:423–429.

22. Rubenfeld GD, McNamara-Aslin E, Rubinson L. The pulmonary artery catheter, 1967–2007: rest in peace? JAMA 2007;298:458–461.

23. Stevenson LW, Perloff JK. The limited reliability of physical signs for estimating hemodynamics in chronic heart failure. JAMA 1989;261:884–888.

24. Drazner MH, Hellkamp AS, Leier CV, *et al.* Value of clinician assessment in advanced heart failure: the ESCAPE trial. Circulation: Heart Failure 2008;1:170–177.

25. Butman SM, Ewy GA, Standen JR, *et al.* Bedside cardiovascular examination in patients with severe chronic heart failure: importance of rest or inducible jugular venous distension. J Am Coll Cardiol 1993;22:968–974.

26. Drazner MH, Hamilton MA, Fonarow G, *et al.* Relationship between right and left-sided filling pressures in 1000 patients with advanced heart failure. J Heart Lung Transplant 1999;18:1126–1132.

27. Stein JH, Neumann A, Marcus RH. Comparison of estimates of right atrial pressure by physical examination and echocardiography in patients with congestive heart failure and reasons for discrepancies. Am J Cardiol 1997;80:1615–1618.

28. Cook DJ. Clinical assessment of central venous pressure in the critically ill. Am J Med Sci 1990;299:175–178.

29. Miller LW, Pagani FD, Russell SD, et al. Use of a continuous-flow device in patients awaiting heart transplantation. N Engl J Med 2007;357:885–896.

30. Costanzo MR, Guglin ME, Saltzberg MT, et al. Ultrafiltration versus intravenous diuretics for patients hospitalized for acute decompensated heart failure. J Am Coll Cardiol 2007;49:675–683.

31. Pappone C, Augello G, Rosanio S, et al. First human chronic experience with cardiac contractility modulation by nonexcitatory electrical currents for treating systolic heart failure: mid-term safety and efficacy results from a multicenter study. J Cardiovasc Electrophysiol 2004;15:418–427.

CHAPTER 7

Impedance Cardiography

Sunthosh V. Parvathaneni[1,2], & Ileana L. Piña[1,2]
[1]Case Western Reserve University, Cleveland, OH, USA
[2]Louis Stokes Cleveland VA Medical Center, Cleveland, OH, USA

Introduction

Clinicians have long sought tools that would help predict impending heart failure (HF) decompensation. The physical examination, although an important tool, can be misleading, particularly in patients with end-stage HF where the classic clinical signs of decompensation may not be present, such as lower extremity edema and rales. The jugular venous pressure has been used as a more reproducible part of the physical examination, but requires some expertise, and unfortunately maybe difficult to interpret in those with large neck circumferences in the more obese patients. As the number of patients with HF grows and clinicians' time with each patient increasingly shrinks, aides are needed to support the delivery of care. To assist with these issues, clinical trials are underway to determine the safety and efficacy of implanted pulmonary artery or left atrial sensors; however, these devices necessitate a surgical placement and hence are invasive. Therefore, an external modality to determine or predict HF decompensation, such as impedance cardiography (ICG), is attractive.

Impedance cardiography

ICG is a noninvasive method to determine cardiac hemodynamics. The device assesses the changes in impedance of the thorax upon application of a constant alternating current, which allows for a mathematical derivation of stroke volume. Because of the device's noninvasive nature, the device allows for many possible clinical uses, such as in the ER, ICU, and/or the outpatient setting [1]. Moreover, it allows for quick assessment of a patient's volume status at a relatively low cost, which could translate to more efficient and accurate patient care.

Development of impedance cardiography

However, to comprehend ICG, it is important to have a sufficient understanding of the underlying physics and mathematical expressions. Calculation of stroke volume is based on a mathematical derivation of Ohm's law:

$$V = IR$$

where V is the voltage, I current, and R resistance.

Because ICG uses the changes in resistance or impedance of an object upon duress of a constant current, the inherent resistivity of the media needs to be known along with the space occupancy of the material; therefore:

$$R = p\left(\frac{L}{A}\right)$$

where L is length, A area, and p resistivity.

Since area is proportional to the length and volume of an object, the equation now changes to:

$$R = p\left(\frac{L^2}{V}\right)$$

where L is length, V volume, and p resistivity.

With the above two suppositions, the mathematical derivation of stroke volume via impedance was possible.

In the 1930s, Cole, among others, examined the conductance of biological tissues, and postulated that the human body can be viewed as both a cylinder and an insulator with cell membranes separating the extracellular fluid and intracellular fluid, thus creating a parallel circuit with both resistance and capacitance [2]. Nyboer, in the 1940s, introduced the use of bioimpedance to evaluate the changes in volume within tissues and eventually extended this concept to include flow [2]. Essentially, Nyboer's concept records a proportional impedance for changes in volume over time and the formula now becomes:

$$\Delta V(t) = p \left(\frac{L^2}{Z^2} \right) \Delta Z(t)$$

where V is volume, L length, Z impedance (resistance), p resistivity [2].

Kubicek [3–7] investigated the measurement of total blood flow through the aorta via bioimpedance. In his original model, Kubicek made the assumption that the human thorax was equivalent to a cylinder which was electronically variable due to underlying composition (see Figure 7.1).

The human thorax is composed mostly of muscle, lung, fat, bone, and air ($R = 200$–$5000\ \Omega$). The inherent resistivities of the above are much larger than blood and plasma, which are 65–$130\ \Omega$, respectively. Because current flows in the path of least resistance, Kubicek postulated that the vena cava and aorta are natural conduits and therefore could assess flow over time via bioimpedance (see Figure 7.2).

By using the first derivative of the impedance waveform, Kubicek was able to mathematically calculate the stroke volume by the use of the peak flow or point of maximum of the first derivative of the impedance waveform as well as ventricular ejection time, and thus the basic ICG formula is:

$$\Delta V = \text{SV} = p \left(\frac{L^2}{Z_0^2} \right) \left(\frac{\delta Z}{\delta t} \right)_{\text{max}} \text{VET}$$

where SV is the stroke volume, p resistivity, Z_0 base impedance, and VET left ventricular ejection time [2]. In addition, from this model, Kubicek was able to calculate timing of the cardiac cycle (see Figure 7.3).

In this formula, the most important factors in determining stroke volume are the first derivative of the maximum impedance waveform (output) and ventricular ejection time (rate). Sramek and Bernstein further modified Kubicek's model by normalizing the mathematical expression to patient size by either height or ideal body weight, the latter being Bernstein's thesis. From this deduction, the derivation of further parameters of cardiac hemodynamics can be done. See Table 7.1 for possible calculations.

Because the stroke volume is a mathematically derived parameter, ICG has limitations. The essence of these limitations lie within the inability of the device to compensate for physiologic changes that cause a change in the impedance wave form or ventricular ejection time, thus allowing for an over- or underestimate of stroke volume. Table 7.2 demonstrates some of those limitations.

Impedance cardiography: comparison to the gold standard

Reproducibility and correlation to hemodynamics

To use a new technology in the clinical HF setting, it must be reproducible, be sensitive to changes in what it measures, and be specific to rule out the existence of a particular syndrome or a decompensation. Reproducibility needs to be present in normal individuals and in patients with disease when there have been no changes in clinical signs and symptoms. In HF, right heart catheterization has been used as the "gold standard" for patient

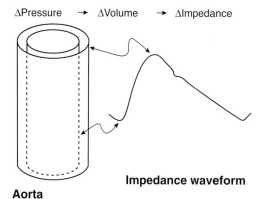

ΔPressure → ΔVolume → ΔImpedance

Impedance waveform

Aorta

Figure 7.1 The human chest was thought to be most similar to a cylinder. The impedance of the cylinder is derived from the mathematical calculation of the change in volume over time along with the object's inherent resistivity.

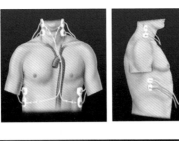

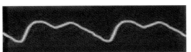

· Four dual sensors with eight lead wires placed on neck and chest.
Outer: transmit—Inner: measure

· Current transmitted and seeks path of least resistance: blood filled aorta

· Baseline impedance (resistance) to signal is measured

· With each heartbeat, blood volume and velocity in the aorta change

· Corresponding change in impedance is measured

· Baseline and changes in impedance are used to measure and calculate stroke volume and cardiac output

Figure 7.2 Noninvasive hemodynamic monitoring: impedance cardiography (ICG). Current flows in the path of least resistance and therefore through the aorta. The current is measured by placing four dual sensor electrodes that measure impedance of the chest (CardioDynamics, Inc., San Diego, CA, USA).

hemodynamic assessment and for monitoring changes, given therapy applications [9–13].

Van de Water et al. prospectively correlated thermodilution measured cardiac output vs ICG derived values in a group of 53 post-bypass patients and found a significant correlation between the two measurements ($r^2 = 0.658$, $r = 0.811$, $p < 0.001$) [14]. However, few patients were at the lower values for cardiac output < 4.0 L/min, which may be closer to the range of patients with impaired left ventricular function.

Drazner et al. determined hemodynamics by right heart catheterization on a group of 50 patients with advanced HF and compared the parameters to bioimpedance values [15]. Tables 7.3 and 7.4 show the sensitivity, specificity, and predictive value of the

impedance values for cardiac index ≤ 2.2 L/min/m^2 measured by thermodilution and Fick. There was no correlation between pulmonary capillary wedge pressure and thoracic fluid content or between right atrial pressure and thoracic fluid content ($r = 0.05$ and $r = 0.08$, respectively).

Table 7.5 summarizes studies comparing ICG to measures of cardiac output by Fick or thermodilution [9,–13,16,17].

From bench to bedside

ICG has many uses even beyond clinical assessment of HF. Research involving the etiology and underlying pathophysiology of HF is rapidly changing from the old paradigm of clinical evaluation and assessment toward structural and conceptual

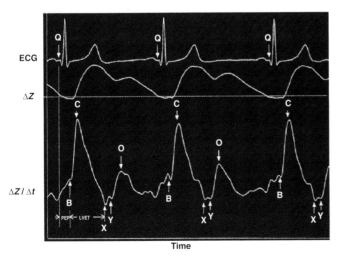

Figure 7.3 ECG and ICG waveforms. Q, ventricular depolarization; B, opening aortic and pulmonic valves; C, maximal slope ΔZ; X, closure aortic valve; Y, closure of pulmonic valve; O, opening mitral valve/rapid filling of ventricles; PEP, preejection period; LVET, left ventricular ejection time. (Adapted from [8].)

Table 7.1 A set of possible calculations that can be made from the calculated stroke volume from impedance cardiography.

Parameter	Formula	Definitions
Cardiac output	CO = HR × SV	CO, cardiac output; HR, heart rate; SV, stroke volume
Cardiac output systemic vascular resistance	CO = (MAP − RA)/SVR	MAP, mean arterial pressure; RA, right atrial pressure; SVR, systemic vascular resistance
Stroke index	SI = SV/BSA	SI, stroke index; SV, stroke volume; BSA, body surface area
Cardiac index	CI = SI × HR CI = CO/BSA	CI, cardiac index; HR, heart rate; CO, cardiac output; BSA, body surface area
Stroke time ratio (contractility)	STR = PEP/LVET	STR, systolic time ratio; PEP, preejection period; LVET, ventricular ejection time
Ejection fraction	EF = 0.84–0.64 (PEP/LVET)	EF, ejection fraction; PEP, preejection period; LVET, ventricular ejection time
Thoracic fluid content (total fluid in thoracic cavity)	TFC = 1/baseline impedance	TFC, thoracic fluid content
Aortic velocity index (contractility)	AVI = First derivative waveform/baseline impedance	AVI, aortic velocity index

Table 7.2 Clinical limitations of impedance cardiography.

Postural changes
Body composition
  Height 4 and/or 7 ft
  Weight 67 and/or 341 lb
Pulmonary edema
Respiratory variations
Significant aortic valve insufficiency
Significant aortic dilation, aneurysm, and coarctation
Intracardiac and pericardiac shunts
Arrhythmias (HR > 250)
Significant hypertension (MAP > 130)
Intra-aortic balloon pump

HR, heart rate; MAP, mean arterial pressure.

Table 7.3 Correlation of impedance cardiography, Fick, and thermodilution as found by Drazner et al. [14].

Comparison	Correlation (r value)	Precision (L/min)	Bias (L/min)	p value
Direct Fick vs thermodilution	0.81	0.95	0.75	<0.001
Direct Fick vs ICG	0.73	1.1	0.74	<0.001
Thermodilution vs ICG	0.76	1.1	0.03	<0.001

Note: $N = 59$ and EF = 25 ± 12%. This table shows that those with higher ICG risk scores are more likely to experience hospitalization for heart failure compared to those with a low risk ICG score. The risk score is a calculated value, incorporating high risk variables, which was derived from the PREDICT trial. ICG, impedance cardiography.
Source: Adapted from [29] with permission.

Table 7.4 Comparison of thermodilution and Fick with cardiac index < 2.2 with impedance cardiography.

	Correlation (r value)	Sensitivity (%)	Specificity (%)	Positive predictive value	Negative predictive value
Cardiac index by thermodilution ≤2.2 L/min/m^2	0.64*	62	79	68	74
Cardiac index by Fick ≤2.2 L/min/m^2	0.61*	56	80	83	50

Source: Adapted from [15].

Note: Asterisk indicates that the correlation was significant.

archetypes. The causes of these changes are largely due to the dynamic nature of the newly processed literature in addition to the notion that there is a phase between deleterious cellular mechanisms that translate into irreversible clinical prodromes as well as the necessity to identify these tribulations in order to make a timely intervention to prevent what clinicians acknowledge as HF. Because ICG can determine stroke volume noninvasively, the mathematical calculation of other hemodynamic variables, such as cardiac output and index as well as contractility, can allow assessment of overall cardiac function. The ability to look at overall cardiac function can prove useful to understand the basic pathological processes involved in HF and the relationship to clinical syndromes and prognosis [18].

Ejection fraction is a key element of prognosis but also can act as a surrogate for interpretation of overall cardiac function. Thompson et al. assessed the basic relationship between ejection fraction (measured by either echocardiography or a gated nuclear scan) and the systolic time ratio (a measure of contractility; preejection period/left ventricular ejection time) [19] and found that ejection fraction was inversely proportional to the systolic time ratio. An ejection fraction ≤ 50% and systolic time ratio ≥ 0.50 had 93% sensitivity and 85% specificity. Therefore, individuals with large systolic time ratio were noted to have associated poor ejection fraction on imaging. This concept was taken one step further to assess whether or not this method could be a cost-effective and noninvasive method to assess response to treatment [20]. Parrot et al. evaluated pre- and posttreatment ejection fractions and cardiac indices and systolic time ratios for patients with ischemic HF , the latter two being derived via ICG. The change in ejection fraction was highly correlated with the change in cardiac index and the systolic time ratio ($r = 0.85$). Furthermore, the systolic time ratio was inversely related to the ejection fraction. Some of these observations should raise the clinician's interest in impedance as a potential tool to manage HF.

Table 7.5 Clinical trials assessing the correlation between impedance cardiography, Fick, and thermodilution; all methods to measure cardiac output.

Study	Author	N	Parameter	Comparison	r value
HF in ICU	Albert et al.	33	CO	ICG vs TD	0.89
HF in catheterization laboratory	Drazner et al.	59	CO	ICG vs Fick	0.73
				TD vs Fick	0.81
				ICG vs TD	0.76
Mechanical Ventilation	Ziegler et al.	52	CO	ICG vs TD	0.89
Post-CABG	Sageman et al.	20	CI	ICG vs TD	0.92
Post-CABG	Van de Water et al.	53	CO	ICG vs TD	0.81

ICG, impedance cardiography; TD, Thermodilution; CO, Cardiac Output; CI, cardiac index; CABG, coronary artery bypass graft; HF, heart failure.

Source: Adapted from [16].

Because ICG is a noninvasive method for measurement of hemodynamics and therefore cardiac function, ICG offers the ability to be a very effective research tool as well. With that in mind, further insights into the known relationships between physiology and laboratory data can be further correlated to optimize patient management.

Impedance cardiography: clinical uses

Heart failure decompensation in clinic or in the emergency department setting

In the setting of acute decompensation, Cotter et al. used total body impedance in several clinical settings, including HF patients [21]. By dividing the cardiac index (CI) into four ranges, they found that in the ranges of CI, where HF patients would likely be included, the relative difference between the thermodilution and the total body impedance increased from 3.28 for $2 < CI < 3$ to 12.99 for $CI < 1.5$ (see Tables 7.6 and 7.7). Therefore, at the lower ranges of output, the technology may not be as accurate.

Pulmonary edema

The early identification and prevention of pulmonary edema continues to be a desirable goal to prevent this significant event in a patient's course. Fein et al. evaluated transthoracic electrical bioimpedance in 33 patients with pulmonary edema and compared them to controls [22]. Only 5 of 11 patients with clinically severe pulmonary edema and 5 of 8 of those with radiographic evidence of pulmonary edema had bioimpedance values outside of normal. Changes in serial measure of bioimpedance were more helpful.

Use with biomarkers

Brain natriuretic peptide (BNP) is emerging as a point of care tool to differentiate dyspnea and to prognosticate HF when patients present acutely or chronically. Many researchers have taken the investigative approach to evaluate the relationship between BNP and ICG. Barcarse et al. assessed this very clinical question in the emergency department scenario [23]. In patients with BNP > 100 pg/mL and CI $= 2.6$ L/min/m^2, ICG was 65% sensitive

and 88% specific for diagnosing ventricular dysfunction, and therefore it was concluded that the addition of ICG to BNP will allow more accurate diagnosis of HF. The above findings were later confirmed by Velazquez-Cecena et al. [24], who stratified a group of HF patients by risk of decompensation and assessed the correlation of hemodynamics derived by ICG, left ventricular end-diastolic pressure by left heart catheterization, echocardiography, and BNP. Patients who were classified as high risk tended to have higher levels of BNP versus their intermediate and low-risk counterparts [24]. Castellanos et al. recently evaluated BNP and ICG to predict future HF events in a nonacute outpatient setting. In total, 524 patients were evaluated, which resulted in 57 HF events [25]. The group found that after regression analysis, BNP and systolic time ratio index (systolic time ratio normalized by body surface area) were the strongest predictors of future HF events. In addition, in patients with known left ventricular dysfunction the relative risk for future HF event increased by 12.5 if both the BNP and systolic time ratio index were high as compared to patients with a low BNP (<100) and systolic time ratio index. These settings indicate a role of BNP in conjunction with ICG in HF.

Patients with hypertension have a high risk for developing left ventricular dysfunction. Bhalla et al. evaluated 193 patients with a history of hypertension and found both BNP and ICG to be significant predictors of left ventricular dysfunction [26]. Similarly, in patients presenting with dyspnea in the emergency department with BNP > 100, a multivariate model along with ICG predicted deaths, readmissions, and emergency department visits within 90 days with an accuracy of 83%. In contrast, in another group of patients presenting to an emergency department with dyspnea, only thoracic fluid content correlated moderately with BNP levels and poorly with cardiac index and systemic vascular resistance [27]. Therefore, two noninvasive tools may in combination improve diagnosis of left ventricular dysfunction and assess prognosis.

Outpatient

ICG has been shown effective in various settings but particularly in the outpatient setting. Of particular interest is the use of ICG to correlate with quality of

Table 7.6 Comparison of methods for deriving cardiac index and whole body impendance.

CI ranges by NICO CI	Result no.	NICO CI (Mean)	Thermodilution CI (Mean)	Relative difference (%)	Significance
CI <1.5	30	1.278 ± 0.16	1.515 ± 0.35	−12.99	0.0002
1.5 < CI < 2	98	1.749 ± 0.14	1.876 ± 0.33	−4.65	<0.0001
2 < CI < 3	220	2.433 ± 0.28	2.392 ± 0.40	3.28	0.0484
CI > 3	70	3.594 ± 0.57	3.449 ± 0.64	5.44	0.0045

CI, cardiac index; NICO, noninvasive cardiac output system/monitor.
Source: Adapted from [21] with permission.

life, functional capacity, and the ability to predict future hospitalizations.

Vijayaraghavan et al. evaluated the correlation between ICG parameters along with BNP and ejection fraction and New York Heart Association (NYHA) classification, 6-minute walk test, visual analog scale (the subjective scale assessing patient dyspnea), and the Minnesota Living with Heart Failure Questionnaire while under treatment for HF [28]. Significant changes in NYHA ($p < 0.05$), 6-minute walk test (from 668 to 874 m), patient visual analog scale, Minnesota Living with Heart Failure Questionnaire along with ICG parameters such as stroke index (from 38 to 41), left ventricular ejection time (from 273 to 291), and systolic time ratio (a correlate for contractility; from 0.56 to 0.52) were strongly correlated. Changes in cardiography parameters were significantly ($p < 0.01$) positively correlated to changes in NYHA ($r = 0.80$), 6-minute walk test ($r = 0.94$), visual analog scale ($r = 0.69$), and Minnesota Living

with Heart Failure Questionnaire score ($r = 0.67$). Vijayaraghavan et al. concluded that ICG can reflect changes in chronic HF along with treatment effectiveness particularly in the outpatient setting. This important groundwork led to the Prospective Evaluation and Identification of Cardiac Decompensation by ICG Test (PREDICT) [29] trial and the currently underway Prevention of Recurrent Venous Thromboembolism-Heart Failure (PREVENT-HF) trial (www.ClinicalTrials.gov, 2007).

Prediction of decompensation

The journey of patients with HF is often marked by repeated hospitalizations due to decompensation. These hospitalizations comprise a large cost to the health care systems. A technology that would identify a priori patients at risk of decompensation would be a welcome adjunct to disease management programs that strive to maintain patients out of the hospital. Nohria et al. have challenged the

Table 7.7 Comparison of the three groups in those after cardiac catheterization, CABG, and heart failure with correlation in whole body impedance.

Group	N	Thermodilution CI ($L/min/m^2$)		NICO CI ($L/min/m^2$)		p value
		Mean	SD	Mean	SD	
Whole sample	418	2.39	0.70	2.38	0.73	NS
Catheterization	40	2.81	0.72	2.81	0.68	NS
CABG	208	2.33	0.72	2.31	0.77	NS
CHF	170	2.35	0.63	2.38	0.66	NS

NS, not significant; NICO, noninvasive cardiac output system/monitor; CABG, coronary artery bypass graft; CHF, congestive heart failure.
Source: Adapted from [21] with permission.

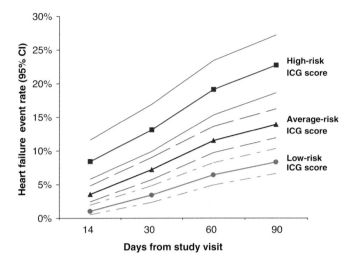

Figure 7.4 Event rate by days from heart failure event ICG score. The figure shows that those with higher ICG risk scores are more likely to experience hospitalization for heart failure versus those with a low ICG risk score. The risk score is a calculated value, incorporating high risk variables, which was derived from the PREDICT trial. $p < 0.0001$ for high vs low; $p < 0.001$ for average vs low; $p < 0.01$ for high vs average. (Adapted from [29].)

development of validated and reproducible noninvasive approaches to maximize care [30]. Packer et al. embarked on an aggressive trial of ICG to identify patients who would be at short-term risk for clinical decompensation [29]. The PREDICT trial evaluated 212 patients with stable chronic HF who had experienced a recent decompensation episode and were assessed clinically and through ICG testing every 2 weeks for 26 weeks. Clinicians were blinded to the impedance data. There were 16 deaths, 78 hospitalizations, and 10 emergency department visits. Three clinical and three ICG parameters were independently associated with an HF event in the following 14 days. A composite score was created using the three ICG parameters, which included velocity index, thoracic fluid content index, and left ventricular ejection time. Patients in the high risk score were 2.5 times as likely to experience an event (see Figure 7.4). This composite score is now being prospectively tested in the PREVENT-HF trial [www.ClinicalTrials.gov, 2007].

Implanted intrathoracic impedance

Because of the promising data concerning ICG and the management of chronic and even acute HF, intrathoracic impedance has come to light. Intrathoracic impedance is a method of invasively measuring thoracic fluid content and its relationship to volume status and its correlate HF. The actual device is placed inside implantable cardioverter-defibrillators and/or cardiac resynchronization therapy/defibrillators. The supposition is that when an electrical current is passed across the lung, accumulation of intrathoracic fluid or pulmonary edema will form a better medium for conductance and therefore will derive a lower impedance than those patients without pulmonary edema. Intrathoracic ICG will allow clinicians to possibly identify HF decompensation at an early stage and therefore provide more effective management and perhaps prevent hospitalizations.

The OptiVol® is a system that incorporates the ideology of intrathoracic impedance and is available through MedTronic devices such as Virtuoso, InSync Sentry, and Concerto. With OptiVol, impedance is measured every 20 minutes from noon to 5 p.m. for a total of 64 measurements over a 5-hour period [31,32]. The device then records the average of the measurements as the daily impedance value; averaging allows minimizing noise, such as respiratory variations [24]. Typically, the measurements start after the ventricular fibrillation detection setting is initiated. These values are then compared to the patient's inherent baseline impedance derived during the first 30 days post-implant [24]. An increase in impedance reflects increased thoracic fluid content and therefore signs of decompensation. Yu et al. in the Medtronic Impedance Diagnostics in Heart Failure Trial (MIDHeFT) found that impedance is inversely correlated with pulmonary capillary wedge pressure ($r = -0.61$, $p < 0.001$) and fluid balance ($r = -0.70$,

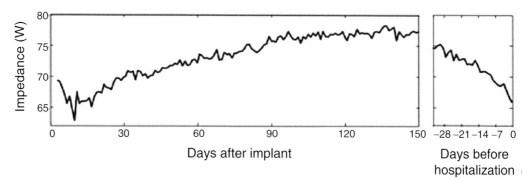

Figure 7.5 Impedance values derived via intrathoracic impedance. A baseline impedance is established within the first 30 days postimplant. The initial dip in impedance is thought to be due to pocket edema. Deviations from the baseline are used to assess increases or decreases in impedance and therefore earlier detection of pulmonary edema or volume overload, reflected by a decrease in impedance. (Adapted from [33].)

p <0.001) [33]. The MIDHeFT also found that the detection of impedance decreases was 76.9% sensitive in detecting future hospitalizations for volume overload. Furthermore, the group found that in the first 34 days of implant, there is actually a decrease in impedance and felt this was actually due to pocket edema surrounding the device (see Figure 7.5).

Because of this, the device does not recognize the first 30 days of implant as the baseline impedance but rather establishes a baseline by averaging the last four daily impedance values after 30 days [28]. Any cumulative deviation of impedance from the reference range is plotted to create the OptiVol fluid index, which represents the magnitude of impedance change versus the reference impedance as well as duration of change. The OptiVol fluid index is measured in unit of ohm-days. These values can then be used to create the OptiVol threshold that the physician determines to be of clinical relevance. The threshold is usually programmed at 60 ohm-days based on the MIDHeFT [33] but can be adjusted to 30–180 ohm-days based on the data surmised by Ypenburg et al. [34].

Because the OptiVol system incorporates the basics of ICG, the system suffers from similar issues and therefore derived inconsistencies from pathology such as pneumonia, pleural effusions, chronic obstructive lung disease, and obesity hypoventilation syndrome (see Table 7.2). In addition, the OptiVol® system mainly detects thoracic fluid content and therefore does not have the capability to assess ascites or lower extremity edema. However, despite these drawbacks, intrathoracic impedance has promising utility in detecting and managing HF.

Conclusions

ICG is a novel technology that can be used to derive a hemodynamic profile. In addition, because ICG is relatively inexpensive and quick, the technology may allow physicians to make better and effective treatment plans. The role of ICG, although shown to be useful in many clinical settings, such as the ICU and ER, seems to be most successful in the outpatient setting where there is much greater difficulty in obtaining invasive hemodynamic measurements. ICG allows for clinical assessment, when done as an adjunct to the physical examination, of chronic HF as well perhaps even predict future hospitalizations and dictate treatment effectiveness. With the continuing evolution of ICG the time may arrive where ICG can be used to tailor therapy just as pulmonary artery catheters are used now in order to provide goal-directed and efficient medical therapy. The ability to predict future decompensations and prevent HF hospitalizations seems to be a lofty and elusive goal. The results of the PREDICT trial are eagerly awaited.

References

1. Forrester JS, Diamond G, Chatterjee K, Swan HJ. Medical therapy of acute myocardial infarction by application of hemodynamic subsets (first of two parts). N Engl J Med 1976;295(24):1356–1362.

2. Summers RL, Shoemaker WC, Peacock WF, Ander DS, Coleman TG. Bench to bedside: electrophysiologic and clinical principles of noninvasive hemodynamic monitoring using impedance cardiography. Acad Emerg Med 2003;10(6):669–680.

3. Kubicek WG. Minnesota impedance cardiograph. Crit Care Med 1995;23(10):1785–1786.

4. Kubicek WG. On the source of peak first time derivative (dZ/dt) during impedance cardiography. Ann Biomed Eng 1989;17(5):459–462.

5. Kubicek WG, Kottke J, Ramos MU, et al. The Minnesota impedance cardiograph—theory and applications. Biomed Eng 1974;9(9):410–416.

6. Kubicek WG, From AH, Patterson RP, et al. Impedance cardiography as a noninvasive means to monitor cardiac function. J Assoc Adv Med Instrum 1970;4(2):79–84.

7. Kubicek WG, Karnegis JN, Patterson RP, Witsoe DA, Mattson RH. Development and evaluation of an impedance cardiac output system. Aerosp Med 1966;37(12):1208–1212.

8. Osypka MJ, Bernstein DP. Electrophysiologic principles and theory of stroke volume determination by thoracic impedance. AACN Clin Issues 1999;10(3):385–399.

9. Albert NM, Hail MD, Li J, Young JB. Equivalence of the bioimpedance and thermodilution methods in measuring cardiac output in hospitalized patients with advanced, decompensated chronic heart failure. Am J Crit Care 2004;13(6):469–479.

10. Moshkovitz Y, Kaluski E, Milo O, Vered Z, Cotter G. Recent developments in cardiac output determination by bioimpedance: comparison with invasive cardiac output and potential cardiovascular applications. Curr Opin Cardiol 2004;19(3):229–237.

11. Pickett BR, Buell JC. Validity of cardiac output measurement by computer-averaged impedance cardiography, and comparison with simultaneous thermodilution determinations. Am J Cardiol 1992;69(16):1354–1358.

12. Rosenberg P, Yancy CW. Noninvasive assessment of hemodynamics: an emphasis on bioimpedance cardiography. Curr Opin Cardiol 2000;15(3):151–155.

13. Sodolski T, Kutarski A. Impedance cardiography: a valuable method of evaluating haemodynamic parameters. Cardiol J 2007;14(2):115–126.

14. Van De Water JM, Miller TW, Vogel RL, Mount BE, Dalton ML. Impedance cardiography: the next vital sign technology? Chest 2003;123(6):2028–2033.

15. Drazner MH, Thompson B, Rosenberg PB, et al. Comparison of impedance cardiography with invasive hemodynamic measurements in patients with heart failure secondary to ischemic or nonischemic cardiomyopathy. Am J Cardiol 2002;89(8):993–995.

16. Yancy C, Abraham WT. Noninvasive hemodynamic monitoring in heart failure: utilization of impedance cardiography. Congest Heart Fail 2003;9(5):241–250.

17. De Maria AN, Raisinghani A. Comparative overview of cardiac output measurement methods: has impedance cardiography come of age? Congest Heart Fail 2000;6(2):60–73.

18. Ventura HO, Pranulis MF, Young C, Smart FW. Impedance cardiography: a bridge between research and clinical practice in the treatment of heart failure. Congest Heart Fail 2000;6(2):94–102.

19. Thompson B, Drazner MH, Dries DL, Yancy CW. Systolic time ratio by impedance cardiography to distinguish preserved vs impaired left ventricular systolic function in heart failure. Congest Heart Fail 2008;14(5):261–265.

20. Parrott CW, Burnham KM, Quale C, Lewis DL. Comparison of changes in ejection fraction to changes in impedance cardiography cardiac index and systolic time ratio. Congest Heart Fail 2004;10(2, Suppl 2):11–13.

21. Cotter G, Moshkovitz Y, Kaluski E, et al. Accurate, noninvasive continuous monitoring of cardiac output by whole-body electrical bioimpedance. Chest 2004;125(4):1431–1440.

22. Fein A, Grossman RF, Jones JG, Goodman PC, Murray JF. Evaluation of transthoracic electrical impedance in the diagnosis of pulmonary edema. Circulation 1979;60(5):1156–1160.

23. Barcarse E, Kazanegra R, Chen A, Chiu A, Clopton P, Maisel A. Combination of B-type natriuretic peptide levels and non-invasive hemodynamic parameters in diagnosing congestive heart failure in the emergency department. Congest Heart Fail 2004;10(4):171–176.

24. Velazquez-Cecena JL, Sharma S, Nagajothi N, et al. Left ventricular end diastolic pressure and serum brain natriuretic peptide levels in patients with abnormal impedance cardiography parameters. Arch Med Res 2008;39(4):408–411.

25. Castellanos LR, Bhalla V, Isakson S, et al. B-type natriuretic peptide and impedance cardiography at the time of routine echocardiography predict subsequent heart failure events. J Card Fail 2009;15(1):41–47.

26. Bhalla V, Isakson S, Bhalla MA, et al. Diagnostic ability of B-type natriuretic peptide and impedance cardiography: testing to identify left ventricular dysfunction in hypertensive patients. Am J Hypertens 2005;18(2, Pt 2):73S–81S.

27. Havelka EG, Rzechula KH, Bryant TO, et al. Correlation between impedance cardiography and B-Type natriuretic peptide levels in dyspneic patients. J Emerg Med 2008 [Epub ahead of print].

28. Vijayaraghavan K, Crum S, Cherukuri S, Barnett-Avery L. Association of impedance cardiography parameters

with changes in functional and quality-of-life measures in patients with chronic heart failure. Congest Heart Fail 2004;10(2, Suppl 2):22–27.

29. Packer M, Abraham WT, Mehra MR, *et al.* Utility of impedance cardiography for the identification of short-term risk of clinical decompensation in stable patients with chronic heart failure. J Am Coll Cardiol 2006;47(11):2245–2252.

30. Nohria A, Mielniczuk LM, Stevenson LW. Evaluation and monitoring of patients with acute heart failure syndromes. Am J Cardiol 2005;96(6A):32G-40G.

31. Wang L. Fundamentals of intrathoracic impedance monitoring in heart failure. Am J Cardiol 2007;99(10A):3G–10G.

32. Ypenburg C, Bax JJ, Van Der Wall EE, *et al.* Intrathoracic impedance monitoring to predict decompensated heart failure. Am J Cardiol 2007;99(4):554–557.

33. Yu CM, Wang L, Chau E, *et al.* Intrathoracic impedance monitoring in patients with heart failure: correlation with fluid status and feasibility of early warning preceding hospitalization. Circulation 2005;112(6):841–848.

34. Ypenburg C, Bax JJ, Van Der Wall EE, Schalij MJ, van Erven L. Intrathoracic impedance monitoring to predict decompensated heart failure. Am J Cardiol 2007;99(4):554–557.

CHAPTER 8

The Use of Echocardiography in Evaluating the Heart Failure Patient and Response to Therapy

John Gorcsan III
University of Pittsburgh, Pittsburgh, PA, USA

Echocardiography plays a major role in the clinical care of the heart failure patient, beginning with establishing a diagnosis, evaluating the severity of disease, and in follow-up determining response to therapy. This was dramatically demonstrated by Senni et al. in an observational study where the use of echocardiography appeared to favorably affect patient survival over 5 years, as compared to patients who did not have echocardiography [1]. Since heart failure patients often present with nonspecific symptoms of dyspnea and fatigue, which may represent many different cardiac, pulmonary, or systemic diseases, an echocardiographic examination plays a critical diagnostic role. Echocardiographic and Doppler imaging may provide information on left ventricular size and function, valvular disease, right ventricular size and function, and pericardial disease, and provide useful noninvasive hemodynamic information all in one complete examination. This chapter will focus selectively on the major roles that echocardiography may play in the management of heart failure patients in a contemporary setting.

Ejection fraction

Left ventricular ejection fraction is perhaps the single-most important measure of left ventricular function because of its widespread clinical use [2].

Ejection fraction, as the ratio of stroke volume to end-diastolic volume, combines information on left ventricular ejection in the numerator and information about left ventricular size and remodeling in the denominator as a powerful prognostic marker (Figure 8.1). Despite its physiological and technical limitations, ejection fraction has been used as a selection criterion for several pharmacological, surgical, and device therapy trials [3–7]. The principal physiological limitation of ejection fraction is its load dependence, being acutely affected by afterload and less affected by alterations in preload [8]. In addition, a common variable that affects ejection fraction is a rapid heart rate, such as new-onset atrial fibrillation with a rapid ventricular response that will acutely, but temporarily depress ejection fraction. In a steady-state clinical scenario, ejection fraction appears to be a robust measure with prognostic clinical significance.

Ejection fraction was historically validated using the radionuclide technique that determines a count ratio reflecting blood volume left ventricular ejection fraction [9]. Although the radionuclide ejection fraction method is generally regarded to have superior reproducibility, two-dimensional echocardiography has become the routine standard for most clinical scenarios because of the additional information that can be obtained and the desire to streamline cardiac testing. Quantitative ejection fraction determination has been most widely advocated from apical four-chamber and apical two-chamber views using the modified Simpson's

Heart Failure: Device Management. Edited by Arthur Feldman.
© 2010 Blackwell Publishing.

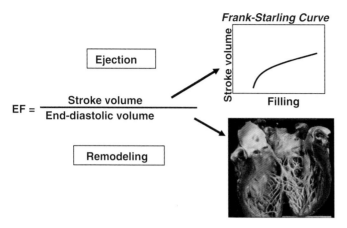

Figure 8.1 Ejection fraction (EF) is the ratio of stroke volume to end-diastolic volume, which combines measures of ventricular function illustrated by the Frank-Starling curve and end-diastolic volume, which is a marker of ventricular remodeling.

formula [10] (Figure 8.2). Quantitative ejection fraction entails manual tracing of the endocardium for end-diastolic and end-systolic frames, which requires training and skill to overcome wall noise and dropout. Tracing of echocardiographic images for ejection fraction has recently become faster and more accurate with digital acquisition and harmonic imaging. However, many laboratories still rely on visual assessment of ejection fraction [11]. "Eye-ball" assessment requires extensive training and experience and appears to be easiest for pa-

tients at the ends of the spectrum with normal ejection fractions or severely reduced (<30%) ejection fractions, and most variability occurs in the 30–40% range [12]. This range contains the ejection fraction threshold for patient selection for several therapies, in particular defibrillator and resynchronization device therapy. Accordingly, the consensus of experts is to perform quantitative echocardiographic ejection fractions on heart failure patients, in particular when making these important therapeutic decisions [10]. A more recent advance

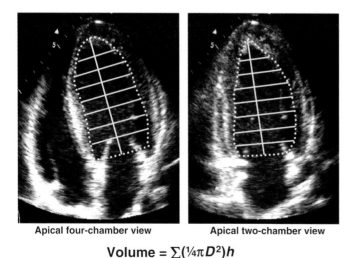

Figure 8.2 The method of determining ejection fraction using biplane Simpson's rule from apical four-chamber (left) and apical two-chamber (right) views and manual tracing of end-diastolic and end-systolic frames.

has been the use of automated computer software programs, such as "auto-ejection fraction," which has the potential to speed quantitative assessment of ejection fraction [12].

A known limitation of two-dimensional echocardiography for determination of ejection fraction is variability in imaging the left ventricular apex. This appears to affect absolute volumes more severely than ejection fractions. The advent of refinements in three-dimensional echocardiography has improved the reproducibility and accuracy of ejection fraction, by including the entire left ventricular blood volume in a pyramidal sector [13,14] (Figure 8.3). Three-dimensional echocardiographic ventricular volume measurements have been shown to correlate favorably with magnetic resonance imaging and have less variability than two-dimensional echocardiography. Although the three-dimensional approaches appear to hold much promise for future applications, the current mainstream of clinical practice still remains two-dimensional techniques, and the consensus is to apply the quantitative technique of endocardial tracing for biplane Simpson's rule [15].

Mitral inflow velocity

The mitral inflow velocity may be readily determined by pulsed Doppler echocardiography. The approach is to place the sample volume at the tips of the mitral valve, usually from the apical four-chamber view (Figure 8.4). Although many important observations have been made from these velocity data regarding diastolic function, the restrictive inflow pattern appears to be of particular prognostic value. A restrictive mitral inflow pattern is defined by the deceleration time from the peak on the mitral inflow E wave to the zero velocity baseline. This is usually reported in terms of absolute time, and no heart rate correction is used. Klein et al. showed that a short deceleration time ≤ 150 milliseconds predicted a poor outcome among patients with cardiac amyloidosis [16]. Xie et al. demonstrated that a deceleration time of ≤ 140 milliseconds was associated with a high mortality rate among a series of cardiomyopathy patients [17]. Accordingly, determination of the deceleration time of the mitral inflow pattern is an important component of the echo-Doppler assessment of the heart failure patient.

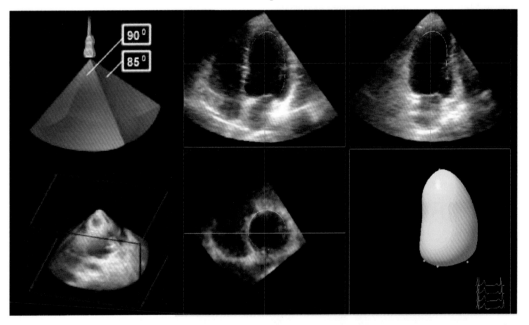

Figure 8.3 An example of three-dimensional echocardiography to determine ventricular volumes and ejection fraction. The left panels demonstrate the pyramid of ultrasound imaging data obtained. The bottom right panel illustrates the three-dimensional determination of the left ventricle. The remaining panels are representative tomographic planes obtained from the three-dimensional data set.

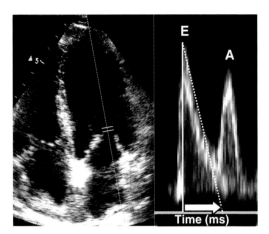

Figure 8.4 An apical four-chamber view with placement of the pulsed Doppler sample volume at the tips of the mitral leaflets (left) to record mitral inflow Doppler velocities (right). The early diastolic E wave and late diastolic A wave are shown. The deceleration time is determined as the time from the peak of the E wave to the zero baseline.

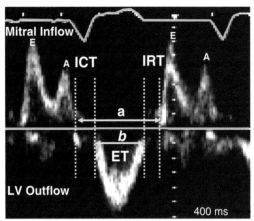

$$\text{Tei index} = \frac{\text{ICT} + \text{IRT}}{\text{ET}} = \frac{a - b}{b}$$

Figure 8.5 The myocardial performance index, also known as the Tei index, determined from mitral inflow and left ventricular (LV) outflow velocities. Interval *a* is measured from the end of the mitral inflow A wave to the beginning of the next inflow E wave. Interval *b* is the left ventricular ejection time measured from pulsed Doppler recordings of the outflow tract. ICT, isovolumic contraction time; IRT, isovolumic relaxation time; ET, ejection time.

Myocardial performance index

A useful index that combines elements of myocardial systolic and diastolic function has been described as the myocardial performance index. Tei et al. used this to determine prognosis in patients with cardiac amyloidosis and heart failure from other causes [18,19]. This dimensionless index is calculated from mitral inflow and left ventricular outflow track velocity data. The Tei index is interval from the end of the mitral inflow A wave to the beginning of the mitral inflow E wave of the next cardiac cycle. This interval is the sum of isovolumic contraction time, isovolumic relaxation time, and ejection time. It is then divided by ejection time (Figure 8.5). This index is useful because diseases that affect systolic function result in increased isovolumic contraction time and decreased ejection time, whereas diastolic dysfunction results in increased isovolumic relaxation time. Accordingly, these three timing events combine to determine global myocardial performance. A Tei index of >0.77 indicates a poor prognosis in patients with cardiac amyloidosis and also dilated cardiomyopathy [18,19].

Mitral annular velocity

Tissue Doppler echocardiography utilizes ultrasound frequency shifts created by tissue motion to calculate myocardial velocities. The favorable Doppler angle of incidence from the apical views combined with the robust signal of mitral annular motion has resulted in the tissue Doppler assessment of mitral annular velocity as a useful index of myocardial function. This was first used as a marker of systolic function where the peak velocity of the S wave during systole was shown to correlate with left ventricular ejection fraction [20] (Figure 8.6). Subsequently, the mitral annular early diastolic E wave has become a standard to assist in the assessment of left ventricular diastolic function. Although nonspecific, it is a marker of active myocardial relaxation and appears to be a sensitive measure of diastolic dysfunction. Nagueh et al. introduced the concept of using the ratio of left ventricular filling velocity (E) to mitral annular velocity (E') as a noninvasive marker of filling pressures [21]. In a series of patients who had invasive hemodynamic

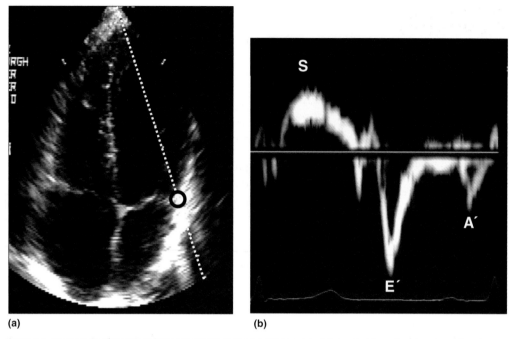

(a)   **(b)**

Figure 8.6 An example of sample volume placement in the lateral annulus of the apical four-chamber view (a) and a pulsed tissue Doppler spectral display of mitral annular velocity (b). S, systolic peak; E', early diastolic peak; A', atrial peak.

correlation, they observed that the E/E' directly correlated with pulmonary capillary wedge pressure. The original description was to use the lateral mitral annulus as a site for tissue Doppler assessment, combined with mitral inflow velocities (Figure 8.7). The simple scheme that was proposed was that the E/E' greater than 10 was indicative of a pulmonary capillary wedge pressure > 15 mmHg, indicating abnormally elevated filling pressures. Ommen et al. later confirmed these observations and added that the tissue Doppler velocity data may be obtained from the medial and lateral annular sites [22]. Furthermore, they demonstrated that E/E' had a high yield in consecutive patients, more so than previous noninvasive markers of filling pressures. A consistent finding has been that there is more variability in the relationship of E/E' with filling pressures in patients with preserved ejection fraction, and the relationship is more predictive in patients with reduced ejection fraction [21,22]. Accordingly, E/E' has emerged as an important noninvasive means to predict filling pressures in heart failure patients with reduced ejection fraction. Clinical scenarios where E/E' does not accurately reflect filling pressures

include mitral stenosis, mitral prostheses, acute hypovolumia, and constrictive pericarditis [23].

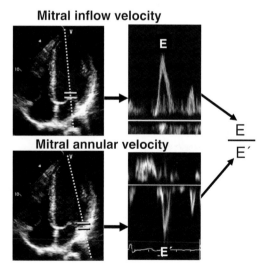

Figure 8.7 Illustration of tissue Doppler mitral annular (E') to pulsed Doppler mitral inflow (E) ratio used to estimate left ventricular filling pressures.

Echocardiographic assessment of dyssynchrony

Interest in assessment of abnormalities of regional mechanical activation, known as dyssynchrony, has emerged with the advent of cardiac resynchronization therapy (CRT). Also known as biventricular pacing, CRT has been shown to improve ventricular function, reduce mitral regurgitation, improve clinical outcomes, and improve survival [3,24–26]. A consistent finding among clinical CRT trials has been that approximately one-third of patients with electrocardiographic QRS widening who undergo CRT do not seem to benefit favorably. Several imaging studies have shown that there is a subset of wide QRS patients who do not have significant mechanical dyssynchrony, and this lack of dyssynchrony is associated with lack of response to CRT. Accordingly, a great deal of effort has been devoted to use a variety of echocardiographic methods to quantify mechanical dyssynchrony as an attempt to refine patient selection for CRT. Although several studies have reported the utility of echocardiographic methods to quantify dyssynchrony, a recent multicenter study evaluating predictors of response to resynchronization therapy, known as PROSPECT, demonstrated that no single echocardiographic method was found to be highly predictive [27]. Accordingly, the value of echocardiographic determination of dyssynchrony is currently controversial for clinical applications, and current guidelines for patient selection using electrocardiographic QRS widening have not been replaced. However, it is appropriate to review the body of literature on dyssynchrony that exists and provide a viewpoint for future clinical applications.

Tissue Doppler assessment of dyssynchrony

The greatest number of published investigations to quantify ventricular dyssynchrony has used the technique of tissue Doppler echocardiography [24,28–37]. As previously described, tissue Doppler can determine regional velocities as markers of mechanical activation and quantify abnormalities in their timing. The most popular methods have been using color-coded tissue Doppler from the apical echocardiographic views to measure longitudinal shortening velocities. This has been useful because

of the favorable Doppler angle of incidence from the apical windows. A simple dyssynchrony approach using the difference in time to peak velocities from septal and lateral walls was originally proposed by Bax et al. [30]. An opposing wall delay cutoff value of ≤65 milliseconds had a favorable balance of sensitivity and specificity to predict acute hemodynamic response, clinical response, and reverse remodeling following CRT [30,31] (Figure 8.8). Most of the patients who did not have significant tissue Doppler dyssynchrony did not appear to respond to CRT. A sensitive, but more complex approach by Yu et al. is time to peak velocities in 12 segments from the basal and mid-ventricular levels of each of three standard apical views (apical four-chamber, apical two-chamber, and apical long axis) [36–38]. Yu et al. calculated standard deviation in time to peak velocities and found a cutoff value of approximately ≥33 milliseconds to be associated with response to CRT [38]. In addition, the maximum difference in time to peak among the 12 segments ≥100 milliseconds was associated with response to CRT [35]. It is important to have a careful systematic approach to tissue Doppler analysis to have reproducible results. This includes an adequately large region of interest and manual adjustment of the region of interest to achieve spatial averaging, described in detail elsewhere [32]. This process can yield reproducible results with training and experience.

Speckle tracking assessment of dyssynchrony

A recent advance in quantitative echocardiography has been speckle tracking, which derives information from routine gray-scale images. This computer program determines the stable speckle patterns from frame to frame in digital echo images and can derive transmural strain, displacement, and velocity data [39]. Myocardial strain is particularly useful because it can determine active thickening mostly independent of passive motion or tethering [40]. Speckle tracking echocardiography has been shown to be a useful means to determine the timing of radial thickening and can be applied to dyssynchrony analysis. Since dyssynchrony is a three-dimensional phenomenon, the addition of speckle tracking radial strain is complementary to the longitudinal velocity information obtained from apical views (Figure 8.9). Several ultrasound manufacturers have

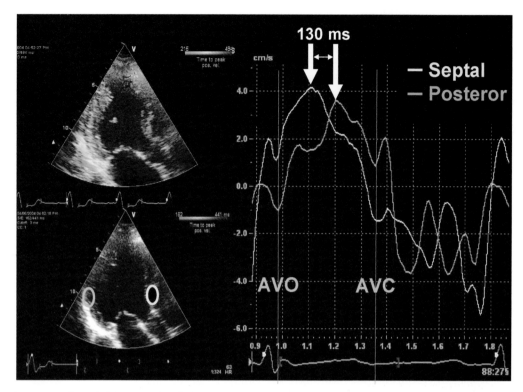

Figure 8.8 Color-coded tissue Doppler of a heart failure patient with left bundle branch block and mechanical dyssynchrony. An apical long-axis view is shown with an early septal time to peak velocity color coded as green and later posterior time to peak velocity color coded as orange (upper left). The septal time velocity curve is shown in yellow and posterior wall time velocity curve shown in turquoise. There is a 130-millisecond delay from septal to posterior wall velocity peaks shown during the ejection interval. AVO, aortic valve opening; AVC, aortic valve closure.

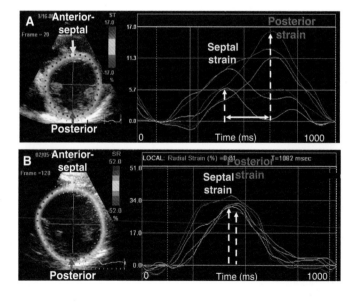

Figure 8.9 Examples of speckle tracking radial strain from the midventricular short-axis views. Patient A (top) had a QRS duration of 150 milliseconds, and significant dyssynchrony (septal to posterior wall peak strain delay of 270 ms). Patient A had a favorable response to resynchronization therapy. Patient B (bottom) had a similar QRS duration of 150 milliseconds, but no significant dyssynchrony (septal to posterior wall peak strain delay of 50 ms). Patient B did not have a favorable response to resynchronization therapy.

recently introduced speckle tracking analysis programs, and this approach appears to be increasing in its clinical usage [41–43]. Suffoletto et al. showed that the application of speckle tracking to midventricular short-axis views can derive radial strain with a high yield from the septal and posterior wall segments [39]. As with other advanced image analysis techniques, training and experience is required to carefully adjust the region of interest on the left ventricular wall to achieve reproducible results. A time to peak strain value of ≥130 milliseconds was associated with response to therapy in patients with routine indications for CRT: widened QRS ≥120 milliseconds, symptomatic heart failure, and reduced ejection fraction. Similar to the tissue Doppler observations, the majority of patients with no significant mechanical dyssynchrony did not demonstrate a response to CRT. A combined approach using both tissue Doppler longitudinal velocities and speckle tracking radial strain

appears to be superior to either method alone in predicting response [33]. Speckle tracking echocardiography is still relatively new, and refinements are ongoing, such as the technological advance of three-dimensional speckle tracking (Figure 8.10).

In summary, no single echocardiographic method has yet replaced the current clinical selection criteria for CRT using the wide QRS [2]. Efforts continue to reduce variability through training and further clinical evaluations to find the appropriate role for echocardiographic assessment of dyssynchrony in clinical practice. A potential current application of echocardiographic and Doppler determination of mechanical dyssynchrony is for patients who meet borderline clinical criteria for CRT, in particular those with a borderline QRS duration between 110 and 130 milliseconds [32]. The dyssynchrony data may serve as an adjunct to assist in clinical decision making regarding CRT implantation. A potential future use of echocardiographic

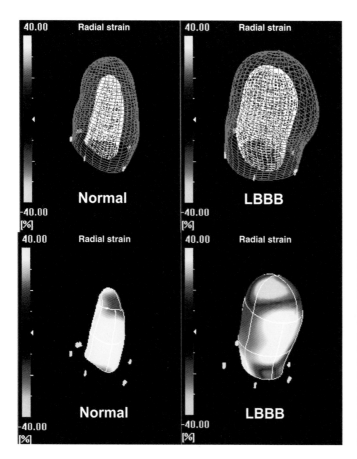

Figure 8.10 Examples of three-dimensional strain by speckle tracking echocardiography. A normal volunteer is shown on the left, and a heart failure patient with left bundle branch block (LBBB) is shown on the right. The wire mesh displays (top panels) and the three-dimensional strain display (bottom panels) are shown at end systole. Strain is color coded, with yellow indicating peak radial thickening and blue radial thinning. The patient with LBBB displays a delay in peak strain to the posterior lateral region of the left ventricle at end systole (right side of the image).

markers of dyssynchrony is to identify the subset of patients with narrow QRS duration who have been observed to have mechanical dyssynchrony [24,44]. This is important because it has the potential to expand the benefits of CRT to a larger group of heart failure patients. However, the first randomized trial of CRT in a narrow QRS population, known as the RethinQ study, showed mixed results [45]. This study randomized 172 heart failure patients with a narrow QRS duration < 130 milliseconds and a low ejection fraction who met inclusion criteria for mechanical dyssynchrony. The primary endpoint of peak myocardial oxygen consumption was not different between groups, and this study did not conclude as positive. However, patients who were randomized to CRT showed improvements in New York Heart Association functional class and 6-minute walk distance in the subgroup with nonischemic disease. In addition, there were only 14 heart failure events (16%) in the CRT-on group compared with 41 heart failure events (22%) in the CRT-off group. Future randomized trials are needed to more clearly define if patients with narrow QRS with mechanical dyssynchrony can benefit from CRT. Current efforts to improve dyssynchrony analysis continue to intensify, and future refinements for clinical applications are ongoing.

Acknowledgments

Dr Gorcsan is supported by National Institutes of Heath Awards 2 K24 HL004503-06, RO1 HL086918-01A1, and RO1 HL073198-01 as well as by research grants from Medtronic and St. Jude Medical Corporations.

References

1. Senni M, Rodeheffer RJ, Tribouilloy CM, et al. Use of echocardiography in the management of congestive heart failure in the community. J Am Coll Cardiol 1999;33:164–170.

2. Hunt SA, Abraham WT, Chin MH, et al. ACC/AHA 2005 Guideline update for the diagnosis and management of chronic heart failure in the adult. A report of the American College of Cardiology/American Heart Association Task Force on Practice Guidelines (Writing Committee to Update the 2001 Guidelines for the Eval-

uation and Management of Heart Failure): developed in collaboration with the American College of Chest Physicians and the International Society for Heart and Lung Transplantation: endorsed by the Heart Rhythm Society. Circulation 2005;112:e154–e235.

3. Abraham WT, Fisher WG, Smith AL, et al. Cardiac resynchronization in chronic heart failure. N Engl J Med 2002;346:1845–1853.

4. Bardy GH, Lee KL, Mark DB, et al. Amiodarone or an implantable cardioverter-defibrillator for congestive heart failure. N Engl J Med 2005;352:225–237.

5. Cleland JG, Daubert JC, Erdmann E, et al. The effect of cardiac resynchronization on morbidity and mortality in heart failure. N Engl J Med 2005;352:1539–1549.

6. Moss AJ. Background, outcome, and clinical implications of the multicenter automatic defibrillator implantation trial (MADIT). Am J Cardiol 1997;80:28F–32F.

7. Moss AJ, Vyas A, Greenberg H, et al. Temporal aspects of improved survival with the implanted defibrillator (MADIT-II). Am J Cardiol 2004;94:312–315.

8. Mandarino WA, Pinsky MR, Gorcsan J III. Assessment of left ventricular contractile state by preload-adjusted maximal power using echocardiographic automated border detection. J Am Coll Cardiol 1998; 31:861–868.

9. Strauss HW, Zaret BL, Hurley PJ, Natarajan TK, Pitt B. A scintiphotographic method for measuring left ventricular ejection fraction in man without cardiac catheterization. Am J Cardiol 1971;28:575–580.

10. Lang RM, Bierig M, Devereux RB, et al. Recommendations for chamber quantification: a report from the American Society of Echocardiography's Guidelines and Standards Committee and the Chamber Quantification Writing Group, developed in conjunction with the European Association of Echocardiography, a branch of the European Society of Cardiology. J Am Soc Echocardiogr 2005;18:1440–1463.

11. Amico AF, Lichtenberg GS, Reisner SA, Stone CK, Schwartz RG, Meltzer RS. Superiority of visual versus computerized echocardiographic estimation of radionuclide left ventricular ejection fraction. Am Heart J 1989;118:1259–1265.

12. Cannesson M, Tanabe M, Suffoletto MS, et al. A novel two-dimensional echocardiographic image analysis system using artificial intelligence-learned pattern recognition for rapid automated ejection fraction. J Am Coll Cardiol 2007;49:217–226.

13. Sugeng L, Mor-Avi V, Weinert L, et al. Quantitative assessment of left ventricular size and function: side-by-side comparison of real-time three-dimensional echocardiography and computed tomography with magnetic resonance reference. Circulation 2006;114:654–661.

14. Mor-Avi V, Lang RM. Echocardiographic quantification of left ventricular volume: what can we do better? J Am Soc Echocardiogr 2008;21:998–1000.

15. Lang RM, Bierig M, Devereux RB, *et al.* Recommendations for chamber quantification. Eur J Echocardiogr 2006;7:79–108.

16. Klein AL, Hatle LK, Taliercio CP, *et al.* Prognostic significance of Doppler measures of diastolic function in cardiac amyloidosis: a Doppler echocardiography study. Circulation 1991;83:808–816.

17. Xie GY, Berk MR, Smith MD, Gurley JC, DeMaria AN. Prognostic value of Doppler transmitral flow patterns in patients with congestive heart failure. J Am Coll Cardiol 1994;24:132–139.

18. Tei C, Dujardin KS, Hodge DO, Kyle RA, Tajik AJ, Seward JB. Doppler index combining systolic and diastolic myocardial performance: clinical value in cardiac amyloidosis. J Am Coll Cardiol 1996;28:658–664.

19. Tei C, Nishimura RA, Seward JB, Tajik AJ. Noninvasive Doppler-derived myocardial performance index: correlation with simultaneous measurements of cardiac catheterization measurements. J Am Soc Echocardiogr 1997;10:169–178.

20. Gulati VK, Katz WE, Follansbee WP, Gorcsan J III. Mitral annular descent velocity by tissue Doppler echocardiography as an index of global left ventricular function. Am J Cardiol 1996;77:979–984.

21. Nagueh SF, Mikati I, Kopelen HA, Middleton KJ, Quinones MA, Zoghbi WA. Doppler estimation of left ventricular filling pressure in sinus tachycardia: a new application of tissue Doppler imaging. Circulation 1998;98:1644–1650.

22. Ommen SR, Nishimura RA, Appleton CP, *et al.* Clinical utility of Doppler echocardiography and tissue Doppler imaging in the estimation of left ventricular filling pressures: a comparative simultaneous Doppler-catheterization study. Circulation 2000; 102:1788–1794.

23. Jacques DC, Pinsky MR, Severyn D, Gorcsan J III. Influence of alterations in loading on mitral annular velocity by tissue Doppler echocardiography and its associated ability to predict filling pressures. Chest 2004;126:1910–1918.

24. Bleeker GB, Holman ER, Steendijk P, *et al.* Cardiac resynchronization therapy in patients with a narrow QRS complex. J Am Coll Cardiol 2006;48:2243–2250.

25. Bristow MR, Saxon LA, Boehmer J, *et al.* Cardiac-resynchronization therapy with or without an implantable defibrillator in advanced chronic heart failure. N Engl J Med 2004;350:2140–2150.

26. Kanzaki H, Bazaz R, Schwartzman D, Dohi K, Sade LE, Gorcsan J III. A mechanism for immediate reduction in mitral regurgitation after cardiac resynchroniza-tion therapy: insights from mechanical activation strain mapping. J Am Coll Cardiol 2004;44:1619–1625.

27. Chung ES, Leon AR, Tavazzi L, *et al.* Results of the predictors of response to CRT (PROSPECT) trial. Circulation 2008;117:2608–2616.

28. Bax JJ, Abraham T, Barold SS, *et al.* Cardiac resynchronization therapy. Part 2: Issues during and after device implantation and unresolved questions. J Am Coll Cardiol 2005;46:2168–2182.

29. Bax JJ, Abraham T, Barold SS, *et al.* Cardiac resynchronization therapy. Part 1: Issues before device implantation. J Am Coll Cardiol 2005;46:2153–2167.

30. Bax JJ, Bleeker GB, Marwick TH, *et al.* Left ventricular dyssynchrony predicts response and prognosis after cardiac resynchronization therapy. J Am Coll Cardiol 2004;44:1834–1840.

31. Gorcsan J III, Kanzaki H, Bazaz R, Dohi K, Schwartzman D. Usefulness of echocardiographic tissue synchronization imaging to predict acute response to cardiac resynchronization therapy. Am J Cardiol 2004;93:1178–1181.

32. Gorcsan J III, Abraham T, Agler DA, *et al.* Echocardiography for cardiac resynchronization therapy: recommendations for performance and reporting—a report from the American Society of Echocardiography Dyssynchrony Writing Group endorsed by the Heart Rhythm Society. J Am Soc Echocardiogr 2008;21:191–213.

33. Gorcsan J III, Tanabe M, Bleeker GB, *et al.* Combined longitudinal and radial dyssynchrony predicts ventricular response after resynchronization therapy. J Am Coll Cardiol 2007;50:1476–1483.

34. Sogaard P, Egeblad H, Kim WY, *et al.* Tissue Doppler imaging predicts improved systolic performance and reversed left ventricular remodeling during long-term cardiac resynchronization therapy. J Am Coll Cardiol 2002;40:723–730.

35. Yu CM, Bax JJ, Gorcsan J III. Critical appraisal of methods to assess mechanical dyssynchrony. Curr Opin Cardiol 2009;24:18–28.

36. Yu CM, Chau E, Sanderson JE, *et al.* Tissue Doppler echocardiographic evidence of reverse remodeling and improved synchronicity by simultaneously delaying regional contraction after biventricular pacing therapy in heart failure. Circulation 2002;105:438–445.

37. Yu CM, Fung JW, Zhang Q, *et al.* Tissue Doppler imaging is superior to strain rate imaging and post-systolic shortening on the prediction of reverse remodeling in both ischemic and nonischemic heart failure after cardiac resynchronization therapy. Circulation 2004;110:66–73.

38. Yu CM, Gorcsan J III, Bleeker GB, *et al.* Usefulness of tissue Doppler velocity and strain dyssynchrony for predicting left ventricular reverse remodeling response

after cardiac resynchronization therapy. Am J Cardiol 2007;100:1263–1270.

39. Suffoletto MS, Dohi K, Cannesson M, Saba S, Gorcsan J III. Novel speckle-tracking radial strain from routine black-and-white echocardiographic images to quantify dyssynchrony and predict response to cardiac resynchronization therapy. Circulation 2006; 113:960–968.

40. Dohi K, Suffoletto MS, Schwartzman D, Ganz L, Pinsky MR, Gorcsan J III. Utility of echocardiographic radial strain imaging to quantify left ventricular dyssynchrony and predict acute response to cardiac resynchronization therapy. Am J Cardiol 2005;96:112–116.

41. Cannesson M, Tanabe M, Suffoletto MS, Schwartzman D, Gorcsan J III. Velocity vector imaging to quantify ventricular dyssynchrony and predict response to cardiac resynchronization therapy. Am J Cardiol 2006;98:949–953.

42. Delgado V, Ypenburg C, van Bommel RJ, et al. Assessment of left ventricular dyssynchrony by speckle tracking strain imaging comparison between longitudinal, circumferential, and radial strain in cardiac resynchronization therapy. J Am Coll Cardiol 2008;51:1944–1952.

43. Tanabe M, Lamia B, Tanaka H, Schwartzman D, Pinsky MR, Gorcsan J III. Echocardiographic speckle tracking radial strain imaging to assess ventricular dyssynchrony in a pacing model of resynchronization therapy. J Am Soc Echocardiogr 2008;21:1382–1388.

44. Yu CM, Chan YS, Zhang Q, et al. Benefits of cardiac resynchronization therapy for heart failure patients with narrow QRS complexes and coexisting systolic asynchrony by echocardiography. J Am Coll Cardiol 2006;48:2251–2257.

45. Beshai JF, Grimm RA, Nagueh SF, et al. Cardiac-resynchronization therapy in heart failure with narrow QRS complexes. N Engl J Med 2007;357:2461–2471.

CHAPTER 9

Revascularization for Left Ventricular Dysfunction

Nicholas J. Ruggiero II, Thomas J. Kiernan,
Juan M. Bernal, & Igor F. Palacios
Massachusetts General Hospital, Boston, MA, USA

It is well known that the prevalence of left ventricular (LV) dysfunction in the United States is increasing. Concomitantly, we know that the state of the left ventricle is a strong predictor of outcome in patients with coronary artery disease (CAD). The revascularization of patients with CAD, LV systolic dysfunction, and symptomatic heart failure has been the subject of much debate and surprisingly little research over the past 30 years [1,2]. Our current understanding of how best to treat these patients stems from subset analyses of the coronary artery bypass grafting (CABG) versus medicine clinical trials performed in the 1970s and early 1980s and analyses of large registries of patients from the same era [3–7]. Although such analyses have generally demonstrated that patients with more advanced CAD and more severe LV dysfunction derive larger benefit from CABG relative to medical therapy, in practice both cardiologists and surgeons have substantial uncertainty about whether these projected benefits are counterbalanced by the increased early risks of the surgical approach. CABG is associated with higher postoperative morbidity and mortality compared with patients with normal LV function [3,8,9]. Percutaneous coronary intervention (PCI) with stent implantation is less invasive than surgical treatment, offers predictable angiographic outcomes, and has a high success and low complications rate but is supported by a paucity of data [9–12].

CABG has been the mainstay of treatment for patients with CAD and LV dysfunction for many years. Randomized trials of CABG surgery enrolling 2234 patients from 1971 to 1979 established the safety of surgical revascularization in patients with preserved LV systolic function and chronic stable angina [5]. Improved survival after CABG compared with medical therapy alone was shown for patients with angina and flow-limiting stenoses of the left main coronary artery or multiple coronary arteries, especially in patients with severe stenosis of the proximal left anterior descending coronary artery. The Coronary Artery Surgery Study (CASS) was the only one of these seven early studies to stratify randomization of the 780 patients enrolled based on left ventricular ejection fraction (LVEF, 35–50% vs >50%), angiographic extent of CAD (1-, 2-, or 3-vessel stenosis), and the presence or absence of angina at the time of enrollment. At the conclusion of 10 years of follow-up, 82 (21%) of 390 patients randomly assigned to receive medical therapy alone had died and 70 (18%) of 390 patients randomly assigned to receive medical therapy plus CABG had died ($p = 0.25$)[13]. The subgroup of patients with an LVEF of 35–50% was the only stratified subgroup in CASS to show a significant survival difference. Of the 160 patients in CASS who had left ventricular systolic dysfunction (LVSD), 32 (38%) of the 82 medically treated patients died, whereas 16 (21%) of the 78 patients who underwent CABG ($p = 0.01$) died. However, the 54-patient subset of CASS who had LVSD but no angina did not derive a statistical survival advantage from CABG ($p = 0.12$).

Heart Failure: Device Management. Edited by Arthur Feldman.
© 2010 Blackwell Publishing.

Since the initial description of the clinical syndrome of ischemic cardiomyopathy more than three decades ago [14], the clinical care of patients with CAD and LVSD has undergone a dramatic evolution. When the last patient was randomized between CABG and medical therapy during the time of CASS enrollment, medical therapy for patients with congestive heart failure (CHF), LVSD, and CAD was limited to digitalis and diuretics, which are medications now known to have a neutral effect on mortality. Current American College of Cardiology/American Heart Association guidelines highlight the major advances in pharmacotherapy and device therapy that have improved the quality of life and survival of patients with CAD, CHF, and LVSD [15]. However, the evidence base remains deficient in identifying which, if any, patients with CAD and LVSD should receive revascularization. Although specific clinical problems in this population, such as severe angina, are used to decide on revascularization strategies, the vast majority of patients with ischemic cardiomyopathy have limited or no angina and fall into a gray zone, where clear evidence for adding CABG to medical therapy is either absent or outdated. Thus, divergent views have evolved among clinicians since the reports of the CASS data as to the most appropriate

diagnostic and management strategy for patients with ischemic cardiomyopathy. Table 9.1 summarizes current guideline recommendations as they relate to the use of CABG as a treatment option for patients with poor LV function [15–19].

The weight of observational data suggests that HF and LVSD remain associated with a higher risk of post-CABG complications and mortality, and although increasing numbers of patients with LVSD and angina are referred to CABG, it might remain underused [19,20]. Of the 24,959 patients screened and entered into the CASS registry from 1975 to 1979, 751 patients had severe LVSD (as defined by an LVEF $< 35\%$), 231 patients underwent CABG, and 420 patients remained on medical therapy [4]. Overall 5-year survival favored medical therapy. However, the subset of patients with an LVEF $< 26\%$ had a survival advantage demonstrated for the 82 patients who received CABG compared with the 172 patients treated medically ($p = 0.006$). The CASS Registry CABG group had more angina and less severe LVSD than the CABG cohort in the randomized trial. The CASS Registry patients undergoing CABG presenting with angina had improved survival free of functional limitation, but patients with predominant CHF did not. A large observational series summarized outcomes for 1391 patients with

Table 9.1 CABG recommendations for patients with poor LV function.

Guideline/indication	Classification of recommendation	Level of evidence
American College of Cardiology/American Heart Association 2004 guideline update for CABG surgery [16]		
CABG should be performed in patients with poor LV function who have significant left main coronary artery stenosis	Class I	B
CABG should be performed in patients with poor LV function who have left main equivalent: significant ($\geq$70%) stenosis of proximal LAD and proximal left circumflex artery	Class I	B
CABG should be performed in patients with poor LV function who have proximal LAD stenosis with 2- or 3-vessel disease	Class I	B
CABG can be performed in patients with poor LV function with significant viable noncontracting, revascularizable myocardium and without the above anatomic patterns	Class IIa	B
CABG should not be performed in patients with poor LV function without evidence of significant revascularizable myocardium	Class III	B

CABG, coronary artery bypass grafting; LAD, left anterior descending coronary artery; LV, left ventricular.

CAD and an LVEF < 40% who underwent diagnostic coronary angiography from 1969 to 1994 [7]. After adjustment for baseline differences, the 339 patients who received CABG had a better survival rate than the 1052 patients who received only medical therapy. However, unlike CASS registry patients, this observed survival advantage occurred in all patients, regardless of LVEF and CHF status. The perspective that CABG use in patients with LVSD should be confined only to the patient subset with ongoing angina continues to influence treatment guidelines today.

In 2002, the National Heart, Lung, and Blood Institute (NHLBI) funded the Surgical Treatment for Ischemic Heart Failure (STICH) trial to address two pressing clinical and policy questions regarding the management of patients with CHF with surgically revascularizable CAD and decreased LV function: (1) Is contemporary CABG surgery superior to contemporary medical/secondary prevention therapy in prolonging survival in these patients? (2) Among patients with significant anterior wall dysfunction, does the addition of surgical ventricular reconstruction to CABG improve hospitalization-free survival [20]. The STICH trial is designed to enroll at least 2000 men and women aged 18 years and older who have CAD amenable to revascularization and LVSD defined by a clinically determined LVEF of 35% or less. Patients awaiting a planned PCI to treat symptomatic CAD within the next 30 days are not eligible, although previous PCI is not an exclusion criterion. Although planned operative treatment of the aortic valve excludes potential candidates, the decision to pursue operative management of any other valves, specifically the mitral valve, is left to the discretion of responsible physicians and surgeons. Should the STICH trial show that revascularization provides survival benefit beyond that of modern medical therapy, not only will CABG be used more aggressively in patients with LVSD and CAD amenable to CABG, but it will also indicate the need to evaluate for CAD in all patients who present with HF and LVSD.

As the cardiovascular patient population becomes more elderly, the percentage of patients in this cohort with systolic LV dysfunction also increases in magnitude. These patients are being referred for percutaneous or surgical revascularization, with a limited amount of data in existence with respect to mortality in this patient group. In the earlier studies that predated use of stents and glycoprotein IIb/IIIa antagonists, results have documented poorer outcomes for patients with LV dysfunction undergoing PCI [21–24].

In an analysis from the NHLBI registry of adverse events 8 years after angioplasty, a history of CHF at baseline was the strongest predictor of outcome among six clinical characteristics evaluated [25]. Anderson et al. took patients from four randomized trials (the Perfusion Balloon Catheter Study Group [PBC] trial, Coronary Angioplasty Versus Excisional Atherectomy Trial [CAVEAT]-I and -II, and Integrelin to Manage Platelet Aggregation to Prevent Coronary Thrombosis-II [IMPACT-II]) and one interventional (Duke) database. These data were collected from April 1989 to August 1991 in the PBC trial, from July 1991 to July 1992 in CAVEAT-I, from March 1992 to September 1993 in CAVEAT-II, from November 1993 to November 1994 in IMPACT-II, and between April 1986 and June 1989 in the Duke data set. The four trials and prospective cohort combined include data from 6602 patients. Of these patients, 5260 had both EF and CHF history available and provide the basis for this analysis [26].

The 30-day and 6-month mortality were higher in patients with a clinical history of CHF than in those without such a history (2% vs <1%, $p = 0.002$ at 30 days; 5% vs 1%, $p = 0.001$ at 6 mo). Heart failure history did not influence the incidence of myocardial infarction (MI), use of angioplasty, or the use of bypass surgery during follow-up. Multivariable analysis revealed that heart failure history added significantly to EF in predicting intermediate-term (6-mo) mortality ($p = 0.01$). Stepwise logistic regression also revealed heart failure history to be an independent predictor of 6-month mortality (OR 1.9, 95% CI 1.1–3.5) [26].

A clinical history of CHF is associated with increased early and intermediate-term mortality in patients undergoing percutaneous revascularization. CHF history appears to provide prognostic information independent of that available from a patient's LV function. These findings suggest that patients with a clinical history of CHF who undergo a percutaneous intervention should be closely monitored, especially those with the lowest EFs [26].

Multiple studies have attempted to stratify risk based upon the degree of LV dysfunction. One study by Keelan et al. evaluated the influence of left ventricular ejection fraction LVEF indexes on in-hospital and 1-year outcomes in 1458 patients within the NHLBI-sponsored Dynamic Registry. Patients ($n = 300$) with acute MI were excluded. The remaining 1158 patients were subdivided into three categories: Group 1, EF < 40% ($n = 166$); Group 2, EF = 41–49% ($n = 126$); and Group 3, EF > 50% ($n = 866$). They looked at the frequency of individual and composite adverse events (death/MI/CABG) at discharge and 1 year. In the Dynamic Registry patients, mean EF in the three groups was 32, 45, and 62% and in-hospital mortality was 3.0, 1.6, and 0.1%, respectively ($p < 0.001$). The composite endpoint of death/MI was also significant, but other in-hospital adverse events did not differ between groups. The respective mortality rates were 11.0, 4.5, and 1.9% ($p < 0.001$) after 1 year. The composite endpoints of death/MI and death/MI/CABG also occurred more frequently in Group 1 patients. Thus, significant LV dysfunction was still associated with increased in-hospital and 1-year mortality in patients having contemporary PCI [11].

A second study by Wallace et al. evaluated the association between the severity of LV systolic dysfunction and hospital mortality in patients who undergo elective PCI. A retrospective cohort study was conducted of all patients who underwent elective PCI in New York State in 1998 and 1999. Patients were stratified into five groups on the basis of their LVEFs before PCI (>55, 46–55, 36–45, 26–35, and <25%). Comparisons of demographic, procedural, and outcome variables were performed, and adjusted odds ratios (ORs) were calculated to evaluate the relation between the EF and hospital mortality. Among 55,709 patients who underwent elective PCI, EFs <25, 26–35, and 36–45% were present in 3.4, 7.6, and 17.4%, respectively. Hospital mortality was 0.3, 0.2, 0.6, 1.2, and 2.7% in the groups with EFs >55, 46–55, 36–45, 26–35, and <25%, respectively ($p < 0.001$). After multivariate adjustment, an increased risk for hospital mortality was significant for EF groups of 36–45% (OR 1.56, 95% CI 1.06–2.30), 26–35% (OR 2.17, 95% CI 1.42–3.31), and <25% (OR 3.85, 95% CI 2.46–6.01) compared with EF > 55%, respectively.

This analysis demonstrates that elective PCI is commonly performed in patients with reduced EFs, and the risk for hospital mortality increases as the EF decreases. For patients who undergo elective PCI, an EF < 45% is associated with higher adjusted hospital mortality. Whether elective PCI in patients with low EFs reduces morbidity and/or mortality over medical therapy alone is unknown [27].

Current notable studies of PCI have either excluded or underenrolled patients with systolic dysfunction [28]. The Clinical Outcomes Utilizing Revascularization and Aggressive Drug Evaluation (COURAGE) trial excluded patients with EFs ≤ 30% and included only 406 patients (17.7%) with EFs of 30–50% [29]. The Medicine, Angioplasty, or Surgery Study (MASS), comparing medical therapy with PCI or CABG surgery in patients with stable angina and multivessel CAD, excluded patients with EFs ≤ 40% from enrollment [30]. The use of PCI in this subset of patients is further complicated by the higher prevalence of other characteristics, including diabetes mellitus and multivessel CAD, which are associated with worse long-term outcomes after PCI [31].

Most recently, PCI in LV dysfunction was validated by Columbo in a study published in the *International Journal of Cardiology*. In his study, 422 consecutive patients with LVEF ≤ 35% (assessed by cineangiography and/or echocardiography) underwent myocardial revascularization by either bare metal stent or drug-eluting stent (DES) implantation. Patients with acute and/or recent (<1 wk) transmural MI ($n = 72$) were excluded from the analysis. All patients suffered from angina and/or had a documented inducible ischemia.

The in-hospital course was uneventful in 322 (95.3%) patients. In-hospital death occurred in 5 patients (1.5%). At 2-year, 83 patients (24.6%) died (nonsurviving group), whereas 254 (75.4%) were alive (surviving group). Sudden death occurred in 65% of cases. An acute MI at follow-up occurred more often in the nonsurviving group (18% vs 5.4%, $p = 0.001$). An implantable cardioverter-defibrillator (ICD) was implanted in 6.7% of patients in the nonsurviving group versus 20.7% of the surviving group ($p = 0.005$). LVEF significantly improved at follow-up only in the surviving group ($29 \pm 6\%$ to $35 \pm 11\%$, $p = 0.001$), whereas remained unchanged in the nonsurviving group (27 ± 5% to 26 ± 7%, $p = 0.30$). The independent predictors of death at follow-up were as follows: acute MI (hazard ratio [HR] 4.94, 95% CI 2.53–9.64, $p < 0.001$), use of β-blockers (HR 0.34, 95% CI 0.18–0.65, $p < 0.001$), ICD implantation (HR 0.16, 95% CI 0.05–0.51, $p = 0.002$), LVEF < 25% (HR 2.16, 95% CI 1.25–3.76, $p = 0.006$), and completeness of revascularization (HR 0.29, 95% CI 0.10–0.82, $p = 0.020$). This study shows that PCI in patients with LVEF ≤ 35% is feasible and safe. Independent predictors of death at 2 years are occurrence of an acute MI, treatment by β-blockers, ICD implantation, LVEF < 25%, and completeness of revascularization [32].

To directly compare CABG with PCI, Hartzler and colleagues performed a retrospective analysis of 100 consecutive patients treated with CABG compared with a matched, concurrent cohort of 100 treated with multivessel percutaneous transluminal coronary angioplasty, with all patients having an EF ≤ 40% [33]. In-hospital mortality rates were similar in the bypass (5%) and angioplasty (3%) groups. Repeat revascularization procedures and late MI occurred more frequently during follow-up in the angioplasty group. During 5-year follow-up, superior relief from disabling angina (99% vs 89%, $p = 0.01$) and a trend toward improved survival (76% vs 67%, $p = 0.09$) were observed in the CABG group as compared with the angioplasty group. Of note, late survival was similar in both groups of patients who were completely revascularized. It must be remembered that this study was performed in the pre-stent era.

Seven-year follow-up data from the Bypass Angioplasty Revascularization Investigation (BARI) suggest that patients with LV dysfunction and diabetes may be better served by CABG [34]. However, no survival benefit was noted for CABG over percutaneous transluminal coronary angioplasty in nondiabetic patients.

A single-center observational study was performed on 117 consecutive patients who had severe LV dysfunction (15% ≤ EF ≤ 30%) and underwent either CABG ($n = 69$) or percutaneous revascularization ($n = 48$) between 1992 and 1997 [35]. More vessels were revascularized, and revascularization was more complete by CABG (84% vs 48%, $p < 0.0001$). Morbidity and mortality at 30 days were similar, and there was no significant difference in

3-year survival (73% vs 67%), although 3-year cardiac event-free survival (52% vs 25%, $p = 0.0011$) and 3-year target vessel revascularization-free survival (71% vs 41%, $p < 0.0001$) were significantly better in the CABG group, and LVEF was significantly improved after CABG. The authors concluded that in clinically selected patients with severe LV dysfunction, CABG compared with PCI achieves more complete revascularization, improved LV function, fewer cardiac events, and fewer target vessel revascularizations, but does not affect mid-term survival.

Angina With Extremely Serious Operative Mortality Evaluation (AWESOME) was a nationwide, prospective, randomized, Department of Veterans Affairs clinical trial designed to compare the long-term survival with CABG versus PCI for patients with medically refractory myocardial ischemia and increased risk of adverse outcomes with CABG. Patients were enrolled only if they had one or more than one of five risk factors for adverse outcomes with CABG (prior CABG, MI within 7 days, LVEF < 35%, age > 70 yr, or intra-aortic balloon required to stabilize). Eligible patients who were deemed by their physicians and by study investigators to be suitable for CABG and PCI were asked to participate in the randomized trial. Eligible patients who were acceptable for either CABG or PCI but who refused randomization were entered into a prospective patient choice registry. Eligible patients who were unacceptable for either CABG or PCI were entered into a physician-directed registry. The study protocol and the 3-year survival and quality of life of patients enrolled in the randomized study and registry have been previously reported [36–38]. EF was reported by the investigator at each site and estimated from contrast ventriculography or echocardiography or calculated by radionuclide ventriculography. Patients with EFs < 35% were a prespecified subgroup for analysis.

There were 2431 patients enrolled in the AWESOME study between 1995 and 2000, including 446 patients with EFs < 35% (94 randomized and 352 randomized study). The registry included more patients with coronary artery narrowings of >70% (39% vs 27%), more patients with prior CABGs (36% vs 23%), more patients with 3-vessel disease (55% vs 40%), and more total occlusions (59% vs 42%) than the randomized study.

The results of the AWESOME study (including the only group of patients with EFs < 35% randomly allocated to therapy with PCI vs CABG) suggest that the outcomes with PCI in the current era are similar to those with CABG for patients with acute coronary syndromes, even in the presence of low LVEFs. Previous studies and published guidelines favor CABG over PCI in the setting of low LVEF [6,11,23,39–47], although previous randomized trials of revascularization have systematically excluded patients with LVEFs < 35% [44–46]. This is important because current practice based on studies that show benefit from an early invasive and interventional strategy for patients with acute coronary syndromes [48,49] favors PCI over CABG. Moreover, the early initiation of antiplatelet therapy with clopidogrel, which has been shown to be beneficial in patients with acute coronary syndromes [50,51] and which is recommended in current guidelines, is associated with an excess risk of bleeding with CABG. This also favors PCI over CABG in the setting of acute coronary syndromes. The results are consistent with the findings of the AWESOME randomized trial and registry and suggest that the conclusions of that study are applicable to the subset of patients with low LVEFs.

The major limitation of the trial was the absence of a core laboratory and the lack of a strict definition of EF. Nevertheless, the study is relevant to clinical practice because EF was evaluated in the manner commonly used for clinical decision making. Another limitation that must be acknowledged is that AWESOME was a Department of Veterans Affairs study and included few women.

Recently, Gioia et al. studied 222 patients (20% women) with severe LV dysfunction (EF ≤ 35%) who underwent revascularization with either PCI with DES implantation or CABG between May 2002 and May 2005. One hundred twenty-eight patients received DES (sirolimus in 72 and paclitaxel in 54) and 92 patients underwent CABG. The primary endpoint was all-cause mortality. A composite endpoint of major cardiac adverse events (MACCE), including all-cause mortality, stroke, MI, and target vessel revascularization, was the secondary endpoint [52]. At 2-year follow-up, both groups had the same survival probability from death (83% in both groups). The 2-year MACCE-free survival rate was 76% in DES group and 79% in the CABG co-

hort. Eight (6%) DES patients needed additional PCI in nontarget vessels during follow-up. It is interesting to note that the magnitude of New York Heart Association class improvement was greater for the CABG than DES patients (0.9 vs 1.5, $p = 0.01$). This study extended the positive results of the ARTS 2 study [53], which showed similar outcomes between sirolimus-eluting stent implantation and coronary bypass surgery in patients with multivessel CAD and a normal LV function, to patients with a very low EF.

To date, this is the first report to compare DES with CABG in a relatively large cohort of patients with severe LV dysfunction. Both techniques were performed at the best of their technological maturity considering that a substantial proportion of CABG patients were offered a thoracic artery mammary graft and a quarter of them underwent off-pump surgery. In fact, the number of diseased vessels was greater and clinical presentation with unstable angina was more frequent in patients referred for CABG. However, most of the other factors known to be predictive of worse outcome, such as low LVEF, history of MI or CHF, and presence of diabetes, were fairly similar between the two groups: 1.3 arteries/patient were treated in the DES cohort with 57% of diseased vessel revascularized (1.3 artery-treated/2.3 mean vessel disease), whereas surgical therapy used 3 grafts/patient, achieving a more complete revascularization. Despite the completeness of revascularization in the surgical group, it did not translate into improved survival or better MACCE rate.

PCI for revascularization in patients with a reduced EF is becoming the norm rather than the obscure. As can be seen, it can be performed safely in the correct patient population, with the appropriate techniques and support devices. It is a problem that is only going to be encountered more and more frequently and we must be prepared to deal with it. To do so, a number of support devices have been produced to aid in the performance of these procedures.

The role of prophylactic intra-aortic balloon pump (IABP) during percutaneous coronary revascularization in patients with depressed LV function has been retrospectively studied by single centers as well as by large nationwide registries. It has been frequently used during high-risk coronary interventions due to complex anatomy and/or LV dysfunction. Despite its wide acceptance and long record use, IABP remains a controversial device. It is extensively used during cardiogenic shock due to MI and/or intrinsic myocardial process as well as in the pre- and postoperative cardiac surgery setting due to low cardiac output and/or refractory hypotension. The beneficial effects of IABP are mostly mediated by a decrease in afterload, augmentation in diastolic aortic pressure, and reduced oxygen consumption [54]. It is important to mention that Kern et al. demonstrated that augmented diastolic pressure did not translate into an augmented coronary blood flow beyond critical stenosis [55] unless successful angioplasty was performed, thus revealing that the mechanistic benefit of IABP in setting of critical coronary stenosis is mediated mostly via decreased afterload.

The first retrospective study of IABP in LV dysfunction by Schreiber et al. [56] analyzed 149 patients that underwent high-risk PCI due to complex coronary anatomy and/or LV dysfunction. The patients were supported by either CPS (percutaneous cardiopulmonary support) or IABP. Ninety-one patients underwent IABP insertion. From this cohort, 62 patients had an LVEF < 35%, with a mean EF of $32 \pm 14\%$. Even though the exact rate of complications for the patients with depressed EF and IABP was not reported, the overall rate of MI, stroke, and death postprocedure for this cohort occurred in 2.2, 1.1, and 8.7%, respectively. Apart from a greater incidence of peripheral vascular complication, IABP and CPS did not differ significantly in any other outcome. The authors concluded that high-risk patients could undergo angioplasty with IABP or CPS.

Whether prophylactic IABP compared to "rescue" IABP insertion improves procedural and clinical outcomes remains an area of research interest. Encouraging data became available for the use of IABP in the setting of LV dysfunction by Briguori et al. [57]. The authors studied 133 patients undergoing elective PCI with high-risk characteristics on the basis of a mean EF of 27% as well as a moderate-to-high myocardial jeopardy score. The study cohorts were selected to have an IABP prophylactically or non-IABP on the basis of the operator's discretion. The group of patients receiving an IABP before the procedure had a significantly higher myocardial jeopardy score (8.0 ± 2.8 vs 6.7 ± 2.4). The study demonstrated that even though the patients selected to have prophylactic IABP had higher risk characteristics, the procedural and in-hospital complications were lower. Indeed, the IABP cohort had no intraprocedural events such as hypotension, lethal ventricular arrhythmias, or cardiac arrest. The rate of events compared to non-IABP was significantly lower (0% vs 15%). Furthermore, in-hospital complications despite being nonstatistically significant were lower in the IABP cohort (5% vs 10%), including a lower rate of vascular complications.

Furthermore, Mishra et al. [58] reviewed retrospectively a contemporary patient cohort for procedural and 6-month outcomes. A total of 115 patients who underwent high-risk PCI with a mean EF of 27% in the absence of cardiogenic shock or acute ST elevation MI were studied. Overall, 69 patients had IABP inserted prophylactically, whereas in 46 patients it was used in a "rescue" fashion.

Patients undergoing prophylactic IABP insertion had a higher incidence of comorbidities such as diabetes mellitus or hypercholesterolemia and a greater use of bivalirudin and glycoprotein IIb/IIIa inhibitors. There was no significant difference in coronary anatomy complexity. There was a statistically significant reduction in the rate of in-hospital and 30-day adverse events. Prophylactic IABP reduced the incidence of in-hospital and 30-day death: 0% vs 22% and 4% vs 27%, respectively.

Moreover, this study provided the only mid-term clinical outcome data available to date for the role of prophylactic IABP in the setting of high-risk PCI. The 6-month follow-up confirmed a lower statistically significant reduction in death (8% vs 29%) as well as a lower but nonsignificant rate of Q wave MI and target vessel revascularization. Unfortunately, no data were reported looking at the changes in LV function.

In conclusion, the IABP has been and still is frequently used during high-risk coronary interventions due to complex anatomy and/or LV dysfunction. It is indisputable that it is simply and rapidly inserted through a relatively small sheath, with extremely low rate of vascular complications, and provides a satisfactory yet not ideal hemodynamic support during high-risk interventions.

However, uncertainties regarding critical issues such as proper augmentation of distal coronary flow in high-grade lesions and hemodynamic support during full circulatory collapse [59,55,60] remain worrisome for the interventional cardiology community and have led to the development of newer percutaneously inserted devices capable of providing full circulatory support for extended periods of time.

TandemHeart®: This percutaneous ventricular assist device is a left atrial to femoral bypass system that can provide a relatively rapid full circulatory support. The device consists of a centrifugal pump suspended by a magnetic force on lubricating fluid, hence reducing heat and friction and providing continuous flow up to 4 L/min. Its cannulation system includes a 22-French (F) transseptal venous cannula with a large 14-F end hole for aspiration of oxygenated blood from the left atrium and a femoral artery perfusion catheter ranging from 9 to 17 F. The device directly unloads the left ventricle, reducing cardiac workload and oxygen demand. Also, the device has been demonstrated to resolve pulmonary edema and metabolic abnormalities associated with cardiogenic shock due to extensive MI [61]. Nevertheless, the device insertion technique requires proficiency in transseptal puncture, which limits its use to trained interventional cardiologists as well as in emergency situations where rapid full circulatory support is mandated.

This device has not been systematically evaluated for its use in high-risk PCI due to decreased LV dysfunction. However, small series evaluating its feasibility and safety are reported. The first series by Vranckx et al. [62] reported 3 patients with severe LV systolic function (mean EF 22%) undergoing high-risk PCI. Prophylactic insertion of a TandemHeart® before PCI of the last remaining patent vessel or multivessel disease was performed with a mean insertion time of 28 minutes. The device provided adequate improvement in cardiac index (2.3 L/min/mm^2 vs 3.2 L/min/mm^2) and a reduction in pulmonary capillary wedge pressure (21 mmHg vs 10 mmHg). The authors reported a 100% procedural success with no device-related complications, including residual shunts at the atrial level and/or hemolysis. Most important, at 7-month follow-up, all the patients were alive and well. The mean duration of pump support was 33 hours. Of note, the TandemHeart® has been reported to provide safe and adequate extracorporeal circulation for up to 8 days [63] in the absence of significant peripheral vascular disease.

Aragon et al. [64] reported 8 cases of high-risk PCI due to combined LV dysfunction (mean EF 30 ± 9%) and high-risk anatomical substrate, and in 1 case severe aortic stenosis. The device was inserted prophylactically at the operator's discretion. The authors reported 100% procedural success and in all the cases the TandemHeart® was removed at the cardiac catheterization laboratory after the intervention. No major vascular complications or device-related death occurred. With an average (189 ± 130)-day follow-up, 6 patients were event-free and 1 patient developed acute renal failure requiring hemodialysis due to underlying chronic kidney disease and outside-the-hospital cardiac arrest.

Al-Husami et al. [65] in a single-center experience retrospectively reviewed the short-term outcomes of 6 patients undergoing high-risk PCI due to LV systolic dysfunction (mean EF 33%) and/or complex coronary anatomy. There was 100% procedural success. There were no device-related complications, and the mean device insertion time was 36.5 minutes comparable to the times reported by Vranckx. One patient died following successful PCI due to multiorgan failure. The overall survival at 30 days was 83%.

Last but not least, to date the largest retrospective study was published by Vranckx et al. In this 6-year, single-center experience, 23 patients underwent TandemHeart® insertion due to emergent or elective high-risk PCI. Of these patients, 70% of them had an EF < 30%. The procedural success rate was 96%. The device was successfully implanted in 100% of the patients, with a mean insertion time of 34 ± 12 minutes. The mean duration of support was 33 ± 49 hours. The device offered adequate circulatory support up to 4 L and reduction in pulmonary capillary wedge pressure in all the patients. Two of these patients presented nonpulsatile blood pressure, with one of these patients recovered pulsatile blood pressure within 24 hours whereas the second patient expired while in the pump. Importantly, device-related complications were infrequent, with systemic hypothermia occurring in 26% of the cases likely due to concomitant anesthetic and/or paralytic use as well as pump exposed to room temperature. Also, bleeding and limb ischemia in patients were reported to occur at a rate of 27 and 4.3%, respectively. No hemolysis was reported. Once more this study highlighted the safety and feasibility of the TandemHeart® for high-risk PCI.

Overall, these small, nonrandomized studies accounting for less than 50 patients in total demonstrated the feasibility of percutaneous left ventricular assist devices (TandemHeart®) in the setting of high-risk PCI and LV dysfunction. Unfortunately, the deficiency of large registries and/or comparative studies, and hence lack of proven clinical benefits, limits its widespread use in the setting of high-risk PCI due to LV dysfunction. Moreover, as mentioned above, the level of expertise to perform a safe transeptal puncture is not present in many centers, confining its potential use to large referral centers.

Impella Recover LP 2.5: The Impella LVAD Recover LP 2.5 is a miniaturized rotary blood pump mounted on a 9-F pigtail catheter which is advanced retrogradely into the left ventricle via the femoral artery. The device is placed via a 13-F sheath. The pump unloads the left ventricle by aspirating blood and expelling directly into the ascending aorta. It can provide up to 2.5 L/min at its maximum speed of 51,000 rpm. Due to ease of insertion, superior hemodynamic support, and few true contraindications, this device has become very attractive in the interventional community. The device reduces end-diastolic pressure and volume, which translates into a lower wall tension and reduced oxygen demand [66]. Moreover, it has been shown to increase mean distal coronary pressure, increase coronary flow reserve, and decrease coronary microvascular resistance. It was first reported to be used in the setting of high-risk PCI by Valgimigli et al. [66]. The authors reported the successful use of the Impella Recover LP 2.5 pump in a 56-year-old patient undergoing a higher risk PCI due to concomitant LV dysfunction. Subsequently, Henriques et al. [67] published a single-center feasibility and safety study of 19 patients undergoing high-risk PCI due to complex anatomy and/or LV dysfunction. All the patients had an LVEF < 40%. Sixty-three percent of those had an LVEF < 25%. Coronary interventions and device insertion were successfully achieved in all the patients. There were no device-related complications or malfunctions. Furthermore, no evidence of hemolytic or device-induced aortic regurgitation was reported. Due to these encouraging results, a more rigorous, multimember US study was recently conducted. The PROTECT I study [68] analyzed 20 patients with severe LV systolic dysfunction (EF < 35%) undergoing high-risk PCI due to unprotected left main or last patent coronary conduit. Patients with recent ST myocardial infraction, cardiogenic shock, aortic stenosis, and moderate-to-severe aortic regurgitation were excluded. The safety endpoint at 30 days was the incidence of major cardiovascular events, defined as death, myocardial infraction, stroke, target vessel revascularization, or emergent bypass. The efficacy endpoint was freedom from hemodynamic compromise during PCI defined as decrease in mean arterial pressure below 60 mmHg for more than 1 minute. The authors reported an incidence of major cardiac events of 20%. There were 2 per procedural MI and 2 device-unrelated deaths. Moreover, there were only 2 cases of transient hemolysis of no clinical consequences. None of the patients developed hemodynamic compromise during the PCI.

The study corroborated the safety and efficacy of the Impella LP 2.5 in the setting of high-risk PCI due to LV dysfunction and/or complex coronary anatomy.

In summary, the Impella LP 2.5 has excellent hemodynamic profile, proven safety, as well as being the only circulatory support device to improve LV systolic function following high-risk PCI. Nonetheless, no randomized data were yet available to make it a class I recommendation in the setting of high-risk percutaneous revascularization.

Currently, the PROTECT II trial is randomizing high-risk patients undergoing PCI of an unprotected left main or last patent conduit to IABP vs Impella. This is a superiority trial, which we hope will provide us with better insight into how to better manage this rapidly growing population of elderly patients with LV systolic dysfunction and/or complex coronary anatomy who will benefit from percutaneous revascularization.

As can be seen from this chapter the revascularization of patients with LV dysfunction has been a challenge for many years and the difficulty is extrapolating the data to fit the patient who is sitting in front of you. However, we hope that it has presented the data in a concise and practical manner to guide management of this complex patient population. In the field of interventional cardiology we are looking at new ways not only to manage the coronary disease of these patients, but also to hopefully develop strategies to deal with the valvular and structural cardiac components in the very near future.

References

1. Charaeonthaitawee P, Gersh BJ, Araoz PA, Gibbons RJ. Revascularization in severe left ventricular dysfunction: the role of viability testing. J Am Coll Cardiol 2005;46:567–574.

2. Jones RH. Is it time for a randomized trial of surgical treatment of ischemic heart failure? J Am Coll Cardiol 2001;37:1210–1213.

3. Passamani E, Davis KB, Gillespie MJ, Killip T. A randomized trial of coronary artery bypass surgery: survival in patients with a low ejection fraction. N Engl J Med 1985;312:1665–1671.

4. Alderman EL, Fisher LD, Litwin P, et al. Results of coronary artery surgery in patients with poor left ventricular function (CASS). Circulation 1983;68:785–795.

5. Yusuf S, Zucker D, Peduzzi P, et al. Effect of coronary artery bypass graft surgery on survival: overview of 10-year results from randomized trials by the Coronary Artery Bypass Graft Surgery Trialists Collaboration. Lancet 1994;344:563–570.

6. Baker DW, Jones R, Hodges J, Massie BM, Konstam MA, Rose EA. Management of heart failure. III: The role of revascularization in the treatment of patients with moderate or severe left ventricular systolic dysfunction. JAMA 1994;V:1528–1534.

7. O'Connor CM, Velazquez EJ, Gardner LH, et al. Comparison of coronary artery bypass grafting versus medical therapy on long-term outcome in patients with ischemic cardiomyopathy (a 25-year experience from the Duke Cardiovascular Disease Databank). Am J Cardiol 2002;90:101–107.

8. Topkara VK, Cheema FH, Kesavaramaujam S, et al. Coronary artery bypass grafting in patients with low ejection fraction. Circulation 2005;112:344–350.

9. Christakis GT, Weisel RD, Fremes SE, et al.; Cardiovascular Surgeons of the university of Toronto. Coronary artery bypass grafting in patients with poor left ventricular function. J Thorac Cardiovasc Surg 1992;103:1083–1091.

10. Sedlis SP, Ramanathan KB, Morrison DA, Sethi G, Sacks J, Henderson W. Outcome of percutaneous coronary intervention versus coronary bypass grafting for patients with low left ventricular ejection fractions, unstable angina pectoris, and risk factors for adverse outcomes with bypass (the AWESOME Randomized Trial and Registry). Am J Cardiol 2004;94:118–120.

11. Keelan PC, Johnston JM, Koru-Sengul T, et al. Comparison of inhospital and one-year outcomes in patients with left ventricular ejection fractions ≤ 40%, 41% to 49%, and ≥ 50% having percutaneous coronary revascularization. Am J Cardiol 2003;91:1168–1172.

12. Stevens T, Kahn JK, McCallister BD, et al. Safey and efficacy of percutaneous coronary angioplasty in patients with left ventricular dysfunction. Am J Cardiol 1991;68:313–319.

13. Alderman EL, Bourassa MG, Cohen LS, et al. Ten-year follow-up of survival and myocardial infarction in the randomized coronary artery surgery study. Circulation 1990;82:1629–1646.

14. Burch GE, Tsui CY, Harb JM. Ischemic cardiomyopathy. Am Heart J 1972;83:340–350.

15. Hunt SA, Abraham WT, Chin MH, et al. ACC/AHA 2005 guideline update for the diagnosis and management of chronic heart failure in the adult. Circulation 2005;112:e154–e235.

16. Eagle KA, Guyton RA, Davidoff R, et al. ACC/AHA 2004 guideline update for coronary artery bypass graft surgery. Circulation 2004;110:e340–e437.

17. Cheitlin MD, Armstrong WF, Aurigemma GP, et al. ACC/AHA/ASE 2003 guideline update for the clinical application of echocardiography—summary article. J Am Coll Cardiol 2003;42:954–970.

18. Klocke FJ, Baird MG, Lorell BH, et al. ACC/AHA/ASNC guidelines for the clinical use of cardiac radionuclide imaging—executive summary. J Am Coll Cardiol 2003;42:1318–1333.

19. Gibbons RJ, Abrams J, Chatterjee K, et al. ACC/AHA 2002 guideline update for the management of patients with chronic stable angina—summary article. J Am Coll Cardiol 2003;41:159–168.

20. Velazquez EJ, Lee KL, O'Connor CM, et al. STICH Investigators. The rationale and design of the Surgical Treatment for Ischemic Heart Failure (STICH) trial. J Thorac Cardiovasc Surg 2007;134(6): 1540–1547.

21. Holmes DR Jr, Detre KM, Williams DO, et al. The NHLBI PTCA Registry. Long-term outcome of patients with depressed left ventricular function undergoing percutaneous transluminal coronary angioplasty. Circulation 1993;87:21–29.

22. Serota H, Deligonul U, Lee WH, et al. Predictors of cardiac survival after percutaneous transluminal coronary angioplasty in patients with severe left ventricular dysfunction. Am J Cardiol 1991;67:367–372.

23. Kohli RS, DiSciascio G, Cowley MJ, Nath A, Goudreau E, Vetrovec GW. Coronary angioplasty in patients with severe left ventricular dysfunction. J Am Coll Cardiol 1990;16:807–811.

24. Lewin RF, Dorros G. Percutaneous transluminal coronary angioplasty in patients with severe left ventricular dysfunction. Cardiol Clin 1989;7:813–825.

25. Holmes DR, Detre K, Weh WL, *et al.* The NHLBI PTCA Registry. Eight year, long term outcome after PTCA: factors associated with adverse events [abstract]. J Am Coll Cardiol 1996;27:361A.

26. Anderson R, Holmes DR, Harrington RA, *et al.* Prognostic value of congestive heart failure history in patients undergoing percutaneous coronary interventions. J Am Coll Cardiol 1998;32:936–941.

27. Wallace T, *et al.* Impact of left ventricular dysfunction on hospital mortality among patients undergoing elective percutaneous coronary intervention. Am J Cardiol 2009;103:355–360.

28. Katritsis DG, Ioannidis JP. Percutaneous coronary intervention versus conservative therapy in nonacute coronary artery disease: a meta-analysis. Circulation 2005;111:2906–2912.

29. Boden WE, O'Rourke RA, Teo KK, *et al.* Design and rationale of the Clinical Outcomes Utilizing Revascularization and Aggressive Drug Evaluation (COURAGE) trial Veterans Affairs Cooperative Studies Program No. 424. Am Heart J 2006;151:1173–1179.

30. Hueb W, Soares PR, Gersh BJ, *et al.* The Medicine, Angioplasty, or Surgery Study (MASS-II). A randomized, controlled clinical trial of three therapeutic strategies for multivessel coronary artery disease: one-year results. J Am Coll Cardiol 200443:1743–1751.

31. Hannan EL, Racz MJ, Walford G, *et al.* Long-term outcomes of coronary-artery bypass grafting versus stent implantation. N Engl J Med 2005;352:2174–2183.

32. Brigouri C, *et al.* Stent implantation in patients with severe left ventricular systolic dysfunction. Int J Card 10 July 2009;135(3): 376–384.

33. O'Keefe JH Jr, Allan JJ, McCallister BD, *et al.* Angioplasty versus bypass surgery for multivessel coronary artery disease with left ventricular ejection fraction < or = 40%. Am J Cardiol. 15 April 1993;71(11):897–901.

34. Detre KM, Lombardero MS, Brooks MM, *et al.* for Bypass Angioplasty Revascularization Investigation Investigators. The effect of previous coronary artery bypass surgery on the prognosis of patients with diabetes who have acute myocardial infarction. N Engl J Med 6 April 2000;342(14):1040–1042.

35. Toda K, Mackenzie K, Mehra MR, *et al.* Revascularization in severe ventricular dysfunction (15% < OR = LVEF < OR = 30%): a comparison of bypass grafting and percutaneous intervention. Ann Thorac Surg December 2002;74(6):2082–2087.

36. Morrison DA, Sethi G, Sacks J, *et al.* Percutaneous coronary intervention versus coronary artery bypass graft surgery for patients with medically refractory myocardial ischemia and risk factors for adverse outcomes with bypass: a multicenter, randomized trial. J Am Coll Cardiol 2001;38:143–149.

37. Morrison DA, Sethi G, Sacks J, *et al.* A multi-center, randomized trial of percutaneous coronary intervention versus bypass surgery in high-risk unstable angina patients. The VA AWESOME Multicenter Registry: comparison with the randomized clinical trial. J Am Coll Cardiol 2002;39:266–273.

38. Rumsfeld JS, Magid DJ, Plomondon ME, *et al.* Health-related quality of life after percutaneous coronary intervention versus coronary bypass surgery in high-risk patients with medically refractory ischemia. J Am Coll Cardiol 2003;41:1732–1738.

39. Elefteriades JA, Tolis G Jr, Levi E, Mills LK, Zaret BL. Coronary artery bypass grafting in severe left ventricular dysfunction: excellent survival with improved ejection fraction and functional state. J Am Coll Cardiol 1993;22:1411–1417.

40. Stahle E, Bergstrom R, Edlund B, *et al.* Influence of left ventricular function on survival after coronary artery bypass grafting. Ann Thorac Surg 1997;64:437–444.

41. Trachiotis GD, Weintraub WS, Johnston TS, Jones EL, Guyton RA, Craver JM. Coronary artery bypass grafting in patients with advanced left ventricular dysfunction. Ann Thorac Surg 1998;66:1632–1639.

42. Ellis SG, Cowley MJ, DiSciascio G, *et al.* The Multivessel Angioplasty Prognosis Study Group. Determinants of 2-year outcome after coronary angioplasty in patients with multivessel disease on the basis of comprehensive preprocedural evaluation. Implications for patient selection. Circulation 1991;83:1905–1914.

43. Eltchaninoff H, Franco I, Whitlow PL. Late results of coronary angioplasty in patients with left ventricular ejection fractions ≤ 40%. Am J Cardiol 1994;73:1047–1052.

44. Killip T, Passamani E, Davis K. Coronary Artery Surgery Study (CASS): a randomized trial of coronary bypass surgery. Eight years follow-up and survival in patients with reduced ejection fraction. Circulation 1985;72:V102–V109.

45. Sharma GV, Deupree RH, Khuri SF, Parisi AF, Luchi RJ, Scott SM; Veterans Administration Unstable Angina Cooperative Study Group. Coronary bypass surgery improves survival in high-risk unstable angina. Results of a Veterans Administration Cooperative Study with an 8-year follow-up. Circulation 1991;84(5 Suppl): III260–III267.

46. Eagle KA, Guyton RA, Davidoff R, *et al.* ACC/AHA Guidelines for coronary artery bypass graft surgery: a report of the American College of Cardiology/American Heart Association Task Force on Practice Guidelines (Committee to Revise the 1991 Guidelines for Coronary Artery Bypass Graft Surgery). J Am Coll Cardiol 1999;34:1262–1347.

47. Braunwald E, Antman EM, Beasley JW, *et al.* ACC/AHA 2002 Guideline update for the management of patients

with unstable angina and non-ST-segment elevation myocardial infarction: a report of the American College of Cardiology/American Heart Association Task Force on Practice Guidelines (Committee on the Management of Patients With Unstable Angina). Available at: http://circ.ahajournals.org/cgi/content/extract/106/14/1893.

48. Cannon CP, Weintraub WS, Demopoulos LA, *et al.* The TACTICS—Thrombolysis in Myocardial Infarction 18 Investigators. Comparison of early invasive and conservative strategies in patients with unstable coronary syndromes treated with the glycoprotein IIb/IIIa inhibitor tirofiban. N Engl J Med 2001;344:1879–1887.

49. FRagmin and Fast Revascularisation during InStability in Coronary artery Disease Investigators. Invasive compared with non-invasive treatment in unstable coronary artery disease: FRISC II prospective randomised multicentre study. Lancet 1999;354:708–715.

50. The Clopidogrel in Unstable Angina to Prevent Recurrent Events Trial Investigators. Effects of clopidogrel in addition to aspirin in patients with acute coronary syndromes without ST-segment elevation. N Engl J Med 2001;345:494–502.

51. Mehta SR, Yusuf S, Peters RJ, *et al.* Clopidogrel in Unstable angina to prevent Recurrent Events trial (CURE) Investigators. Effects of pretreatment with clopidogrel and aspirin followed by long-term therapy in patients undergoing percutaneous coronary intervention: the PCICURE study. Lancet 2001358:527–533.

52. Gioia G, Matthai W, Gillin K, *et al.* Revascularization in severe left ventricular dysfunction: outcome comparison of drug-eluting stent implantation versus coronary artery bypass grafting. Catheter Cardiovasc Interv 2007;70(1):26–33.

53. Serruys PW, Morice MC, Kappetein AP, *et al.* Arterial revascularization therapies study II: Sirolimus-eluting stents for the treatment of patients with multivessel de novo coronary artery lesions (ARTS II). Presented at the 2005 ACC 54th Annual Scientific Session, Orlando, FL, March 2005.

54. Powell WJ Jr, Daggett WM, Magro AE, *et al.* Effects of intra-aortic balloon counterpulsation on cardiac performance, oxygen consumption, and coronary blood flow in dogs. Circ Res 1970;26(6):753–764.

55. Kern MJ, Aguirre F, Bach R, *et al.* Augmentation of coronary blood flow by intra-aortic balloon pumping in patients after coronary angioplasty. Circulation 1993;87(2):500–511.

56. Schreiber TL, Kodali UR, O'Neill WW, *et al.* Comparison of acute results of prophylactic intraaortic balloon pumping with cardiopulmonary support for percutaneous transluminal coronary angioplasty (PCTA). Cathet Cardiovasc Diagn 1998;45(2):115–119.

57. Briguori C, Sarais C, Paolo P, *et al.* Elective versus provisional intra-aortic balloon pumping in high-risk percutaneous transluminal coronary angioplasty. Am Heart J 2003;145(4):700–707.

58. Mishra S, Chu WW, Torguson R, *et al.* Role of prophylactic intra-aortic balloon pump in high-risk patients undergoing percutaneous coronary intervention. Am J Cardiol 2006;98(5):608–612.

59. DeWood MA, Notske RN, Hensley GR, *et al.* Intraaortic balloon counterpulsation with and without reperfusion for myocardial infarction shock. Circulation 1980;61(6):1105–1112.

60. Nanas JN, Moulopoulos SD. Counterpulsation: historical background, technical improvements, hemodynamic and metabolic effects. Cardiology 1994;84(3):156–167.

61. Thiele H, Lauer B, Hambrecht R, *et al.* Reversal of cardiogenic shock by percutaneous left atrial-to-femoral arterial bypass assistance. Circulation 2001;104(24): 2917–2922.

62. Vranckx P, Foley DP, de Feijter PJ, *et al.* Clinical introduction of the TandemHeart, a percutaneous left ventricular assist device, for circulatory support during high-risk percutaneous coronary intervention. Int J Cardiovasc Intervent 2003;5(1):35–39.

63. Pavie A, Leger P, Nzomvuama A, *et al.* Left centrifugal pump cardiac assist with transseptal percutaneous left atrial cannula. Artif Organs 1998;22(6): 502–507.

64. Aragon J, Lee MS, Kar S, *et al.* Percutaneous left ventricular assist device: 'TandemHeart' for high-risk coronary intervention. Catheter Cardiovasc Interv 2005;65(3):346–352.

65. Al-Husami W, Yturralde F, Mohanty G, *et al.* Single-center experience with the TandemHeart percutaneous ventricular assist device to support patients undergoing high-risk percutaneous coronary intervention. J Invasive Cardiol 2008;20(6):319–322.

66. Valgimigli M, Steendijk P, Sianos G, *et al.* Left ventricular unloading and concomitant total cardiac output increase by the use of percutaneous Impella Recover LP 2.5 assist device during high-risk coronary intervention. Catheter Cardiovasc Interv 2005;65(2):263–267.

67. Henriques JP, Remmelink M, Baan J Jr, *et al.* Safety and feasibility of elective high-risk percutaneous coronary intervention procedures with left ventricular support of the Impella Recover LP 2.5. Am J Cardiol 2006;97(7):990–992.

68. Dixon SR, Henriques JP, Mauri L, *et al.* A prospective feasibility trial investigating the use of the Impella 2.5 system in patients undergoing high-risk percutaneous coronary intervention (The PROTECT I Trial) initial U.S. experience. JACC Interv 2009;2(2):91–96.

CHAPTER 10

Minimally Invasive Treatment of Mitral Valve Disease

Andra M. Popescu, & Paul J. Mather
Jefferson Medical College, Philadelphia, PA, USA

Introduction

In the United States, mitral regurgitation (MR; acute and chronic) affects approximately 5 in 10,000 people, associated independently with female sex and advanced age. Mitral valve disease is the second most common valvular lesion, preceded only by aortic stenosis. Acute or chronic MR can be caused by a multitude of disorders. The most common cause of MR in the Western society is mitral valve prolapse (MVP). Other common causes of MR are rheumatic heart disease, infective endocarditis, and annular calcification, while less common etiologies include trauma, collagen vascular diseases, carcinoid, the hypereosinophilic syndrome, and exposure to phentermine, fenfluramine, and other appetite-suppressants drugs.

Mitral valve disease is often complex because it involves the entire mitral valve apparatus (Figure 10.1), composed of mitral valve leaflets, chordae tendineae, papillary muscles, and mitral annulus. Any of these structures can be affected, resulting in mitral regurgitation. The most common *leaflet abnormalities* are seen in MVP (with both leaflets being affected), chronic rheumatic heart disease, and infective endocarditis. The *chordae tendineae* also play an important role in the MVP syndrome. Their rupture, whether spontaneous or secondary to infectious endocarditis, trauma, or rheumatic heart disease, can result in acute, subacute, or chronic mild-to-severe MR, depending on the number of

chordae involved in the pathology. *Coronary perfusion* can also affect MV function. Terminal branches of the coronary arteries vascularize the papillary muscles and therefore ischemia may affect their function. If transient, ischemia may cause transitory episodes of MR, but when severe and prolonged, chronic MR will be seen. One of the most common causes of mitral valve regurgitation is the dilatation of the coronary annulus that accompanies cardiac dilatation and heart failure. This abnormality has been associated with a worsened functional capacity and a poorer prognosis.

A *submitral aneurysm* due to a congenital defect of the posterior aspect of the annulus has also been described as a cause of annular dilatation. Calcification of the annulus can also cause MR, although usually this is less severe.

Management

Medical management of MR is currently limited to a few drug classes. Although there is no doubt that afterload reduction therapy with angiotensin-converting enzyme inhibitors, nitroprusside or nitroglycerin, may be salutary in acute MR, there is varying degrees of evidence that they are as valuable in chronic MR.

There are yet no randomized trials to compare medical management to surgical therapy in patients with severe chronic MR who meet indications for corrective surgery. In asymptomatic patients with preserved systolic function, angiotensin-converting enzyme inhibitors did not prove to affect significantly left ventricular (LV) volumes or ejection fraction (EF) significantly in the absence of symptoms

Heart Failure: Device Management. Edited by Arthur Feldman.
© 2010 Blackwell Publishing.

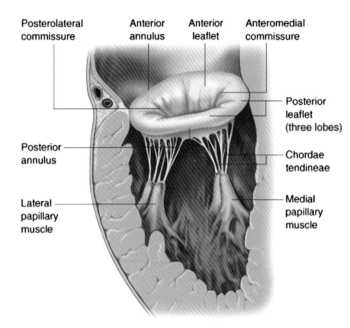

Posterolateral commissure · Anterior annulus · Anterior leaflet · Anteromedial commissure · Posterior leaflet (three lobes) · Posterior annulus · Chordae tendineae · Lateral papillary muscle · Medial papillary muscle

Figure 10.1 Continuity of the mitral apparatus and the left ventricular myocardium. Mitral regurgitation (MR) may be caused by any condition that affects the leaflets or the structure and function of the left ventricle. Similarly, a surgical procedure that disrupts the mitral apparatus in an attempt to correct MR has adverse effects on left ventricular geometry, volume, and function. (From [1].)

or hypertension. The American College of Cardiology/American Heart Association (ACC/AHA) guidelines published in 2006 [2] recommend *surgical treatment* for symptomatic patients with severe acute or chronic MR and for asymptomatic patients or mildly symptomatic patients with progressively worsening EF or increasing LV dimensions (class Ia).

Evolution of mitral valve surgery

From the introduction of the cardiopulmonary bypass in 1953 by Gibbon [3–5] to the first artificial valve prosthesis used in 1961 by Starr [6] and the first biologic prosthesis introduced in 1970s by Hancock and Carpentier-Edwards, valve surgery has continued to evolve in a dynamic fashion. According to the 2006 ACC/AHA guidelines [2], mitral valve surgery is recommended for symptomatic patients with acute MR, symptomatic patients with severe MR in the absence of severe LV dysfunction, as well as for asymptomatic patients with severe chronic MR and EF of 30–60% and/or end-systolic dimension ≥ 40 mm (class Ia). Class IIa recommendation includes asymptomatic patients with severe chronic MR and preserved LV systolic function who have new-onset atrial fibrillation or pulmonary hypertension. Mitral valve repair is recommended in

asymptomatic severe chronic MR with preserved LV systolic function (EF ≥ 60% and end-systolic dimension < 40%) if likelihood of successful repair without residual MR is greater then 90% (class IIa) [2,7].

Success depends on patient's clinical and hemodynamic status, the presence of comorbidities (renal failure, hepatic disease, pulmonary disease), and the experience of the surgical team [8]. In the early stages of mitral valve surgery, replacement was considered a standard treatment option. Currently, repair is the preferred intervention and constitutes class Ia recommendation according to the ACC/AHA guidelines [2].

Mitral valve repair (valvuloplasty) consists of reconstruction of the mitral valve including an annuloplasty with a flexible or rigid ring (Figure 10.2). Repair is often successful in children and young adults with MVP and in those with MR due to annular dilatation, papillary muscle ischemia or rupture, chordae tendineae rupture, and leaflet perforation due to infective endocarditis. Older patients with rigid, calcified rheumatic valves or severe subvalvular thickening and mitral annular calcifications, as well as patients who previously underwent mitral valve surgery, usually require *mitral valve replacement* (MVR) because repair results can be suboptimal. One disadvantage of MVR is the prosthesis

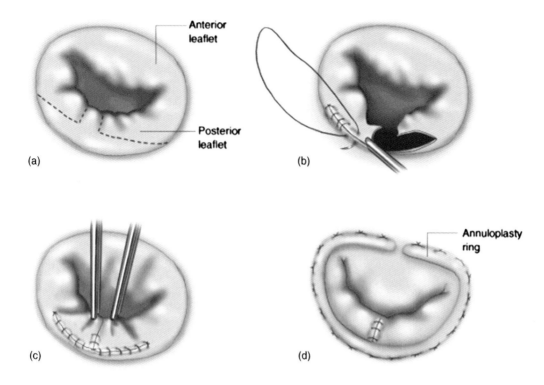

Figure 10.2 Mitral valve repair employing reduction excision and reattachment of the posterior leaflet with implantation of an annuloplasty ring: (a) reduction excision of posterior leaflet, (b) reattach posterior leaflet (sliding valvuloplasty), (c) repair posterior leaflet, and (d) completed supported repair. (From [9].)

itself. It can increase the risk of thromboembolic events or hemorrhage (due to anticoagulation required with mechanical prosthesis), delayed mechanical dysfunction (seen with bioprothesis), or increased risk of infective endocarditis (with both mechanical and bioprosthesis). Excellent outcomes are obtained with both repair and replacement, but repair tends to have slightly better results when successful [10–13]. It has been noted that systolic function preservation is superior with mitral valve repair and this has been attributed partially to the preservation of annular-chordal-papillary muscle continuity. Currently when performing MVR, preservation of the subvalvular apparatus is considered critical and is attempted whenever possible [14,15].

The Society of Thoracic Surgeons National Database Committee reported an operative mortality rate of <2% in 3309 patients undergoing isolated mitral valve repair in 2002 [16,17]. This compares favorably to the 6% operative mortality for the 4069

patients undergoing isolated MVR. Although many centers in the United States are now performing repair in the majority of their cases, overall MVR is performed more often than mitral valve repair due to an increase in technical difficulty seen with the latter.

Recently, there is an increasing interest for the development and improvement in less traumatic techniques and minimally invasive approach for mitral valve disease.

Minimally invasive techniques

While standard mitral valve surgery with a median sternotomy approach has long established excellent clinical outcomes [17], the newly developed minimally invasive approach has yet to match the high-quality results of this conventional surgical therapy, likely due to a continuing learning curve on the part of cardio-surgeons. The idea of less trauma with minimally invasive surgery is thought to be more attractive to the patient. Smaller incisional scars and subsequent quicker recovery as well as shorter length of stay, less intensive care unit days, and fewer blood products are also very attractive—especially for patients with heart failure.

Minimally invasive refers to the small surgical access site since there obviously remains a need for temporary perioperative support using extracorporeal circulation and cardiac arrest. Although the incisional approach is different, the actual technique for mitral valve repair and replacement and the need for cardiopulmonary bypass and cardioplegia remain similar to the conventional method.

The advances in minimally invasive mitral valve surgery within the past decade are primarily an evolution toward an optimal approach. With the current modern techniques the outcomes in minimally invasive mitral valve surgery, whether repairing or replacing the valve, are similar to those obtained with conventional surgery [18]. In the past several years, minimally invasive mitral valve surgery has gained more and more clinical acceptance among surgeons, and even more, there is an increasing interest shown by the patients to be treated in a minimally invasive fashion.

We will focus this chapter on the current indications for minimally invasive surgery, the evolution of the techniques, the current clinical practice, and the use of telemanipulators and robotic surgery.

Indications

Surgery or minimally invasive intervention is indicated in patients who have severe symptomatic disease or in those with moderate disease if there is a good chance that repair will be successful. The success of repair with the minimally invasive approach in specialized centers is comparable to conventional surgery and reaches 70%. Initially, it was considered that certain high-risk patients should undergo a conventional approach, but it is now believed that the safety and reliability of the two approaches are similar [19].

The evolution of minimally invasive mitral valve surgery

The classical median sternotomy was not the first type of incision used for mitral valve surgery. The first mitral valve operations were performed using a lateral thoracotomy with femoral access for extracorporeal circulation. More than a decade ago, as the minimally invasive approach increased in prevalence, a lateral minithoracotomy with direct visualization of the valve became more popular. Among the first to publish their results, Arom and Navia came to conclusion that the mitral valve is accessible with this lateral minithoracotomy and that the mortality was low with this new approach [20,21]. The next step in the evolution of the minimally invasive approach was the creation of specialized surgical tools. The Stanford group introduced direct visualization using the Port-Access intra-aortic balloon occlusion and cardioplegia. They published their initial results in dogs and then later in humans [22–24]. In the following years the Port-Access intra-aortic balloon technique had developed and had been used by many different groups [25–27]. Unfortunately, despite the widespread interest and quickly gained technical experience, an increased risk in aortic dissection as well as severe complications due to retrograde perfusion limited the overall acceptance of the intra-aortic balloon pump (endoclamp). The failure of Port-Acces system to satisfy surgeon's expectations translated into an intense search for a better, safer, and less expensive way to clamp the aorta. Finally, in 1997 Chitwood first introduced the percutaneous transthoracic aortic clamp [28,29]. It is a simple, cost-effective, and relatively safe device, which is currently used widely at many centers that perform minimally invasive mitral valve surgery.

The next step in the evolution of minimally invasive mitral valve surgery was the use of endoscopes to improve visualization. Initially, two-dimensional and then three-dimensional *videoscopes* were introduced by Chitwood, Carpentier, and Falk [29–31].

The current standard used in many centers involves a right lateral minithoracotomy in the submammary fold, with access inside the chest through the fifth intercostal space [32]. The endoscopic camera is introduced via a stab incision in the right axillary line through the third intercostal space (Figures 10.3 and 10.4). The lung is deflated and the pericardium entered anterior to the phrenic nerve. The transthoracic aortic clamp is introduced via a stab incision in the right posterior axillary line through the third intercostal space. A special 35-cm-long steel cannula is used for cardioplegia and intro-

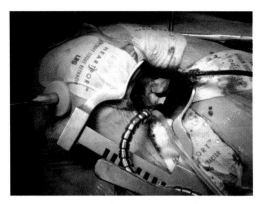

Figure 10.3 Lateral minithoracotomy access for minimally invasive mitral valve surgery. (Reproduced with permission from [32], copyright Elsevier (2006)).

duced before clamping the aorta. A left atrial vent is introduced via left atriotomy and used to enhance exposure of the mitral valve and decrease any distension of the left ventricle. This way, mitral valve surgery can be performed in a standard fashion with excellent exposure using a direct trans-incision view or the endoscopic view.

However, there are alternative approaches, as described by Detter et al. in their review on different techniques for minimally invasive mitral valve surgery [34]. As the endo-clamp (Port-Acces) technique discussed above has been now abandoned due to the increased risk for retrograde aortic dissection, other groups developed different techniques. Angoular and Mischer described a direct aortic clamping technique and direct cannulation of the vessel but they used an 8-cm-long anterolateral thora-

cotomy with direct aortic clamping and superior vena cava cannulation through the third intercostal space, thus avoiding groin cannulation [35].

Ngaage et al. [36] proposed a left atrial roof incision to expose the mitral valve. At the Cleveland Clinic, a partial sternotomy with direct cannulation is used [37]. Grossi and colleagues at New York University proposed a left posterior minithoracotomy. They published their data on 40 patients and concluded that the left posterior minithoracotomy approach can be safely used, especially in complicated reoperative mitral valve procedures [38]. Cohn and colleagues at Brigham and Women's Hospital used a lower ministernotomy with excellent results as well [39].

Although the right lateral minithoracotomy with femoral cannulation is currently the standard for minimally invasive mitral valve surgery, alternative techniques are available depending on surgeon's preference and patient's necessities, and all these approaches have proven to have excellent outcomes.

Use of telemanipulators in minimally invasive mitral valve surgery

The next step in the evolution of minimally invasive mitral valve surgery was introduction of telemanipulators (Figure 10.5). While Carpentier and

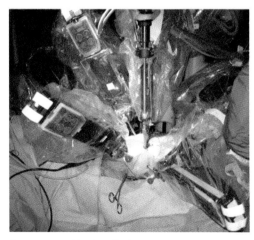

Figure 10.5 Positioning of robotic instrument arms and endoscope for totally endoscopic mitral valve repair. Starting clockwise from the transthoracic aortic cross-clamp are the left robotic arm, the endoscope inserted through a combined access/camera port, and the right robotic arm. (Reproduced with permission from [33], copyright Elsevier (2006).)

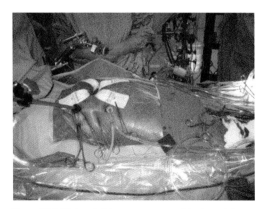

Figure 10.4 Right minithoracotomy—positioning of the surgical instruments and transthoracic aortic clamp. (Reproduced with permission from [33], copyright Elsevier (2006).)

Falk were the first to perform and publish their results with robotic surgery, Chitwood and colleagues have methodically adopted and developed the technique, and their reviews on telemanipulators are very optimistic [40–43]. Two other groups [32,44] published data on small series of patients (26 and 25 respectively), but despite these good outcomes, Walther et al. [32] seem to believe that a completely endoscopic approach, although very attractive, is less feasible. In their opinion the need for an annuloplasty device or even replacement dictates a small thoracotomy in most of the cases and a complete endoscopic approach while extremely tempting is probably not feasible in many cases.

The question that rises with the minimally invasive surgery in general is whether this approach is feasible to all types of repair or replacement. According to Walther et al. [32], whose opinion is shared by many surgeons, any type of repair can be performed using minimally invasive mitral valve surgery. In their experience, repair was successful in over 70% of more than 1000 patients who underwent minimally invasive mitral valve surgery at their center [32]. The minimally invasive approach had a significant success with MVR as well, with either mechanical valves or stented or stentless xenografts with papillary muscle reattachment [45,46].

Percutaneous repair

Trials are underway for percutaneous mitral valve repair, and animal models have already demonstrated that such an approach is feasible [47,48]. Appropriate candidates for percutaneous interventions should not have a severely dilated annulus and the mitral valve leaflets should be relatively normal [47]. Important questions will need to be addressed, such as relative efficacy compared to open repair and, if efficacy is less, how much less efficacy is acceptable compared to avoidance of surgery [47].

Results of the safety and midterm durability of a percutaneous mitral valve repair using the edge-to-edge technique were recently published in JACC. [49]. Results of EVEREST trial involving 107 patients with moderate-to-severe MR (3+ to 4+) followed for at least 12 months and up to more than 3 years are now available.

A clip device (Evalve) is delivered to the MV via percutaneous femoral venous transseptal access. The device grasps the mitral leaflet edges to create a double orifice with better leaflet coaptation. There are certain criteria that need to be fulfilled for percutaneous interventions: the flail leaflet segment width has to be less than 15 mm, the flail gap less than 10 mm, the coaptation depth less then 11 mm, and the coaptation length less than 2 mm. Also, the regurgitant jet had to originate from within the central two-thirds of the line of leaflet coaptation. One hundred and seven patients underwent Evalve implantation attempt, 23 of them with functional MR (21%). Median age was 71, which is higher compared to the median age of 59 seen in MV surgical repair registries or 61 seen in surgical MVR registries. 96 patients (90%) had the Evalve implanted, 79 (74%) with immediate success. No clip embolization has occurred at any time point. Ten partial clip detachments occurred, only one after 30 days. There was only one death, not related to the the procedure though. Thirty two patients had mitral valve surgery (repair or replacement) after Evalve attempt and the clip proved not to interfere with the surgical success. Clinical symptoms were improved in 74% patients, implying a clinical benefit achieved along with MR reduction (at 12 months 66% of patients had MR <2+). These results are certainly promising and a randomized comparison of percutaneous repair with the MitraClip device to surgical repair or replacement is underway. Percutaneous MVR using a double-crowned valved stent is also under rapid developement.

Safety and efficacy of minimally invasive mitral valve surgery

Because minimally invasive mitral valve surgery is already an established technique at many centers, it is difficult to conduct at this point a prospective study looking at minimally invasive versus conventional mitral valve surgery. Despite the lack of prospective comparative studies there is a multitude of minimally invasive data published by different groups, many of them with large patient series over several years. Cohn et al. published their results on 353 patients receiving minimally invasive mitral valve surgery over a period of 5 years [50]. They found a shorter intensive care unit stay, shorter length of in-hospital stay, and thus lower costs with minimally invasive approach. They also found a lower incidence of postoperative atrial fibrillation, lower amount of blood transfusions, and lower posthospital rehabilitation requirements. They concluded that minimally invasive valve surgery is a safe approach, with mortality similar to that of conventional valve surgery. In 2002 Grossi and his group from New York University reported their 6-year experience with minimally invasive mitral valve surgery in 714 patients [51], with in-hospital mortality being 1.1 and 5.8% for isolated mitral valve repair and replacement, respectively. The follow-up echocardiography showed that almost 90% of the patients had none or only trace residual mitral valve insufficiency, and therefore they concluded that minimally invasive mitral valve surgery is reproducible with low perioperative morbidity and mortality and with late outcomes comparable with conventional surgery. Onnasch et al. [52] also reported their experience in 2002. Their series of 449 patients had a mean survival of 96.4% at a mean follow-up of 2 years, and thus they concluded that minimally invasive mitral valve surgery is safe and reliable and can possibly replace conventional sternotomy. In a later review on minimally invasive mitral valve surgery, Walther from the same group stated that their 2006 data on more than 1000 patients showed an 83% survival at 6.8-year follow-up and 93% of the patients had none or only trivial MR [32]. Cohn et al. [39] published their excellent outcomes again in 2003 and this time included their follow-up data. More than 90% of their patients were free from MR and reoperation at 5-year follow-up. Vanermen's group also reported in several papers [53–55] exceptional results with the minimally invasive technique and this is even more remarkable since his group is using a truly videoscopic approach almost without any rib retraction. Half of their patients were back at work in less than 4 weeks and 93% of them stated they would choose the same procedure again.

Overall, minimally invasive mitral valve surgery showed results similar to those of conventional surgery in the early postoperative stage as well as at follow-up. The positive aspects are higher patient's satisfaction, shorter intensive care unit and in-hospital stay, lower need for blood transfusion, and overall lower costs. Postoperative pain and quality of life were addressed in studies done by Walther's and Yamada's groups, who concluded that patient's satisfaction is higher with the minimally invasive approach [56,57].

There are certain circumstances where the minimally invasive approach was considered less feasible initially due to redo surgery, low EF, or different comorbidities.

Current data published by Burfeind et al. at Duke and Walther et al. in Germany demonstrate that minithoracotomy is a safe approach in patients who require a second cardiothoracic surgery [19,58]. Walther et al. also describe excellent results with minimally invasive mitral valve surgery in 79 patients with a dilated cardiomyopathy with low EF (21 ± 8%), half of whom had severe pulmonary hypertension [32]. This suggests that minimally invasive mitral valve surgery can be now safely used in almost any circumstances, no matter how complex the patient is.

Due to these technical improvements minimally invasive mitral valve surgery is currently performed routinely in many specialized centers with excellent results.

Conclusions

Minimally invasive mitral valve surgery has evolved within the last 15 years and is currently standard of care in many specialized centers. However, there is a learning curve that surgeons are expected to achieve when deciding to start using the minimally invasive approach. Although initially the limited access may seem difficult, the visualization of mitral valve is at least as good with lateral minithoracotomy as with the conventional sternotomy. Minimally invasive mitral valve surgery in experienced hands is now as safe as the conventional surgery, with the positive aspect that patient's satisfaction is higher given better cosmesis and quicker recovery. Last but not least, the costs can be kept lower when using a minimally invasive approach. With the future use of flexible annuloplasty devices, currently being clinically tested, minimally invasive procedures can be performed using a true endoscopic technique or telemanipulators.

Percutaneous approaches for mitral valve repair and replacement are certainly very interesting especially in heart failure population. Recent published data on safety and midterm durability of percutaneous mitral repair with the MitraClip system looks promising, and randomized trials comparing the MitralValve device to surgical valve repair or replacement are underway.

In summary, mitral valve surgery has evolved from a standard sternotomy approach toward the minimally invasive approach. Both repair and replacement can be performed safe and with increased patient satisfaction and decreased hospital costs. This approach is expected to extend from specialized centers to other surgical centers once surgeons gain experience by training at specialized centers and will be of particular importance for patients with heart failure who are far less able to tolerate the rigors of a median sternotomy and routine valve replacement surgery.

Percutaneous MitraClip as well as self expended valved stents are certainly raising interest especially in heart failure population and further randomized trials are expected to answer concerns regarding safety and durability.

References

1. Otto CM. Evaluation and management of chronic mitral regurgitation. N Engl J Med 2001;345:740.
2. Bonow RO, Carabello BA, Chatterjeede K, et al. ACC/AHA Guidelines for the management of patients with valvular heart disease. A report of the American College of Cardiology/American Heart Association Task Force on Practice Guidelines (Writing Committee to Revise the 1998 Guidelines for the Management of Patients with Valvular Disease). J Am Coll Cardiol 2006;48:e1.
3. Gibbon JH Jr. Artificial maintenance of the circulation during experimental occlusion of the pulmonary artery. Arch Surg 1937;341107–1108.
4. Gibbon JH Jr. The application of a mechanical heart and lung apparatus to cardiac surgery. Minn Med 1954;37:176.
5. Gibbon JH Jr. The development of the heart–lung apparatus. Am J Surg May 1978;135(5):608–619.
6. Starr A, Edwards ML. Mitral replacement: late results with a ball valve prosthesis. J Cardiovasc Surg 1963;4:435–447.
7. Iung B, Gohlke-Barwolf C, Tornos P, et al. Recommendations on the management of the asymptomatic patient with valvular heart disease. Eur Heart J 2002;23:1253.
8. Edwards FH, Peterson ED, Coombs LP, et al. Prediction of operative mortality after valve replacement surgery. J Am Coll Cardiol 2001;37:885.
9. Doty DB, editor. Cardiac Surgery: Operative Technique. St. Louis: Mosby-Year Book; 1997:259.
10. Krayenbuehl HP. Surgery for mitral regurgitation: repair versus valve replacement. Eur Heart J 1986;7:638.
11. Enriquez-Sarano M, Schaff HV, Orszulak TA, Tajik AJ, Bailey KR, Frye RL. Valve repair improves the outcome of surgery for mitral valve regurgitation: a multivariate analysis. Circulation 1995;91(4):1022–1028.
12. Lee EM, Shapiro LM, Wells FC. Superiority of mitral valve repair in surgery for degenerative mitral regurgitation. Eur Heart J 1997;18(4):655–663.
13. Moss RR, Humphries KH, Gao M, et al. Outcomes if mitral valve repair or replacement: a comparison by propensity score analysis. Circulation 2003;108(Suppl 1):II90–II97.
14. Rozich JD, Carabello BA, Usher BW, Kratz JM, Bell AE, Zile MR. Mitral valve replacement with and without chordal preservation in patients with chronic mitral regurgitation. Circulation 1992;86(6):1718–1726.
15. Goldman ME, Mora F, Guarino T, Fuster V, Mindich BP. Mitral valvuloplasty is superior to valve replacement for preservation of left ventricular function: an intraoperative two-dimensional echocardiographic study. J Am Coll Cardiol 1987;10(3):568–575.
16. Society of Thoracic Surgeons National Database Committee. STS National Database Spring 2003 Executive Summary—Contents. 2003. Available at: http://www.ctsnet.org/file/STSNationalDatabaseSpring2003ExecutiveSummary.pdf.
17. Savage EB, Ferguson BT Jr, DiSesa VJ. Use of mitral valve repair: analysis of contemporary United States experience reported to the Society of Thoracic Surgeons National Cardiac Database. Ann Thorac Surg 2003;75820–825.
18. Grossi EA, LaPietra A, Ribakove GH, et al. Minimally invasive versus sternotomy approaches for mitral reconstruction: comparison of intermediate-term results. J Thorac Cardiovasc Surg 2001;121:708–713.
19. Onnasch JF, Schneider F, Falk V, et al. Minimally invasive approach for redo mitral valve surgery: a true benefit for the patient. J Card Surg 2002;17:14–19.
20. Arom KV, Emery RW. Minimally invasive mitral operations. Ann Thorac Surg 1997;63:1219–1220.
21. Navia JL, Cosgrove DM. Minimally invasive mitral valve operations. Ann Thorac Surg 1996;62:1542–1544.
22. Pompili MF, Stevens JH, Burdon TA, et al. Port-Access mitral valve replacement in dogs. J Thorac Cardiovasc Surg 1996;112:1268–1274.
23. Fann JI, Pompili MF, Stevens JH, et al. Port-Access cardiac operations with cardioplegic arrest. Ann Thorac Surg 1997;63(Suppl 6):S35–S39.
24. Fann JL, Pompili MF, Burdon TA, et al. Minimally invasive mitral valve surgery. Semin Thorac Cardiovasc Surg 1997;9:320–330.
25. Mohr FW, Falk V, Diegeler A, et al. Minimally invasive Port-Access mitral valve surgery. J Thorac Cardiovasc Surg 1998;115:567–574.
26. Cosgrove DM, Sabik JF. Minimally invasive ap-

proach for aortic valve operations. Ann Thorac Surg 1996;62:596–597.

27. Spencer FC, Galloway AC, Grossi EA, *et al.* Recent developments and evolving techniques of mitral valve reconstruction. Ann Thorac Surg 1998;65:307–313.

28. Chitwood WR, Elbeery JR, Moran JM. Minimally invasive mitral valve repair: using a minithoracotomy and transthoracic aortic occlusion. Ann Thorac Surg 1997;63:1477–1479.

29. Chitwood WR, Elbeery JR, Chapman WH, *et al.* Video-assisted minimally invasive mitral valve surgery: the "micro-mitral" operation. J Thorac Cardiovasc Surg 1997;113:413–414.

30. Carpentier A, Loulmet D, Carpentier A, *et al.* Chirurgie a Coeur overt par video-chirurgie at mini-thorocatomie, premier cas (valvulaplastie mitrale) opera avec success. CR Acad Sci III 1996;319:219–223.

31. Falk V, Walther T, Autschbach R, *et al.* Robot-assisted minimally invasive solo mitral valve operation. J Thorac Cardiovasc Surg 1998;115:470–471.

32. Walther T, Falk V, Mohr FW. Minimally invasive surgery for valve disease. Curr Probl Cardiol 2006;31(6):399–437.

33. Woo YJ, Rodriguez E, Atluri P, *et al.* Minimally invasive, robotic and off-pump mitral valve surgery. Thorac Cardiovasc Surg 2006;18(2):139–147.

34. Detter C, Boehm DH, Reichenspurner H. Minimally invasive valve surgery: different techniques and approaches. Expert Rev Cardiovasc Ther 2004;2:239–251.

35. Angoular DC, Mischer RE. An alternative surgical approach to facilitate minimally invasive mitral valve surgery. Ann Thorac Surg 2002;73:673–674.

36. Ngaage DL, Nair UR. The left atrial roof incision: an asset for minimally invasive mitral valve surgery. Heart Surg Forum 2002;5(Suppl 4):S421–S430.

37. Gilinov AM, Banbury MK, Cosgrove DM. Hemisternotomy approach for aortic and mitral valve surgery. J Card Surg 2000;15:15–20.

38. Saunders PC, Grossi EA, Sharony R, *et al.* Minimally invasive technology for mitral valve left thoracotomy: experience in forty cases. J Thorac Cardiovasc Surg 2004;12:58–63.

39. Greelish JP, Cohn LH, Leacche M, *et al.* Minimally invasive mitral valve repair suggests earlier operations for mitral valve disease. J Thorac Cardiovasc Surg 2003;126:365–371.

40. Felger JE, Nifong LW, Chitwood WR Jr. The evolution of and early experience with robot-assisted mitral valve surgery. Surg Laparosc Endosc Percutan Rech 2002;12:58–63.

41. Kypson AV, Nifong LW, Chitwood WR Jr. Robotic mitral valve surgery. Semin Thorac Cardiovasc Surg 2003;15:121–129.

42. Kypson AV, Nifong IW, Chitwood WR Jr. Robotic

mitral valve surgery. Surg Clin North Am 2003;83: 1387–1403.

43. Kypson AP, Felger JE, Nifong LW, *et al.* Robotics in valvular surgery: 2003 and beyond. Curr Opin Cardiol 2004;19:128–133.

44. Tatooles AP, Pappas PS, Gordon PJ, *et al.* Minimally invasive mitral valve repair using the da Vinci robotic system. Ann Thorac Surg 2004;77:1978–1984.

45. Walther T, Walther C, Falk V, *et al.* Early clinical results after stentless mitral valve implantation and comparison to conventional valve repair or replacement. Circulation 1999;100(Suppl II):78–83.

46. Walther T, Walther C, Falk V, *et al.* Midterm clinical results after stentless mitral valve replacement. Circulation 2003;108(Suppl II):85–89.

47. Block PC. Percutaneous mitral valve repair: are they changing the guard? Circulation 2005;111:2154.

48. Daimon M, Shiota T, Gillinov Am, *et al.* Percutaneous mitral valve repair for chronic ischemic mitral regurgitation: a real-time three-dimensional echocardiographic study in an ovine model. Circulation 2005;111(17):2183–2189.

49. Feldman T, Kar S, Rinaldi M, *et al.* Percutaneous Mitral Valve Repair with the MitraClip System. Safety and Midterm Durability in the Initial EVEREST (Endovascular Valve Edge-to-Edge Repair Study) Cohort. J Am Coll Cardiol 2009;54(8): 686–694.

50. Cohn LH. Minimally invasive valve surgery. J Card Surg 2001;16:260–265.

51. Grossi EA, Galloway AC, LaPietra A, *et al.* Minimally invasive mitral valve surgery: a 6-year experience in 714 patients. Ann Thorac Surg 2002;74:660–663.

52. Onnasch JF, Schneider F, Falk V, *et al.* Five years of less invasive mitral valve surgery: from experimental to routine approach. Heart Surg Forum 2002;5:132–135.

53. Schroeyers P, Wellens F, DeGeest R, *et al.* Minimally invasive video-assisted mitral valve repair: short and mid-term results. J Heart Valve Dis 2001;10:579–583.

54. Schroeyers P, Wellens F, DeGeest R, *et al.* Minimally invasive video-assisted mitral valve surgery: our lessons after a 4-year experience. Ann Thorac Surg 2001;72:S1050–S1054.

55. Casselman FP, VanSlycke S, Wellens F, *et al.* Mitral valve surgery can now routinely be performed endoscopically. Circulation 2003;108(Suppl II):II-48–II-54.

56. Walther T, Falk V, Metz S, *et al.* Pin and quality of life after minimally invasive versus conventional cardiac surgery. Ann Thorac Surg 1999;67:1643–1647.

57. Yamada T, Ochiai R, Takeda J, *et al.* Comparison of early postoperative quality of life in minimally invasive versus conventional valve surgery. J Anesth 2003;17:171–176.

58. Burfeind WR, Glower DD, David RD, *et al.* Mitral valve surgery after prior cardiac operation: Port-Access versus sternotomy or thoracotomy. Ann Thorac Surg 2002;74:S1323–S1325.

CHAPTER 11

Percutaneous Mechanical Assist Devices

Suresh Mulukutla[1], Lawrence Schneider[2], & Howard A. Cohen[2]

[1]University of Pittsburgh Medical Center, Pittsburgh, PA, USA
[2]Lenox Hill Heart and Vascular Institute, New York, NY, USA

Introduction

It is now more than a half-century since the concept of "diastolic augmentation" was first introduced [1] and four decades since the use of the intra-aortic balloon pump or IABP [2] in the setting of cardiogenic shock and acute myocardial infarction (MI) was first reported. Although first conceived of and inserted surgically by the cardiovascular surgeons, once the IABP could be inserted percutaneously, it became widely adopted by the "invasive" and subsequently by the "interventional" cardiologist. Today, the IABP is the most widely employed mechanical cardiac "assist" device now used in a wide variety of clinical scenarios, including cardiogenic shock, unstable acute coronary syndromes such as MI, acute and chronic congestive heart failure (CHF) of multiples etiologies, high-risk percutaneous coronary intervention (PCI), and as a prelude to high-risk open heart surgery. Furthermore, studies have demonstrated that the aggressive use of the IABP in selected patient is cost-effective due to decreased lengths of stay and reduction of complications [3].

Since the introduction of the IABP, other percutaneous assist devices have come and gone, including the cardiopulmonary support system or CPS and the Hemopump™. Although CPS was instrumental in saving some lives, the difficulties with insertion and the complications associated with its use resulted in the abandonment of this method of mechanical support. Similarly, the Hemopump™ proved to be a clinically effective assist device for some patients, but the vascular complications and the significant incidence of hemolysis associated with its use led again to its abandonment as a left ventricular (LV) support device. The concept, however, persisted and subsequently led to the development of the Impella 2.5™ device that recently received Food and Drug Administration (FDA) approval. The Impella 2.5™ device is now being investigated in the United States in randomized clinical trials versus the IABP. The larger Impella 5.0™ device provides increased level of support but must be surgically placed due to its large size. The TandemHeart® is a percutaneous left ventricular assist device (LVAD) that first received FDA approval in 2003, although the concept for the device had been in place for more than four decades [4]. As of January 2009, the TandemHeart® has been used in more than 1500 cases worldwide, with approximately one-third of the cases done in the setting of cardiogenic shock, one-third in high-risk PCI, and one-third in high-risk surgery (data on file at CardiacAssist, Incorporated, Pittsburgh, PA, USA).

The IABP, the TandemHeart®, and the Impella 2.5™ are the three percutaneous devices that are currently clinically available in the United States and will be further discussed in detail in the remainder of this chapter. The Cancion® device is a novel device that will also be reviewed, although it is not truly an LVAD but may have a role in

Heart Failure: Device Management. Edited by Arthur Feldman.
© 2010 Blackwell Publishing.

treating patients with CHF. Prior to discussing the specifics of each device, a brief discussion of what we would consider to be the "ideal" percutaneous LVAD would be worthwhile. The very first consideration, of course, should be the safety and efficacy of the device. To achieve wide acceptance, any device will have to achieve a high degree of safety first and hopefully a high degree of efficacy second. Any device that lacks safety is doomed to failure. A device that is very safe but lacks a high degree of efficacy may achieve some acceptance as long as the complication rate remains low. The efficacy of these devices may be judged by the level of support they provide. Hemodynamically, the efficacy can be simply assessed using parameters such as cardiac output, cardiac power, and LV filling pressure. More sophisticated assessments have been employed as well using LV pressure–volume loops, for example. Clinically, the efficacy can be judged by short- and long-term outcomes. Improved survival is hard to prove, given the difficulty in enrolling cardiogenic shock patients in randomized clinical trials as demonstrated in the landmark SHOCK (SHould we emergently revascularize Occluded coronaries for Cardiogenic shocK) trial [5]. The CPS system is an example of a device that was highly effective in the very short term, but not very safe and thus abandoned. The major complications of *implantable* LVADs have been well documented and include infection, thromboembolism, bleeding, device failure, and hemolysis, which occur with a disturbing frequency in end-stage heart failure patients [6]. To achieve a high degree of safety, these complications need to be obviously avoided in the percutaneously inserted devices as well. The percutaneously inserted devices have the additional potential complication of peripheral vascular compromise. This is particularly important, as these devices are comparatively large and are being used in patients prone to have significant peripheral vascular disease.

In addition to safety and efficacy issues, the ease of insertion, cost, and availability all need to be addressed as well. A device that is comparatively safe and effective but too difficult to insert may not achieve widespread acceptance. Similarly, a device that proved to be very safe, effective, and easy to insert but was too costly would also have difficulty achieving widespread acceptance, particularly in the current environment of cost constraints.

Finally, the availability of a device remains important as well, although this criterion tends to be a function of safety, efficacy, cost considerations, and ultimately FDA approval. None of the devices discussed are "ideal" and each has advantages and disadvantages with regard to these issues. The reader should keep this in mind during the ensuing description and discussion of the various devices.

Intra-aortic balloon pump

Origins of the IABP—a historical overview

In 1953, the Kantrowitz brothers introduced the concept of diastolic augmentation [1]. This was followed by the seminal work of Birtwell, Claus, and Harken at Harvard University where they studied the concept of counterpulsation [7,8]. These two components led to the understanding of how to affect blood flow in increasing diastolic coronary flow while also decreasing afterload. These critical foundations ultimately led Kantrowitz's group to the first clinical use of the IABP in patients with cardiogenic shock in 1968 [2]. A new age of circulatory support was born. Early experience with the IABP showed physiological benefits, with an improvement in cardiac function and diastolic blood pressure and a reduction in systemic acidosis [9].

The initial IABP catheter size was a 15-French (F) gauge and required surgical insertion and removal. Because of these limitations, in the early years of the IABP, it was a device largely limited to the surgical community. The earliest studies, therefore, were largely performed in postoperative patients, such as those who required surgical revascularization or those who could not be weaned off of cardiopulmonary bypass [10]. In 1979, Datascope Corporation introduced the first percutaneous IABP, and with continued technological advances, several changes ensued. The indications and applications for the IABP expanded broadly, and it became a mainstay in the cardiac catheterization laboratory. Since the introduction of the percutaneous IABP and the improved safety of these devices, the number of IABPs placed in the catheterization laboratory has increased steadily while those placed in the surgical intensive care units has declined.

Hemodynamic and physiologic efficacy of the IABP

Many hemodynamic parameters are affected by IABP counterpulsation and diastolic augmentation. The key physiological principles involve a rapid decrease in intra-aortic pressure in synchrony with LV ejection followed by a rapid increase in aortic pressure during isovolumic relaxation. The reduction in intra-aortic pressure during systole results in afterload reduction, while the diastolic increase in aortic pressure with balloon inflation improves diastolic coronary flow. Balloon pump deflation translates into decreased afterload, increased stroke volume, decreased end-diastolic volume, and decreased myocardial consumption while IABP inflation results in increased coronary flow and oxygen supply, improved cardiac output, decreased end-diastolic volume, and decreased end-diastolic pressure, which again results in decreased myocardial consumption.

Several studies have reported on the degree of hemodynamic benefit of the IABP. Cardiac output in some studies is increased by as much as 50%, though other studies show much more modest improvements [11–13]. Myocardial oxygen consumption is reduced with IABP use [14,15]. Myocardial tension time index, a measure of LV workload, is reduced with counterpulsation by 20–40% [15,16]. From a physiologic standpoint, the IABP also has a number of beneficial effects. Coronary and cerebral blood flow may increase by as much as 15%, though this is controversial [17–19].

Despite the hemodynamic and physiological benefits of the IABP, the ejection fraction has not been shown to increase with its use. Moreover, whether these benefits translate into improved clinical outcomes has been a subject of intense research. Unfortunately, as will be discussed, for many conditions the IABP has not been shown to substantially improve outcomes when used independently.

IABP indications—cardiogenic shock

Cardiogenic shock, secondary to acute MI, remains the most common indication for IABP use. Since 1990, the American College of Cardiology/American Heart Association Task Force has suggested that cardiogenic shock is a class I indication for IABP [20]. However, these initial recommendations seem to have been made predominantly because of the hemodynamic and phys-

iological benefits of the IABP, rather than upon clinical information from observational or randomized data that show a benefit. Cardiogenic shock is the leading cause of death among patients hospitalized for acute MI. Two randomized controlled trials in the pre-reperfusion era failed to show any benefit of the IABP in patients presenting with acute MI and shock [21,22]; nonetheless, the device gained widespread acceptance based upon physiological principles. In the reperfusion era with thrombolytic therapy, several observational studies suggested a modest but significant clinical benefit of IABP use in decreasing mortality [23,24]. However, the benefit of IABP use may largely be limited to those individuals who also underwent revascularization. In fact, in the GUSTO (Global Utilization of Streptokinase and Tissue plasminogen activator for Occluded coronary arteries) study, after adjustment for cardiac catheterization status and revascularization, there was no significant relationship between IABP use and mortality [25]. A recent meta-analysis of several studies evaluating the impact of IABP use in cardiogenic shock failed to show any significant difference between those patients treated with an IABP and those who were not [26].

Still, given the poor survival rates in this sick and often unstable patient population, IABP is still considered a class I recommendation, and there is still clear evidence that the hemodynamic parameters do improve with IABP use. Moreover, the relative ease of the placement of the IABP and its relative safety as compared to other devices have enhanced its utility. It has become an essential therapy in patients who suffer from mechanical complications of acute MI, including acute mitral regurgitation and rupture of the ventricular septum [27,28]. In these particular scenarios, the use of an IABP may provide substantial acute benefit and studies show a 30% improvement in cardiac output and cerebral blood flow [27].

IABP indications—postoperative low cardiac output syndrome

One of the most effective uses of the IABP is in the setting of those who require support due to postcardiotomy low cardiac output syndrome. Kantrowitz's group initially suggested this as a major indication for the IABP in their 1968 article [2]. Buckley was the first to clinically validate the use of the IABP for this clinical entity [10,29]. Postcardiotomy low cardiac output syndrome is a multifactorial process resulting from inadequate myocardial protection during the perioperative period. Without IABP support, mortality is as high as 90%; however, with support, survival may dramatically improve to 40–70% [30–33]. Still, approximately 1% of cardiac surgical patients cannot be weaned from bypass in spite of inotropic and IABP support [33], and in these patients other support devices may be required to provide a bridge to recovery, assist device, or transplantation.

IABP indications—refractory heart failure and cardiac transplantation

The role of IABP therapy in patients with CHF but without cardiogenic shock is controversial. Hagemeijer studied class III–IV heart failure patients after a recent MI and reported significant hemodynamic improvement in 80% of patients with 56% hospital survival [34], but more recent studies suggest that the survival rates in this population may be poorer and that IABP use may not alter long-term therapy [35]. Currently, IABP therapy is used only as an adjunctive therapy in those with refractory heart failure and as a bridge to a more definitive therapy.

Cardiac transplantation is becoming a widely accepted and utilized approach to treating those with severe, chronic heart failure. In the earlier era of transplantation, IABP was used widely as a bridge to cardiac transplantation [36–38]. However, in the current era, given the advancements with ventricular assist devices, the use of IABP is limited in this patient population.

IABP indications—high-risk cardiac procedures

Patients undergoing high-risk cardiac procedures may benefit from preoperative insertion of an IABP. High-risk characteristics include decreased LV function, severe coronary artery disease, and hemodynamic compromise. A retrospective analysis from Christenson determined that factors associated with increased mortality and need for placement of IABP include preoperative unstable angina, redo-coronary artery bypass grafting, LV ejection fraction < 40%, diffuse coronary artery disease, and left main coronary stenosis [39]. These criteria

are also often utilized to determine individuals who may benefit from support prior to high-risk percutaneous coronary interventions, though data to support this is lacking. There appears to be no consensus upon how long to treat patients with intra-aortic counterpulsation. Given the advent of drug-eluting stents, higher risk percutaneous coronary interventions are being performed. This has been largely driven by the recent evidence of increased efficacy and safety of these stents in patients with complex coronary artery disease, including diabetic patients and those treated for off-label indications [40,41].

IABP-related complications

While there has been wide variation in the reported complication rate associated with the IABP, the most recent studies suggest a rate of about 15% [42,43]. Major complications occur with an incidence of 5–15%, while minor complications occur in 30% of cases [42,43]. Vascular complications constitute the majority of IABP-related complications, ranging from mild ischemia of the lower extremity to arterial thrombosis and limb loss. Therefore, whenever possible, it is paramount that patients in whom an IABP is placed are deemed suitable for this intervention from a vascular standpoint. This is even more critical with other support devices given their larger size. Imaging of the distal aorta, iliac, and femoral vessels with angiography, computed tomography, or magnetic resonance imaging are all options. As this is often not possible in many patients receiving an IABP, it is then imperative to perform frequent vascular evaluations while patients remain on IABP therapy. Risk factors that may predispose patients to IABP-related complications include peripheral vascular disease, female sex, and diabetes [42–45]. In a prospective study of over 1100 patients on IABPs, Cohen found that a history of peripheral vascular disease increases the risk of vascular complications by four times [42]. Female gender is associated with a twofold risk for vascular complications [42]. Diabetes is also an important independent risk factor for vascular complications [42,46]. Other factors that predispose to vascular complications are method of insertion, larger catheter size, longer duration of support, advanced age, hemodynamic instability, and emergent IABP insertion [47–49]. Still, the IABP remains among the safest support devices, and the significant decrease in vascular complications over the last two decades can largely be explained by the use of catheters with smaller diameters and better patient selection in avoiding IABP placement in those with severe peripheral vascular disease.

Vascular complications associated with IABP therapy carry a high morbidity and mortality. These complications include arterial thrombosis and occlusion, compartment syndrome, arterial dissection, hematoma, and retroperitoneal bleeding. As many as 25% of patients who experience vascular complications may require surgical intervention, and the mortality from ischemic vascular complications is as high as 60% [50]. Surgical interventions that may be required include thromboembolectomy, profundaplasties, infrainguinal bypasses, fasciotomies, and amputations.

Major bleeding occurs in about 5% of IABP patients [42,51]. Infectious complications, occurring in 10–20% of patients, also contribute significantly to morbidity and mortality. This occurs most frequently when the IABP is used for longer durations or is placed in environments that are less sterile, such as in the cardiac or surgical intensive care units [42–44,52].

While the overall complication rate appears to be declining due to increased experience and improved technology, a high degree of awareness and a careful approach to IABP use is required to help avoid some of the devastating complications associated with this and other mechanical assist devices.

Contraindications to IABP utilization

The major contraindications to IABP are aortic insufficiency and aortic dissection. Peripheral vascular disease is a relative contraindication to IABP placement, but as reviewed earlier, great care is required when placing mechanical devices in patients with peripheral arterial disease.

Percutaneous transseptal left ventricular assist

The TandemHeart®, manufactured by CardiacAssist in Pittsburgh, PA, USA, first obtained FDA approval in 2003. The device allows for partial left heart bypass consists of three main components: a centrifugal continuous flow pump, a microprocessor-based controller, and a 21-F transseptal cannula (Figure 11.1). The pump is a compact, lightweight device that is designed for

TandemHeart PVAD system components

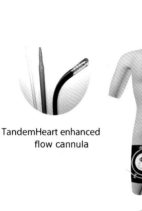

TandemHeart enhanced
flow cannula

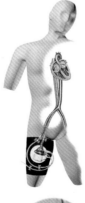

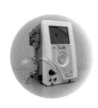

TandemHeart Escort™
controller

TandemHeart pump

Figure 11.1 A drawing demonstrating the extracorporeal placement of the TandemHeart® pump. Also pictured are the 21-F wire wound cannula, obturator and dilator, the controller and the pump. PVAD, percutaneous left ventricular assist device.

paracorporeal placement. It requires only 60 cc of saline to prime the system. Depending on the size of the arterial cannula used, the pump can provide up to 5 L of flow/min. There is a single moving part, the impellar, which is electromagnetically driven and suspended on a novel lubricating and cooling system of heparinized normal saline. The controller is a small microprocessor-based unit that has touch screen display and "instructions for use" built into the system. The pump flow is controlled by a single rheostat that dials up or down the rpm's of the impellar and thus controls the flow. The flow is measured by the controller that is a close approximation of the actual flow, and the flow can be directly measured by an external flow probe placed on the arterial cannula and connected to the controller for digital readout.

The pump withdraws blood from the left atrium that is accessed by standard transseptal technique. Once the left atrium is entered, an Inoue transseptal stainless wire is inserted and coiled in the body of the left atrium (Figure 11.2). A tapered, 14–21-F graduated progressive dilator is then inserted over the wire to dilate the intra-atrial septum. The dilator is then withdrawn and the 21-F transseptal wire-

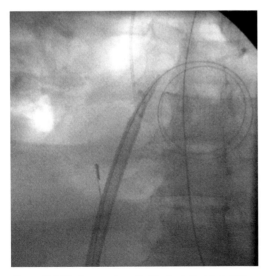

Figure 11.2 The Inoue wire coiled in the left atrium. The graduated 14–21-F dilator is being advanced across the intra-atrial septum. The pigtail catheter marks the level of the aortic valve. An intracardiac echo probe that was used to guide the transseptal puncture in a fully anticoagulated patient can also be seen in the right atrium.

wound cannula with 14 side holes and a large end hole is inserted into the left atrium, with the operator ensuring that all the side holes are in the left atrium in an effort to avoid right to left shunting once the pump is activated. The transseptal cannula has four tantalum markers at the end that allows for tracking of the tip of the catheter, which itself is not radiopaque. Once the transseptal cannula is well positioned and secured, the wire and dilator are withdrawn, making sure not to entrain air into the system. In this regard, volume loading of the patient is advisable, even if the starting pulmonary capillary wedge (PCW) and LA (left atrial) pressures are high, as the cannulae are large and volume loss can be a problem particularly early on in an operator's experience. Centimeter markers are noted at the groin insertion site, and every precaution must be taken to secure the cannula in order to be certain that it is not inadvertently advanced or withdrawn. The transseptal cannula is clamped with a large surgical line clamp as the femoral arterial line is being inserted. The femoral arterial cannula may vary in size from 12 to 17 F, depending on the size of the patient and the degree of peripheral arterial disease. In this regard, all patients should have an abdominal aortogram and runoff study in order to be certain that severe peripheral vascular disease does not preclude insertion of the device. Furthermore, the side for the arterial cannula that is most favorable can be chosen depending on the degree of disease and tortuosity of iliofemoral vessels. The system is primed with saline in both cannulae, with care being taken to completely remove any air. Left heart bypass can then be initiated by removing the clamps and starting the pump. LV filling pressures (PCW) should be monitored with a right heart catheter to be certain that there is adequate volume. Typically, the PCW should be maintained in 18–20 mmHg range to allow for adequate filling and pump flow. In general, patients should be maintained on systemic anticoagulation with heparin and an ACT (activated clotting time) in the 200–250 second range. Patients in whom the TandemHeart® is being used postopen heart surgery cannot be anticoagulated until postoperative bleeding has stopped. Anticoagulation can then be instituted if LV assist is still required at that time.

When the use of the TandemHeart® is being terminated, anticoagulation is discontinued and hemostasis can be achieved with direct manual pressure. In patients with severe peripheral vascular disease, the cannulae may be removed via surgical cut down with local anesthesia. In patients in whom the device is to be used short-term as in high-risk PCI with anticipation of removal immediately post-procedure, the artery and vein can be "preclosed" with hemostasis achieved with suture closure. In patients in whom the device use is anticipated to be longer, the vessels should not be "preclosed" as this increases the risk of infection.

Thiele et al. first reported the use of percutaneous transseptal LV assist with the TandemHeart® in 18 consecutive patients with acute MI and cardiogenic shock [53]. Five of the 18 patients had ventricular septal rupture. The mean duration of support was 4 ± 3 days. Survival at 30 days was 56%. Not including the 5 patients with acute MI complicated by ventricular septal defect, 10 of 13 patients (77%) survived. This is a small study but the findings are suggestive of an important role that the TandemHeart® could play in patients with cardiogenic shock secondary to acute MI. This study also documented significant increase in cardiac output (3.5 to 4.8 L/min), increase in mean arterial pressure (63 to 80 mmHg), and significant decrease in PCW (21 to 14 mmHg). In addition, serum lactate fell significantly (4.7–3.0 μm/mL). Percutaneous transseptal LV assist with the TandemHeart® was therefore successful in reversing the hemodynamic and metabolic abnormalities in this series of patients with acute MI and cardiogenic shock. The same investigators in a subsequent paper comparing the TandemHeart® to the IABP in a randomized clinical trial of patients with acute MI and cardiogenic shock [54] concluded that the ventricular assist device was more effective than the IABP in reversing the hemodynamic and metabolic parameters of cardiogenic shock. The use of the ventricular assist device and extracorporeal support, however, was associated with more complications. Several issues regarding this study are worth mentioning. There was a high percentage of patients in both groups having received thrombolytic therapy as well as glycoprotein IIb/IIIa receptors antagonists. Furthermore, although patients with severe peripheral vascular disease were excluded, no screening aortogram with runoff was performed prior to insertion of the devices. Although this was a randomized trial, patients in the ventricular assist device group by definition had much larger cannulae utilized and would be expected to have higher complication rates (bleeding and peripheral ischemia) if the patients were not appropriately selected (excluded from) for the trial in the first place. The study was not powered to detect a difference in survival.

In a subsequent paper, Burkoff and associates reported on a randomized, multicenter clinical trial of the TandemHeart® versus the IABP in patients with cardiogenic shock [55]. The LVAD was significantly more effective in increasing cardiac index and mean arterial pressure and in decreasing PCW pressures compared to the IABP. There was no difference in the 30-day mortality, but the trial was not powered to detect a difference in mortality. These investigators concluded that in patients presenting within 24 hours of the development of CGS, the TandemHeart significantly improves hemodynamic parameters, even in patients failing IABP, but that larger scale trials are required to assess the influence of improved hemodynamics on survival.

The group at the Texas Heart Institute has had the largest experience with the TandemHeart® and have reported on its use as a bridge to transplant [56], as a bridge to an implantable LVAD (bridge to bridge) [57], as treatment for post-pericardiotomy CHF unresponsive to IABP [58], and as a bridge to recovery in patients with therapy-resistant acute fulminant myocarditis [59]. Others have reported application of the TandemHeart® in the pediatric population [60].

Additional potential applications of the Tandem-Heart® include its use in high-risk PCI [13], high-risk cardiac surgical procedures [61], large non-shock acute MI in an effort to reduce infarct size (trial design on file with CardiacAssist, Pittsburgh, PA, USA), hemodynamically unstable ventricular tachycardia ablation [62], aortic valvuloplasty and percutaneous aortic valve replacement [63,64], and in right ventricular dysfunction as an RVAD in acute MI and in perioperative patients [65]. These are all "off-label" uses of the device and its potential safety and efficacy in these various scenarios remain to be determined.

Potential complications of TandemHeart® insertion include distal limb ischemia, bleeding, and anemia requiring blood transfusion, tamponade due to perforation at the time of transseptal puncture, thromboembolism, air embolism at the time of insertion of the large transseptal cannula, and infection. In general, complications can be avoided by meticulous technique and attention to details at the time of insertion and appropriate screening tests to be certain that the patient is a candidate for the device. Patients with severe peripheral vascular disease, for example, should not receive the device unless provision is made for peripheral perfusion. This can be accomplished by stenting proximally and/or placing a perfusion cannula distally to provide antegrade flow to the lower extremity. Bleeding can be avoided by carefully monitoring the activated clotting time on a regular basis and avoiding excessive anticoagulation. Tamponade can be avoided by meticulous transseptal technique. Only operators who are skilled and experienced with the transseptal technique should insert this device. In patients in whom there is anticipation of prolonged support, prophylactic antibiotics should be administered to avoid infection. Furthermore, these patients should not have the arteriotomy "preclosed" as this markedly increases the risk of infection.

Exclusion criteria for device insertion include antecedent thrombolytic therapy with persistent abnormalities of coagulation. Similarly, patients with known coagulopathy or known thrombophilia should be avoided. As with the IABP, patients with severe aortic regurgitation should be avoided. Patients with septic shock or severe systemic infection should not be subjected to a TandemHeart®. Those patients with severe left and right ventricular dysfunction will not benefit from the TandemHeart® on the left side alone. Clearly, any patient with a "bleeding problem" or who cannot receive systemic anticoagulation should not receive the device. Patients who cannot receive heparin due to allergy can receive alternative antithrombin treatment.

Impella

The latest percutaneous assist device that is available and currently being investigated is the Impella 2.5™ manufactured by Abiomed (Danvers, MA, USA). The device received 510(k) approval from the FDA in 2008. The device consists of a catheter-mounted miniature axial flow pump that is inserted through a 12-F sheath over a guidewire and placed retrograde across the aortic valve (Figure 11.3). The pump rotates as 32,000 rpm and can achieve an output of approximately 2.5 L/min, with blood withdrawn from the left ventricle through a caged inlet

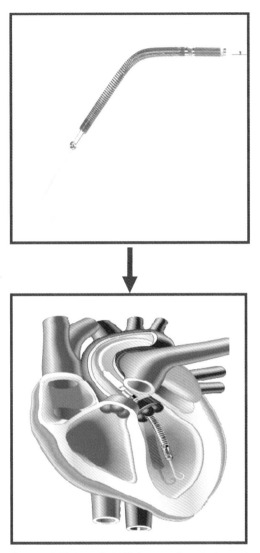

Figure 11.3 The Impella 2.5™ (top panel) can be inserted into the left ventricle via a standard guidewire through the femoral artery, into the ascending aorta, across the valve and into the left ventricle. The tip of the catheter contains a "pigtail" that crosses the patient's heart valve and rests in the left ventricle (bottom panel), generating flows of up to 2.5 L/min.

and expelled into the ascending aorta. The axial flow pump is connected to a small control device that is maintained at the bedside.

During use of the Impella device, anticoagulation should be utilized with an ACT of about 250. After discontinuation of anticoagulation, the device can be removed with hemostasis achieved with manual pressure. As with the TandemHeart®, the artery may be "preclosed" with hemostasis achieved with suture closure. However, again, if the device is to be left in place for more than a day, preclosure is not recommended given the infection risk.

Animal and human studies have documented that during severe acute LV failure, the Impella pump is capable of more effective cardiac unloading and circulatory support than IABP based upon hemodynamic and physiologic measures [66]. From a hemodynamic perspective, this device results in effect LV unloading, resulting in LV end-diastolic pressure and volume reduction and improvement in cardiac output. The Impella device has been utilized across a broad variety of indications. Although most of the studies are relatively small to date, they are promising. Siegenthaler et al. studied the use of the Impella 5.0 device among patients with postcardiotomy failure and described improved survival with the Impella device compared with the IABP [67]. It has been successfully used to help with ventricular unloading in patients with cardiorespiratory failure and in those undergoing mitral valve surgery [68]. Notably, animal data using the Impella device suggest that the device may help to limit infarct size if used at the time of reperfusion therapy (Figure 11.4) [69].

Seyfarth et al. recently reported a randomized two-center clinical trial to assess the safety and efficacy of the Impella 2.5™ compared to the IABP in 25 patients with cardiogenic shock due to acute MI [70]. The primary endpoint of the trial was the cardiac power index at 30 minutes postinsertion of the device and was significantly higher in the Impella 2.5™ group than the IABP, although the differences were no different at 4 and 30 hours. There was a trend but no significant difference in mean arterial pressure and no difference in PCW pressure measured. Serum lactate levels were lower and plasma hemoglobin levels (as a measure of hemolysis) were higher in the Impella 2.5™ group. There was no difference in survival, but the trial was obviously not powered to detect a difference.

Recent studies have reported on the safety and efficacy of the Impella device in high-risk PCI, characterized by poor LV function and high-risk coronary artery disease [71,72]. In the PROTECT (Prophylaxis of Thromboembolism in Critical Care) I trial [72], the device was utilized in 20 patients for a mean of 1.7 ± 0.6 hours. Procedural success using the device was achieved in all patients. Mean

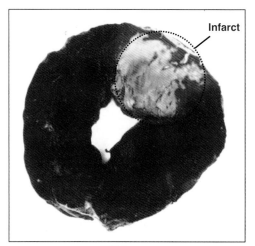

Without Impella support

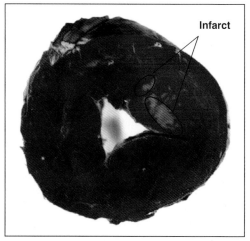

With Impella support

Figure 11.4 The picture on the left shows an area of myocardial necrosis in an animal model when infarction and reperfusion was performed without Impella support. The picture on the right shows a smaller infarct when the infarction was created during support with the Impella device [69].

pump flow was 2.2 ± 0.3 L/min. None of the patients developed hemodynamic compromise during coronary intervention. There was no impact upon the aortic valve with the use of the Impella system nor were there any significant arrhythmias while the device was being used. Mild hemolysis was observed in 2 patients but without clinical sequelae. Overall, the Impella 2.5™ system was regarded to be safe and to provide effective hemodynamic support.

The PROTECT II trial currently recruiting in the United States is a multicenter prospective randomized control trial comparing the Impella 2.5™ to the IABP in patients undergoing high-risk PCI, with the primary endpoint being 30% reduction in a combined endpoint of intra- and postprocedural major adverse clinical events in the Impella patients. The planned enrollment is 654 patients. The RECOVER II study has recently begun and aims to compare the Impella® Recover LP 2.5™ system to the IABP in patients with acute MI and hemodynamic instability/cardiogenic shock. The planned enrollment in RECOVER II is 384 patients. Overall, the indications for use of the Impella device may broaden significantly; the safety and efficacy of this device in these clinical scenarios, however, still require extensive research.

Cancion® system

The Cancion® system (Orqis Medical Corporation, Lake Forest, CA, USA) is an extracorporeal pump that utilizes the concept of continuous aortic flow augmentation (CAFA) in patients with chronic CHF and chronic CHF with acute decompensation. The system is quite simple and consists of a miniature extracorporeal pump that augments aortic flow continuously throughout the cardiac cycle and inflow and outflow cannulae. The pump, driven by an electromagnetic motor, withdraws blood from the iliac artery via the 15-cm-long 12-F inflow cannula and returns the blood to the contralateral iliac artery via a 60-cm-long 12-F cannula, with both cannulae inserted percutaneously. A controller regulates the flow through the system. The pump is designed to recirculate blood from the iliac artery on one side to the descending aorta in a nonpulsatile manner via a cannula placed via the contralateral femoral artery. There is no "gating" of

the cardiac cycle. Pump speeds of 2000–5400 rpm can achieve a flow rate of up to 1.1–1.5 L/min. The blood capacity of the system is approximately 100 cm^3. Hemolysis is described to be in the acceptable range, with plasma-free hemoglobin of <40 mg/dL on two consecutive measurements when the pump has been used up to 5 days [73]. Anticoagulation is required with the partial thromboplastin time maintained within a therapeutic range. In an initial study performed in 24 patients with CHF exacerbation resistant to medical therapy, Konstam et al. reported significant reductions in the PCW pressure and systemic vascular resistance as well as a significant increase in the cardiac index [73].

In a subsequent study, Greenberg et al. [74] reported a multicenter trial of CAFA versus medical therapy alone in 166 patients hospitalized with heart failure, reduced ejection fraction and cardiac index, elevated PCW pressure, and renal impairment or substantial diuretic requirement despite intravenous inotropes/vasodilators. The primary composite endpoint of the study included PCW pressure at 72 and 96 hours and days alive out of hospital off support beyond 35 days. Enrollment was discontinued early because of an inability to demonstrate a significant benefit in the primary composite endpoint ($p = 0.45$) in the face of excess device bleeding. There was a trend ($p = 0.074$) in an improvement in the PCW in the device group compared to the control group, but this did not reach significance. A significant improvement in the cardiac index was noted in the device group compared to the controls (2.05 ± 0.53 to 2.44 ± 0.52 L/min device group, $p < 0.0001$). Through 65 days, no significant differences were noted in all-cause mortality, death, or heart failure hospitalization. Major bleeds, however, were noted in 16.5% (7.3% treatment related) in the device group compared to 5.1% in the control group ($p = 0.05$). The authors concluded that in a group of exceptionally sick patients with chronic CHF that was inadequately responsive to medical therapy, CAFA resulted in short-term hemodynamic improvement. This did not translate, however, into long-term clinical benefit. Further recommendations included investigation in attempts to reduce bleeding and to better identify those patients that might benefit from this type of approach [74].

Summary

In summary, a new group of devices that can support cardiac function and that can be placed percutaneously have now arrived in the marketplace and can be added to the clinician's armamentarium for treating patients with severe and hemodynamically unstable LV dysfunction. These devices can serve as bridges to intervention, recovery, LVADs, or transplantation. Each has risks and rewards and each requires slightly different technological skills. How best to use each of these devices will hopefully be clarified by ongoing and planned clinical trials.

References

1. Kantrowitz A. Experimental augmentation of coronary flow by retardation of the arterial pressure pulse. Surgery 1953;34:678–687.

2. Kantrowitz A, Tjonneland S, Freed PS, et al. Initial clinical experience with intraaortic balloon pumping in cardiogenic shock. JAMA 1968;203:113–118.

3. Mehlhorn U, Kröner A, de Vivie ER, et al. 30 years clinical intra-aortic balloon pumping: facts and figures. Thorac Cardiovasc Surg 1999;47(Suppl 2):298–303.

4. Dennis C, Hall DP, Moreno JR, et al. Reduction of the oxygen utilization of the heart by left heart bypass. Circ Res 1962;10:298–305.

5. Hochman JS, Sleeper LA, Webb JG, et al. SHOCK (Should We Emergently Revascularize Occluded Coronaries for Cardiogenic Shock) Investigators. Early revascularization in acute myocardial infarction complicated by cardiogenic shock. N Engl J Med 1999;341:625–634.

6. Rose EA, Gelijns AC, Moskowitz AJ, et al. Long-term mechanical left ventricular assistance for end-stage heart failure. N Engl J Med 2001;345:1435–1443.

7. Harken DE. Counterpulsation: foundation and future, with tribute to William Clifford Birtwell (1916–1978). In: Unger F, editor. Assisted Circulation. New York: Springer-Verlag; 1979:20–23.

8. Claus RH, Birtwell WC, Albertal G, et al. Assisted circulation. I: The arterial counterpulsator. J Thorac Cardiovasc Surg 1961;41:447–458.

9. Scheidt S, Wilner G, Mueller H, et al. Intra-aortic balloon counterpulsation in cardiogenic shock: report of a cooperative clinical trial. N Engl J Med 1973;288:979–984.

10. Buckley MJ, Craven JM, Gold HK. IABP assist for cardiogenic shock after cardiopulmonary bypass. Circulation 1972;46(Suppl):II76.

11. Talpins NL, Kripke DC, Goetz RH. Counterpulsation and intraaortic balloon pumping in cardiogenic shock. Circ Dyn Arch Surg 1968;97:991–999.

12. Kantrowitz A, Krakauer J, Zorzi G, et al. Current status of intraaortic balloon pump and initial clinical experience with aortic patch mechanical auxiliary ventricle. Transplant Proc 1971;3:1459–1471.

13. Hedayat N, Sherwood JT, Schomisch SJ, Carino JL, Cmolik BL. Circulatory benefits of diastolic counterpulsation in an ischemic heart failure model after aortomyoplasty. J Thorac Cardiovasc Surg 2002;123:1067–1073.

14. Chatterjee S, Rosensweig J. Evaluation of intraaortic balloon counterpulsation. J Thorac Cardiovasc Surg 1971;61:405–410.

15. McDonald RH Jr, Taylor RR, Cingolani HE. Measurement of myocardial developed tension and its relation to oxygen consumption. Am J Physiol 1966;211:667–673.

16. Mueller H, Ayres SM, Conklin EF, et al. The effects of intraaortic counterpulsation on cardiac performance and metabolism in shock associated with acute myocardial infarction. J Clin Invest 1971;50:1885–1900.

17. Shaw J, Taylor DR, Pitt B. Effects of intraaortic balloon counterpulsation on regional coronary blood flow in experimental myocardial infarction. Am J Card 1974;34:552–556.

18. Kimura A, Toyota E, Songfang L, et al. Effects of intraaortic balloon pumping on the septal arterial blood flow velocity waveform during severe left main coronary artery stenosis. J Am Coll Cardiol 1996;27:810–816.

19. Bhayana JN, Scott SM, Sethi GK, Takaro T. Effects of intraaortic balloon pumping on organ perfusion in cardiogenic shock. J Surg Res 1979;26:108–113.

20. Antman EM, Hand M, Armstrong PW, et al. 2007 focused update of the ACC/AHA 2004 guidelines for the management of patients with ST-elevation myocardial infarction: a report of the American College of Cardiology/American Heart Association Task Force on Practice Guidelines (Writing Group to Review New Evidence and Update the ACC/AHA 2004 Guidelines for the Management of Patients with ST-Elevation Myocardial Infarction). J Am Coll Cardiol 2008;51. Available at: www.acc.org/qualityandscience/clinical/statements.htm.

21. O'Rourke MF, Norris RM, Campbell TJ, Chang VP, Sammel NL. Randomized controlled trial of intraaortic balloon counterpulsation in early myocardial infarction with acute heart failure. Am J Cardiol 1981;47:815–820.

22. Flaherty JT, Becker LC, Weiss JL, et al. Results of a randomized prospective trial of intraaortic balloon counterpulsation and intravenous nitroglycerin in patients with acute myocardial infarction. J Am Coll Cardiol 1985;6:434–446.

23. Waksman R, Weiss AT, Gotsman MS, Hasin Y. Intra-aortic balloon counterpulsation improves survival in cardiogenic shock complicating acute myocardial infarction. Eur Heart J 1993;14:71–74.

24. Stomel RJ, Rasak M, Bates ER. Treatment strategies for acute myocardial infarction complicated by cardiogenic shock in a community hospital. Chest 1994;105:997–1002.

25. Berger PB, Holmes DR Jr, Stebbins AL, et al. Impact of an aggressive invasive catheterization and revascularization strategy on mortality in patients with cardiogenic shock in the Global Utilization of Streptokinase and Tissue Plasminogen Activator for Occluded Coronary Arteries (GUSTO-I) trial: an observational study. Circulation 1997;96:122–127.

26. Sjauw KD, Engstrom AE, Vis MM, et al. A systematic review and meta-analysis of intra-aortic balloon pump therapy in ST-elevation myocardial infarction: should we change the guidelines? Eur Heart J 2009;30:459–468.

27. Dekker AL, Reesink KD, Van Der Veen FH, et al. Intra-aortic balloon pumping in acute mitral regurgitation reduces aortic impedance and regurgitant fraction. Shock 2003;19:334–338.

28. Bouchart F, Bessou JP, Tabley A, et al. Urgent surgical repair of postinfarction ventricular septal rupture: early and late outcomes. J Cardiac Surg 1998;13:104–112.

29. Torchiana DF, Hirsch G, Buckley MJ, et al. Intraaortic balloon pumping for cardiac support: trends in practice outcome, 1968–1995. J Thorac Cardiovasc Surg 1997;113:758–769.

30. McGee NG, Zillgitt SL, Trono R, et al. Retrospective analyses of the need for mechanical circulatory support (intraaortic balloon pump/abdominal left ventricular assist device or partial artificial heart) after cardiopulmonary bypass. A 44 month study of 14168 patients. Am J Cardiol 1980;46:135–142.

31. Norman JC, Cooley DA, Igo SR, et al. Prognostic indices for survival during postcardiotomy intra-aortic balloon pumping: methods of scoring and classification, with implications for left ventricular assist device utilization. J Thorac Cardiovasc Surg 1977;74:709–720.

32. Lund O, Johansen G, Allermand H, et al. Intraaortic balloon pumping in the treatment of low cardiac output following open heart surgery—immediate results and long-term prognosis. Thorac Cardiovasc Surg 1988;36:332–337.

33. Campbell CD, Tolitano DJ, Weber KT, et al. Mechanical support for postcardiotomy heart failure. J Cardiac Surg 1988;3:181–191.

34. Hagemeijer F, Larid JD, Haalebos MMP, Hugenholtz PG. Effectiveness of intra-aortic balloon pumping without cardiac surgery for patients with severe heart failure secondary to a recent myocardial infarction. Am J Cardiol 1977;40:951–956.

35. Moulopoulos S, Stametelopoulos S, Petrou P. Intraaortic balloon assistance in intractable cardiogenic shock. Eur Heart J 1986;7:396–403.

36. Hardesty RL, Griffith BP, Trento A, et al. Mortally ill patients and excellent survival following cardiac transplantation. Ann Thorac Surg 1986;41:126–129.

37. O'Connell JB, Renlunnd DG, Robinson JA, et al. Effect of preoperative hemodynamic support on survival after cardiac transplantation. Circulation 1988;78(Suppl III):78–82.

38. Kavarana MN, Sinha P, Naka Y, Oz MC, Edwards NM. Mechanical support for the failing cardiac allograft: a single-center experience. J Heart Lung Transplant 2003;22:542–547.

39. Christenson JT, Simonet F, Schmuziger M. The effect of preoperative intra-aortic balloon pump support in high risk patients requiring myocardial revascularization. J Cardiovasc Surg 1997;38:397–402.

40. Marroquin OC, Selzer F, Mulukutla SR, et al. A comparison of bare-metal and drug-eluting stents for off-label indications. N Engl J Med 2008;358:342–352.

41. Mulukutla SR, Vlachos HA, Marroquin OC, et al. Impact of drug-eluting stents among insulin-treated diabetic patients: a report from the NHLBI Dynamic Registry. JACC Cardiovasc Interv 2008;1:139–147.

42. Cohen M, Dawson MS, Kopistansky C, McBride R. Sex and other predictors of intra-aortic balloon counterpulsation-related complications: prospective study of 1119 consecutive patients. Am Heart J 2000;139:282–287.

43. Cook L, Pillar B, McCord G, Josephson R. Intra-aortic balloon pump complications: a five-year retrospective study of 283 patients. Heart Lung 1999;28:195–202.

44. Gottlieb SO, Brinker JA, Borkon AM, et al. Identification of patients at high risk for complications of intraaortic balloon counterpulsation: a multivariate risk factor analysis. Am J Cardiol 1984;53:1135–1139.

45. Arafa OE, Pedersen TH, Svennevig JL, et al. Vascular complications of the intraaortic balloon pump in patients undergoing open heart operations: 15-year experience. Ann Thorac Surg 1999;67:645–651.

46. Wasfie T, Freed PS, Rubenfire M, et al. Risk associated with intraaortic balloon pumping in patients with and without diabetes mellitus. Am J Cardiol 1988;61:558–562.

47. Scholz KH, Ragab S, von zur Muhlen F, et al. Complication of intra-aortic balloon counterpulsation: the role of catheter size and duration of support in a multivariate analysis of risk. Eur Heart J 1998;19:458–465.

48. Miller JS, Dodson TF, Salam AA, Smith RB III. Vascular complications following intra-aortic balloon pump insertion. Am Surg 1992;58:232–238.

49. Curtis JJ, Bolan M, Bliss D, et al. Intra-aortic balloon cardiac assist: complication rates for the surgical and percutaneous insertion techniques. Am Surg 1988;54:142–147.

50. Sirbu H, Busch T, Aleksic I, *et al.* Ischaemic complications with intraaortic balloon counter-pulsation: incidence and management. Cardiovasc Surg 2000;8:66–71.

51. McEnany MT, Kay HR, Buckley MJ, *et al.* Clinical experience with intraaortic balloon pump support in 728 patients. Circulation 1978;58(Suppl I):124–132.

52. Kantrowitz A, Wasfie T, Freed PS, *et al.* Intraaortic balloon pumping 1967 through 1982: analysis of complications in 733 patients. Am J Cardiol 1986;57:976–983.

53. Thiele H, Lauer B, Hambrecht R, *et al.* Reversal of cardiogenic shock by percutaneous left atrial-to-femoral arterial bypass assistance. Circulation 2001;104(24):2917–2922.

54. Thiele H, Sick P, *et al.* Randomized comparison of intraaortic balloon support with a percutaneous left ventricular assist device in patients with revascularized acute myocardial infarction complicated by cardiogenic shock. Eur Heart J 2005;26(13):1276–1283.

55. Burkhoff D, Cohen H, Brunckhorst C, *et al.* A randomized multicenter clinical study to evaluate the safety and efficacy of the TandemHeart percutaneous ventricular assist device versus conventional therapy with intraaortic balloon pumping for treatment of cardiogenic shock. Am Heart J 2006;152(3):469.e1–e8.

56. Bruckner BA, Jacob LP, Gregoric ID, *et al.* Clinical experience with the TandemHeart percutaneous ventricular assist device as a bridge to cardiac transplantation. Tex Heart Inst J 2008;35(4):447–450.

57. Gregoric ID, Jacob LP, La Francesca S, *et al.* The TandemHeart as a bridge to a long-term axial-flow left ventricular assist device (bridge to bridge). Tex Heart Inst J 2008;35(2):125–129.

58. Pitsis AA, Dardas P, Mezilis N, *et al.* Temporary assist device for postcardiotomy cardiac failure. Ann Thorac Surg 2004;77(4):1431–1433.

59. Khalife WI, Kar B. The TandemHeart pVAD in the treatment of acute fulminant myocarditis. Tex Heart Inst J 2007;34(2):209–213.

60. Aragon J, Lee MS, Kar S, *et al.* Percutaneous left ventricular assist device: "TandemHeart" for high-risk coronary intervention. Catheter Cardiovasc Interv 2005;65(3):346–352.

61. Cohn WE, Morris CD, Reverdin S, *et al.* Intraoperative TandemHeart implantation as an adjunct to high-risk valve surgery. Tex Heart Inst J 2007;34(4):457–458.

62. Friedman PA, Munger TM, Torres N, *et al.* Percutaneous endocardial and epicardial ablation of hypotensive ventricular tachycardia with percutaneous left ventricular assist in the electrophysiology laboratory. J Cardiovasc Electrophysiol 2007;18(1):106–109.

63. Berry C, Oukerraj L, Asgar A, *et al.* Role of transesophageal echocardiography in percutaneous aortic valve replacement with the CoreValve Revalving system. Echocardiography 2008;25(8):840–848.

64. Tanaka K, Rangarajan K, Azarbal B, *et al.* Percutaneous ventricular assist during aortic valvuloplasty: potential application to the deployment of aortic stent-valves. Tex Heart Inst J 2007;34(1):36–40.

65. Arora HS, Loyalka P, Kar B, *et al.* Devices for heart failure: the future is now. Congest Heart Fail 2008;14(3):141–148.

66. Reesink K, Dekker A, van Ommen V, *et al.* Miniature intracardiac assist device provides more effective cardiac unloading and circulatory support during severe left heart failure than intraaortic balloon pumping. Chest 2004;126:896–902.

67. Siegenthaler MP, Brehm K, Strecker T, *et al.* The Impella Recover microaxial left-ventricular-assist-device reduces mortality for postcardiotomy failure—a three center experience. J Thor Cardiovasc Surg 2004;127:812–922.

68. Onorati F, Cristodoro L, Borrello F, *et al.* Ventricular assistance with microaxial flow pump following mitral repair for dilated cardiomyopathy. Int J Artif Organs 2006;29:591–595.

69. Meyns B, Stolinski MD, Leunens V, Verbeken E, Flameng W. Left ventricular support by catheter-mounted axial flow pump reduces infarct size. J Ann Coll Cardiol 2003;41:1087–1095.

70. Seyfarth M, Sibbing D, Bauer I, *et al.* A randomized clinical trial to evaluate the safety and efficacy of a percutaneous left ventricular assist device (Impella LP2.5) versus intra-aortic balloon pumping for treatment of cardiogenic shock caused by myocardial infarction. J Am Coll Cardiol 2008;52:1584–1588.

71. Ramondo A, Napodano M, Tarantini G, *et al.* High risk percutaneous coronary intervention using the intracardiac microaxial pump Impella Recover. J Cardiovasc Med 2006;7:149–152.

72. Dixon SR, Hernriques J, Mauri L, *et al.* A prospective feasibility trial investigating the use of the Impella 2.5 system in patients undergoing high-risk percutaneous coronary intervention (The PROTECT I Trial): initial US experience. JACC Cardiovasc Interv 2009;2:91–96.

73. Konstam MA, Czerska B, Böhm M, *et al.* Continuous aortic flow augmentation: a pilot study of hemodynamic and renal responses to a novel percutaneous intervention in decompensated heart failure. Circulation 2005;112(20):3107–3114.

74. Greenberg B, Czerska B, Delgado RM, *et al.* Effects of continuous aortic flow augmentation in patients with exacerbation of heart failure inadequately responsive to medical therapy: results of the Multicenter Trial of the Orqis Medical Cancion System for the Enhanced Treatment of Heart Failure Unresponsive to Medical Therapy (MOMENTUM). Circulation 2008;118(12):1241–1249.

CHAPTER 12

Left Ventricular Assist Devices for Acute and Chronic Heart Failure

Daniel Marelli[1], Louis Stein[1], &
Abbas Ardehali[2]
[1]Jefferson Medical College, Philadelphia, PA, USA
[2]University of California, Los Angeles, CA, USA

Overview

Left ventricular assist devices (LVADs) support the circulation when the left ventricle is no longer able to meet the body's systemic perfusion needs. This presumes that the right ventricle will be able to support adequately a normal volume load. This is typical of the most common types of chronic heart failure in which the right ventricle has adapted to chronically elevated preload and in many cases afterload as well. Three general strategies using LVADs are employed to treat patients with congestive heart failure (CHF). "Bridge to recovery" is used for patients who demonstrate sufficient recuperation in heart function with mechanical assistance; they can be weaned from the device with subsequent explantation. Early uses of mechanical assist were limited to assisting patients with postcardiac surgery heart failure to recovery. Contemporary uses of "bridge to recovery" have evolved to include treatment of patients with acute viral myocarditis, or, in selected cases, chronic dilated cardiomyopathy [1–3]. Second, "bridge to transplant," is used in patients with advanced CHF on maximal medical treatment in whom orthotopic heart transplantation (OHT) is indicated. Such patients have impending end-organ compromise and marginal hemodynamics. The third strategy, "destination therapy," is indicated for those patients with intractable CHF who are ineligible for heart transplantation [4].

The successful implementation of the heart–lung machine in the early 1950s was significant for its direct application to numerous procedures. With this came the observation that a number of patients in cardiogenic shock (presumably due to poor myocardial protection during surgery) could be weaned from the heart–lung machine after a period of "assisting" the heart. This strategy was not effective in all patients, but it was postulated that longer support could help these patients. Researchers then began pursuing longer mechanisms of support—beginning the quest for an LVAD [5]. Such a device was first reported in 1961 by Dennis et al., who used a roller pump to off-load the left ventricle by receiving blood from the left atrium and returning it to the femoral artery. This device supported 12 patients for 4–17 hours, although no patients were supported to recovery [6]. In 1963, DeBakey reported the first implanted pulsatile VAD, which used unidirectional ball valves and bypassed the heart between the left atrium and the descending thoracic aorta [5]. The implanted VAD consisted of two coaxial tubes: the blood flowed through an inner compliant Dacron tube surrounded by a rigid outer tube. Blood was pumped by pneumatically increasing the transluminal pressure causing the flexible inner tube to narrow [5]. A second patient, supported for 10 days with an extracorporeal version of this device, became the first patient to be supported to recovery with a VAD [7]. In 1969, Cooley et al. performed the first successful bridge to transplant using a total artificial heart [8]. This demonstrated the possibility to support the patient's circulation until a donor heart became possible. In light of these advances, the US government formed the Medical Devices Applications Branch of the National Heart Blood and Lung Institute in 1970 [9]. This agency produced a series of requests for proposals that fueled the development of some of the currently used assist devices.

Through the 1970s and 1980s, advancements in technology and refinements in implantation technique ignited the development of increasingly novel devices. The first LVAD bridge to transplant was performed in 1978 [10]. The introduction of cyclosporine broadened the application of heart transplantation by improving the prognosis of rejection while sparing the innate immune system. This kindled a concomitant growth in the application of LVADs as a "bridge to transplantation." In the early to middle 1990s, US and European regulatory agencies ultimately approved the use of an LVAD for the indication of "bridge to transplant." Current adult pumps generally have a stroke volume of 60–70 mL at an ejection pressure of about 100–120 mmHg. They respond to both preload and afterload similar to a normal human ventricle. Unique challenges for adapting these for the pediatric population are hypertension and lower physiological flows. The former increases the risk of intracranial bleed and the latter increases the risk of thrombus formation.

Indications, patient, and device selection

Universal Algorithm and hemodynamic criteria

While demonstrating lifesaving ability, devices are generally best used to prevent end-organ damage. A risk score predicting poor outcome due to extensive end-organ damage has been proposed. Preoperative LVAD score can be calculated using five clinical variables: postcardiotomy shock, previous LVAD use, ventilatory status, central venous pressure > 16 mmHg, and prothrombin time > 16 seconds [11,12]. In addition to these factors, other important preoperative risk factors include use of an intra-aortic balloon pump (when it reflects prolonged shock) and age, particularly patients older

than the fifth decade of life who generally have decreased end-organ reserve [13]. Preimplant renal dysfunction alone has not been consistent as a predictor of outcome.

Timing of insertion is therefore an important determinant of outcome [14]. As experience with VADs in the last decade has grown, there is general comfort with earlier insertion than in the past. One can therefore envision what can be termed a "Universal Algorithm" for the selection of patients for whom VAD therapy is indicated (Figure 12.1). This simplifies the decision for VAD therapy regardless of diagnosis, chronicity, or goal of therapy. Patients who require VADs usually present with hemodynamic indices indicative of persistent CHF, which have failed to respond to usual medical treatment including volume unloading and which require treatment with continuous infusion of one or two inotropic agents [15]. Symptoms of heart failure should be consistent with NYHA (New York Heart Association) class IV or in selected cases IIIb. Objective hemodynamic indices of CHF indicating VAD therapy generally comprise a cardiac index less than 2 L/min/m^2 associated with normal or slightly elevated ventricular filling pressures [16]. This is often associated with impending renal failure, reflecting poor peripheral perfusion.

Once it is established that a patient requires device therapy, the decisions will then be on what type of device to be used, the need for biventricular support, and, in the case of destination therapy, appropriateness of device therapy. Devices range from the simple percutaneous intra-aortic balloon pump to totally implantable (internal) complex device systems. One should keep in mind that many devices lend themselves easily to a "bridge-to-bridge" strategy. The most basic example of such a strategy can be an intra-aortic balloon pump to stabilize a patient prior to going to the operating room for a more definitive device. In such a case, one should avoid supramaximal doses of pressor agents, particularly norepinephrine, in order to prevent ischemia to lower limb in which the balloon is placed.

Typically, patients with either chronic or acute CHF are considered for VAD implantation. In addition to criteria indicative of refractory heart failure, patients must be carefully selected for their ability to tolerate the surgery as well as benefit from device

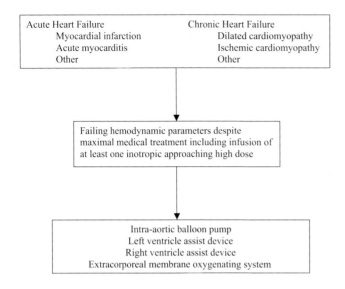

Acute Heart Failure	Chronic Heart Failure
Myocardial infarction	Dilated cardiomyopathy
Acute myocarditis	Ischemic cardiomyopathy
Other	Other

Failing hemodynamic parameters despite maximal medical treatment including infusion of at least one inotropic approaching high dose

Intra-aortic balloon pump
Left ventricle assist device
Right ventricle assist device
Extracorporeal membrane oxygenating system

Figure 12.1 Universal Algorithm leading to the decision for mechanical circulatory support.

therapy. Factors such as sepsis and age are of primary concern: the former due to a plan to implant a foreign body and the latter due to the presence of comorbidities, suggesting significant compromise in end-organ reserve.

As stated above, it is generally easier to prevent end-organ damage than to reverse it. This raises the question: Is earlier implant a possibility? Two factors may be considered in answering this: the risk of mortality resulting from CHF and the risk of complications resulting from VAD placement. VAD implementation is indicated when the severity of the risk of death from CHF exceeds the risks of implanting an assist device. The current standard for this severity is inotropic therapy with worsening congestion [17]. As LVAD technology and safety improve and outcome prediction becomes more reliable, the validity of this standard may be questioned. This would potentially lead to randomized trials evaluating VAD therapy.

Prognosis, mechanical support strategy, and device choice

Chronic heart failure

The most common form of chronic heart failure in adults is systolic left ventricular failure due to ischemic or dilated cardiomyopathy. Such patients typically require bridge-to-transplant therapy. They are typically waiting as urgent status and may have

a trial of an intra-aortic balloon pump for a few days while trying to obtain a donor organ. Such patients usually have adequate right ventricular function, which has adapted to chronically elevated pulmonary artery pressures. These patients do not necessarily have elevated pulmonary vascular resistance, but rather have left ventricle congestion with normal right-sided filling pressures. They also have dilated left ventricles, ideally conformable to apical implantation of a device inflow conduit. Given that taller, larger body surface area potential recipients tend to wait for donor organs longer, this category of patients is suited for implantable (internal) pulsatile LVAD therapy. Current devices for this purpose are true left ventricle "replacement" devices (Figure 12.2a,b) [9]. The distinction of "replacement" device is because these devices are capable of high flow (>7–8 L/min) and total left ventricle decompression, even in large individuals. These devices are electrically powered. The drawback of these pumps is that they require the creation of a large pocket in the abdomen and therefore can generally only be used in patients with a body surface area (BSA) > 1.6 m^2. Driveline exit sites are also a potential source of infection. The driveline is used to connect the pump to its electrical supply and its microprocessor that regulates a Frank-Starling physiology, and provides for an air vent to account for pump displacement during pump diastole. Early satiety may occur after implant due

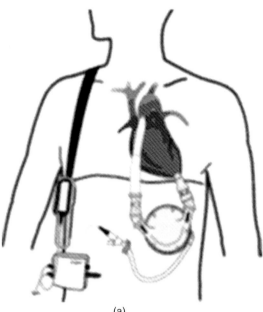

(a)

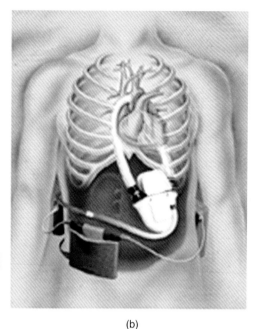

(b)

Figure 12.2   Implantable pulsatile left ventricle assist devices. These devices weigh about 1 kg and have bioprosthetic valves to ensure unidirectional flow. Shown are the device shells containing the pump mechanism. (a) The HeartMate XVE contains a rigid diaphragm that is pushed by an inclined plane mechanism, causing the pump to have a slight rotation during systole. There is a textured inner surface, and it therefore usually requires only antiplatelet agents for anticoagulation. Pump durability is usually 1.5–3 years. (b) The Novacor contains a push plate mechanism and is relatively motionless during systole. It has a built-in sensor to detect wear on moving parts, which can last over 4 years. It requires warfarin therapy in addition to antiplatelet agents for anticoagulation. (Reprinted with permission from the Thoratec and World Heart Corporations.)

to device size and location immediately anterior to part of the stomach. However, because the pump is internal, patients can enjoy maximum mobility, and in many cases outpatient treatment. Prolonged right ventricular support is not possible with these. As with all assist devices, patent foramen ovale must be repaired at surgery so that right to left shunting is avoided.

If patients are smaller, or require prolonged biventricular support, then paracorporeal pulsatile devices are the usual choice. The most commonly used long-term paracorporeal pumps are the Thoratec and Berlin Heart Excor (Figure 12.3a,b). These are typically capable of flows of about 4–6 L/min, and are therefore true "assist" devices that do not decompress the left ventricle as much as the above noted devices, especially in large BSA patients. As mentioned above, lower flow pumps are more prone to thrombus formation due to less vigorous washout. These devices are powered by pneu-

matic energy that compresses a diaphragm against a soft bladder and require larger consoles compared to the electrical devices. Mechanical valves ensure unidirectional flow, and warfarin therapy is needed in addition to antiplatelet agents. The Thoratec pump has recently been modified and is available in a smaller intracorporeal version that allows both right and left pumps to be placed in the abdomen (see below). The Excor is coated with a heparin derivative (Carmeda AB, Sweden). This raises the possibility of heparin-induced thrombocytopenia; however, recipients of these devices have not had increased incidence of heparin/platelet factor 4 antibodies [18,19].

Patients with restrictive cardiomyopathy present a unique challenge. Absence of left ventricle dilatation can cause difficulty during creation of the apical conduit for an implantable device. In the worst-case scenario, the conduit will point toward the septum and will be partially obstructed. This will

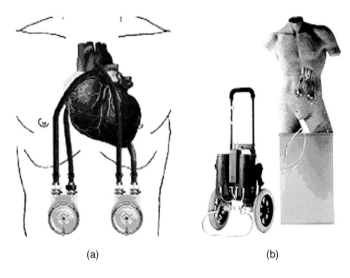

(a)   (b)

Figure 12.3 Long-term paracorporeal pneumatic devices. A portable pneumatic drive is necessary for ambulation during treatment with these devices. (a) The Thoratec biventricular assist device system. (b) The Berlin Heart Excor is available in smaller sizes for infants and children. (Reprinted with permission from the Thoratec and Berlin Heart Corporations.)

cause chronically elevated left atrial pressures and low device flows. This may also increase the risk of thrombus formation. Such patients are therefore often treated with paracorporeal devices. These have smaller apical conduits and, if need be, have the option of left atrial cannualation to avoid the left ventricle apex.

Acute heart failure

Excluding postcardiac surgery, assist device therapy for acute heart failure is less frequent than for chronic heart failure. The two most common indications are acute myocardial infarction with cardiogenic shock and rapidly progressive fulminant viral or giant cell myocarditis. For the purposes of this chapter, postcardiac surgery failure will be considered as acute myocardial infarction. Both of these have in common rapid onset and in extremis presentation. Such patients therefore often require biventricular support, particularly if there is a history of cardiac arrest [20]. The pulsatile pneumatically driven Abiomed BVS 5000 (ABIOMED Inc., Danvers, MA, USA) has been particularly useful for these patients [21,22]. It is commonly available in secondary care centers, and in many cases can be placed without the use of cardiopulmonary bypass. Like the Thoratec, it is paracorporeal, but it differs in that the pump is deaired off the operative field and long tubing is handed to the surgeon to connect to the cannulae exiting the heart. This allows for simple and rapid deployment. In the case

of myocarditis a biopsy is often helpful and can be obtained at surgery from the epicardial aspect of the right ventricle. The disadvantage of this device is that it does not permit ambulation beyond the sitting position. This device is commonly used as a bridge to another bridge or recovery, which can be possible after either of these diagnoses. More recently, an additional device has become available so that the BVS cannulae can be adapted to a more conventional paracorporeal device, the Abiomed AB 5000 [23]. This bridge to bridge has the advantage of being carried out without the need to open the chest (Figure 12.4a,b,c). Hemodynamic stabilization using inotropes is needed during the conversion, which can leave a patient unsupported for 10–20 minutes. The AB 5000 has been used as a prolonged bridge to recovery, short bridge to transplant, or bridge to an implantable internal device.

Although not as commonly used for this purpose, the Thoratec pump has also been used in the setting of acute heart failure, particularly for bridge to recovery after acute myocarditis [24].

Controversies and complications in LVAD therapy

Right ventricle failure

LVAD therapy presupposes that the most common cause of right ventricular failure is left ventricular failure. While this is generally true in many instances of chronic heart failure, this is not always

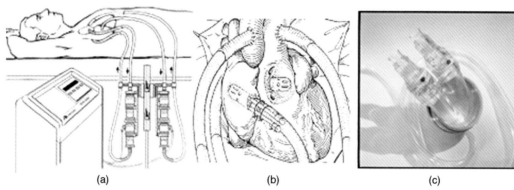

(a)   (b)   (c)

Figure 12.4   The Abiomed paracorporeal assist devices. A synthetic polyurethane makes up the bladder and valves that is encased in a rigid polycarbonate housing. Anticoagulation therapy with heparin, a thrombin inhibitor or Coumadin, as well as an antiplatelet agent is required. (a) The rapidly deployable BVS 5000 is filled by gravity. When the pump displaces 80 mL of air in the driveline, a sensor in the console triggers compressed air to be returned to the pumping chamber, causing the bladder to eject its volume. (b) The intracardiac cannulae can be placed in a variety of ways to avoid the left ventricle apex, which can be friable after myocardial infarction. These same cannulae can be used for the AB 5000 device. (c) The AB 5000 device requires a slight vacuum to fill. The same console can be used for either of these devices, and conversion can be done without opening the chest, allowing transition to a device that will permit greater patient mobility and longer term support. (Reprinted with permission from the ABIOMED, Inc.)

predictable. This is especially true in patients who present in extremis requiring mechanical ventilation and who have abnormal biochemical markers of liver function [25]. Such patients more often require a right ventricle assist device. One must keep in mind that in an LVAD patient the function of the right ventricle is to accept the venous return from the LVAD and to deliver it forward. Although this seems obvious, it is not always recognized. This is because prior to LVAD insertion the right ventricle was "handling" flows of 3–4 L/min (typical index 1.8–2 L/min/m^2). After LVAD insertion, the total body cardiac output can double, unmasking a poorly functioning right ventricle, which cannot "handle" such a load. Under such circumstances, one should avoid the mind trap of volume overloading the right ventricle, simply thinking that the LVAD is underfilled. Cardiac echo is helpful to assess right ventricular filling in such situations. Equally important is to consider pulmonary vascular resistance.

One can further classify the problem into transient right ventricular dysfunction which occurs after LVAD implantation and true chronic right ventricle failure. The former is attributed to elevated pulmonary vascular resistance due to the inflammatory effects of cardiopulmonary bypass and blood product transfusions. This supports the use of the combination of milrinone and low-dose vasopressin (usually 0.04 U/min in adults) in the early postoperative period after LVAD implantation. Of all agents, which can be used to treat the vasodilatory effects of cardiopulmonary bypass and anesthesia, vasopressin is the one that most spares the pulmonary vascular bed [26]. Side effects at low dose are limited to cool extremities, which responds to dose reduction or discontinuation of infusion. Low-dose epinephrine is a good alternative. Inhaled nitric oxide (20 ppm in adults) and dobutamine are also commonly used.

Prior to the availability of nitric oxide, temporary right ventricle mechanical support was often required after LVAD implantation [27]. Many surgeons try to avoid insertion of a temporary right ventricle assist device using these or similar other modalities and sometimes require echocardiogram and direct visualization (before and after LVAD implant) to decide on the need for right-sided support. Nitroglycerine infusion can also decrease both right ventricle preload and afterload, optimizing function. A central venous pressure of <14 mmHg is optimal. This should be complemented by a mean blood pressure of 70–80 mmHg in order to optimize coronary as well as cerebral and splanchnic blood flows. Temporary pacing can also be used to increase heart rate to 90–95, preventing right ventricle overfilling while optimizing output. Typically, one would accept LVAD flows >5–5.5 L/min depending on BSA.

More permanent right ventricle dysfunction can be due to existing pathology (e.g., sarcoidosis) or chronic arrhythmia, which would not respond to left ventricle decompression. In addition, patients with acute myocarditis or postpartum cardiomyopathy usually have pathology that can affect both ventricles. Such patients are therefore usually treated with biventricular support. Still, for these patients, the difficult question remains: If a high enough flow LVAD is used, will the left atrial pressure fall enough so that a right ventricle assist device will not be needed if the pulmonary vascular resistance is normal? One can speculate that severe right ventricle dilatation would dictate the need for prolonged right ventricle assist.

Aortic valve function and mechanical valve in the aortic position

Essential to proper LVAD function is a competent aortic valve. This is because insufficiency would lead to inefficient forward flow. Device flowmeters may show a normal output in such instances. Certainly, patients with greater than mild aortic insufficiency should be considered for repair or replacement at the time of LVAD implant [28]. Mechanical valves are generally considered incompatible with LVADs for two reasons: they have a finite regurgitation, and, perhaps more importantly, may not open regularly during LVAD function and would therefore run the risk of thrombus formation despite anticoagulation. Such thrombus could embolize as VAD ejection rate is asynchronous to that of the native heart. Patients with previously placed mechanical aortic valve prostheses should be considered for valve replacement with a tissue valve at the time of LVAD implant, especially if long-term support is contemplated [29].

Bleeding

Bleeding complications after LVAD implant can occur both early and late. Typically, patients have coagulopathy perioperatively due to previous liver congestion and the effects of cardiopulmonary bypass. Intraoperative use of aprotinin, an antifibri-

nolytic agent, and meticulous surgical technique have contributed to minimize these [30]. Blood products are generally used specifically to correct measured parameters postoperatively. Use of these must be weighed against the tendency for these to cause transient increases in pulmonary vascular resistance. Thromboelastography has been used to guide therapy and to allow a smooth transition to anticoagulation for devices that require this [31]. Late bleeding in the pericardium or intra-abdominal device pocket can occur as a result of necessary anticoagulation. The former can cause tamponade physiology and the latter may cause fever, pain, and possibly infection.

Thrombosis and stroke

Device-related thromboembolism is a significant risk of LVADs. Overall risk for any event ranges from 6 to 23%, depending on the device [32,33]. Many of these events are minor and full recovery is often possible. All VAD patients are treated with aspirin. Except for the HeartMate XVE, all other devices require warfarin anticoagulation. Heparin is used until patients are therapeutic on warfarin. Based on our current practice, it is possible that in the future, direct thrombin inhibitors (which are not dependent on renal clearance) may prove to be superior to heparin, especially since it has been observed that assist device patients may be more prone to heparin-induced thrombocytopenia [34]. Argatroban, which is not dependent on renal clearance, has been our first choice for intravenous anticoagulation since 2006.

The Novacor has undergone modifications, which have greatly improved thromboembolic rates. Interestingly, the textured surface of the HeartMate has not eliminated risk of thrombus formation, pointing to the fact that cause is multifactorial. This is problematic in the face of a risk of intracranial bleed, as patients may have hypertension after LVAD implantation. Hypertension also prevents complete device systole and therefore may cause thrombus formation within the device-pumping chamber. Paracorporeal devices have the advantage of being made of a clear polycarbonate shell which permits device inspection. As already noted, thromboelastography has been used to assess the balance thrombosis and fibrinolysis in VAD patients and is likely to be used more commonly to guide anticoagulation therapy in the future.

Infection

Sepsis related to device insertion is a major concern with implantable devices. Perioperatively various prophylactic antibiotic regimens are used, including antifungals. Chronic driveline and pocket infections can be treated with long-term antibiotics. This may not eradicate the infection but usually will prevent systemic sepsis. Implantation of aminoglycoside and vancomycin eluting beads has also been carried out successfully. Once controlled, these chronic infections generally do not preclude heart transplantation, as device removal is usually curative [35,36].

Liver and kidney dysfunction

Transient liver and kidney dysfunction is not uncommon in the early postoperative period after assist device insertion. When persistent, such multiorgan failure can limit long-term survival.

Liver dysfunction can manifest itself as chronic elevation of total bilirubin level, with minimal disturbance in other biochemical markers. This is the result of a combination of preoperative hypoperfusion and congestion, reperfusion injury, cardiopulmonary bypass-related inflammatory response, and persistent congestion due to residual right ventricular failure. Prolonged preimplant hypoperfusion can be minimized with timely decision making before end-organ damage occurs. Total parenteral nutrition should be avoided postoperatively, as it is generally considered liver toxic.

Immune system sensitization

Multiple resultant transfusions may result in increased antibody development. There is also the interaction between device surface and the immune system. As an example, the textured surface of the HeartMate has been shown to increase the Th2 bias in the immune system [37]. This bias occurs in the context of increased apoptosis of certain populations of T cells [38]. Increased risk of fungal infection may also be a result of increased T-cell death. B-cell hyperreactivity was found to be due to CD40–CD40 ligand interaction between B and T cells, suggesting a potential pretransplant role for calcineurin inhibitors or mono-

clonal antibodies against either CD25 or CD40 [39]. Some studies have indicated that using LVADs as a bridge to transplant increases the panel of reactive antibodies; however, this does not necessarily result in an increase in allograft rejection [40–42]. The requirement for a prospective cross-match in recipients with assist devices undergoing transplant is preferable but remains controversial. Such a requirement is best individualized as certain panel reactive antibodies may be transient and related to the early post-VAD implant period.

Goals of device therapy

Bridge to transplant

LVADs have proven to be an effective means of stabilizing patients, which allow them to potentially leave the hospital while awaiting heart transplant [43]. These devices promote the remission of CHF-associated end-organ damage, improving posttransplant prognosis [44]. Among 655 devices included in the 2005 report of the Mechanical Circulatory Support Device Database (MCSD), 78.3% were reported to be implanted as a "bridge to transplant." This database compared the outcomes of LVAD patients younger than 30 years and older than 50 years. In the younger group, approximately 75% (vs 50%) of patients received a heart transplant while 25% of patients expired or remained too ill to undergo transplant [33]. One can infer that improved timing (and preimplant risk factors) will certainly yield improved results [45,46].

Bridge to transplantation affords advantages in addition to facilitating patient survival to transplant. LVAD implantation has also been demonstrated to improve some instances of pulmonary hypertension before transplantation [47–49]. After heart transplantation, patients who were bridged with a device have comparable outcomes to those supported with inotropic therapy.

Bridge to recovery

LVADs were first implemented to stabilize patients with postcardiotomy shock. Survival outcomes for emergent implantation of LVAD for postcardiotomy shock have remained at 20–40% [50]. Some studies have suggested this low survival may be due in part to the need for right ventricular assistance in some situations [51]. Short-term use of LVAD is also indicated for other forms of acute cardiogenic shock, such as viral myocarditis and myocardial infarction that have the potential for recovery [52].

More recently, implantation of LVADs has expanded to allow a small number of patients with CHF to sufficiently recover and permit explanation of the device [53]. This strategy has been most successful in patients with nonischemic cardiomyopathy such as idiopathic dilated cardiomyopathy [54]. Physiologic indicators attest to the clinical improvement seen in some patients. Functional improvements in the heart are manifested in improved left and right ventricular function, ejection fraction, and left ventricular end-diastolic diameter. Early studies have suggested that the concomitant treatment with clenbuterol improves myocyte performance [55]. Changes in myocyte phenotype-related mechanical support include a decreased cellular hypertrophy [56], susceptibility to apoptosis [57], and alteration in cytoskeletal gene expression [58]. Functional myocyte change associated with recovery include improved contractile strength [59], decreased action potential duration, and increased sarcoplasmic reticulum Ca^{2+} concentration [56].

Destination therapy

In spite of the advances in medical therapy for advanced heart failure, annual mortality for patients in this population remains approximately 20–50% depending on subgroup. OHT has become the most effective therapy for heart failure, with a 1-year survival of >80% and a 10-year survival of ≥50%. OHT is compromised by several factors. In addition to tolerating the actual surgical procedure, heart recipients must withstand long-term immunosuppression with risks of infection and malignancy. Transplanted hearts may eventually become compromised by graft coronary artery disease.

The gap between the number of organ donors and those in whom transplantation is indicated (approximately 2200 and 3300 listed [3]) remains a significant limiting factor. LVADs may be used to stabilize the recipient until they are able to undergo the transplantation procedure when an organ becomes available. As described above, LVADs have demonstrated their capability to "bridge" the entire circulation and establishing the rationale for exploring the use of LVAD as a form of long-term therapy. This of course raises the issue of device durability. Initial trials have therefore been mostly in heart failure patients who were not offered transplant due to advanced age.

The REMATCH trial

In 2002 United States Food and Drug Administration (FDA) approved the HeartMate VE Left Ventricular Assist Device System (Thoratec Inc., Pleasanton, CA, USA) for destination therapy in patients judged ineligible for OHT [60]. This decision was based upon the results of the Randomized Evaluation of Mechanical Assistance for the Treatment of Congestive Heart Failure (REMATCH) trial, which compared use of LVAD to optimal medical management (OMM) in heart failure patients ineligible for OHT [61]. Contraindications to transplantation were mostly due to advanced age, but also included pulmonary hypertension, chronic obstructive pulmonary disease, malignancy, diabetes mellitus, and end-organ failure. The average age of the study cohort was about 67 years. Outcome revealed that while LVADs demonstrated improved survival when compared to OMM, these were associated with a higher rate of various other complications. The particular population studied in this trial is presumed to number 5000–10,000 [3]. It is unclear if this trial will have an impact on the decision making for the treatment of heart failure. One may therefore explore the question: What effect has the approval of LVADs as "destination" had to date?

The REMATCH trial was carried out at 20 cardiac transplantation centers. Patients were diagnosed as NYHA class IV heart failure for 60 of the previous 90 days, which has been deemed refractory to treatment with angiotensin-converting enzyme inhibitors, diuretics, and digoxin. Inclusion criteria also indicated an ejection fraction of ≤25%, peak O_2 consumption ≤12 mL × kg-1, and dependence on inotropes. Subjects were randomized into LVAD and OMM groups in a 1:1 fashion. In total, 129 patients were first enrolled between 1998 and 2001: 68 received LVADs while 61 received OMM. Average age was 66 ± 9.1 years for the LVAD group and 68 ± 8.2 years for the OMM. Age was the most common reason for transplantation ineligibility [4]. One-year survival analysis showed a significant reduction (48%) in all-cause mortality risk in the LVAD group when compared to the OMM group. One-year survival was 25 and 52% for OMM and LVAD groups, respectively, and 2-year survival was 8 and 23%. The most common cause of mortality in the OMM group was left ventricular dysfunction, while sepsis was the most common cause of mortality in those patients implanted with LVADs. OMM median survival time was 150 days, with 106 of these days out of the hospital, while LVAD group had a median survival time of 408 days, 340 of which were out of the hospital [4]. LVAD group had a significantly (2.3 times) higher frequency of adverse events. The stroke rate was 0.19 per year amount in the LVAD group and 0.052 in the OMM group [62]. The risk of sepsis was also higher among LVAD recipients with 0.53 events per patient-year compared to 0.26 events per patient-year [63]. In spite of the survival advantage imparted by LVADs, the higher risk of adverse events with current devices may dissuade their use as destination therapy.

The voluntary MCSD includes 60 participating institutions. The goals of the database is to catalog implantation and outcome for LVADs implanted for $\geq$30 days to better identify risk factors, improve patient management, and develop predictive models of outcomes. In the 2005 report of the MCSD, 78 of 655 LVAD recipients received their device as destination therapy [33]. The two most common causes

for transplant ineligibility were advanced age ($n = 38$) and comorbidity ($n = 28$). Other causes for exclusion to transplant were fixed pulmonary hypertension ($n = 8$), contraindication to immune suppression ($n = 2$), and patient refusal of transplant ($n = 2$). Survival data revealed that 65 and 34% of patients were alive at 6 months and 1 year, respectively. Two percent of the destination patients opted to receive transplants at 6 months and 11% opted for transplant at 1 year. No patients demonstrated sufficient improvement in hemodynamic function as to have their LVAD removed, or so-called bridge to recovery [33]. The MCSD demonstrates age to be a significant risk factor for mortality during LVAD destination therapy. Of 78 patients receiving destination therapy, 41 were older than 65 years. One-year survival for patients receiving LVAD therapy was 26% for those older than 65 years and 41% for patients younger than 65 years [33]. A summary of the data of these studies of LVAD destination therapy is listed in Table 12.1.

Possible impact of regulatory approval of LVAD destination therapy

There are at least four potential consequences of permanent LVAD implantation on heart failure

Table 12.1 Comparison of destination therapy data from randomized trial and voluntary registry.

Study	REMATCH trial	Mechanical circulatory support device database
Study type	Randomized clinical trial	Nonrandomized cohort
Study size	Total = 129 OMM = 61 LVAD destination = 68	Of 655 patients receiving LVAD therapy, 78 were indicated for destination therapy
Most common reason for contraindication to OHT/indication for destination therapy	Advanced age ($n = $ not available)	Advanced age ($n = 38$) Comorbidity ($n = 28$) Fixed pulmonary HTN ($n = 8$) Contraindication to immunotherapy ($n = 2$) Patient refuses transplant ($n = 2$)
Average age	OMM = 66 ± 9.1 LVAD = 68 ± 8.2	Not available
One-year survival	LVAD: 52% OMM: 23%	Overall: 34% Age > 65 yr ($n = 41$): 26% Age < 65 yr ($n = 37$): 41%

HTN, hypertension; LVAD, left ventricle assist device; OHT, orthotopic heart transplantation; OMM, optimal medical management.

therapy: (i) increased LVAD implants, (ii) shorter waiting time for heart transplant, (iii) limited impact, and (iv) stimulation for the development of novel and improved devices.

Increased LVAD implants

This new indication of LVAD implantation may be used as a supplemental therapy to those already utilized for end-stage heart failure. This would predict an increase in total procedures for implantation of LVADs.

Corporate data demonstrate a progressive increase in the use of LVADs. In 2003, Thoratec reported the HeartMate was implanted 42 times as destination therapy. The number of implants grew to 171 in 2004, and in 2005 Thoratec reported a 21–23% increase in device sales over each commensurate quarter in 2004. Similarly, World Heart investor data reported 104 Novacor devices were sold in 2002, which grew to 118 devices sold in 2003 [64]. This increase in the number of devices sold is indicative of increased volume of implantation. Disagreement between Thoratec data reporting 171 implants for destination therapy and the MCSD report of 78 implants for destination therapy suggests insufficient use of this valuable database.

Shorter waiting time for heart transplant

One of the hoped for uses of the LVAD is as an alternative to transplant. If the REMATCH trial results persuaded physicians to use assist devices in this regard, less patients would remain on the wait list, resulting in shorter wait times for these patients. Since 1994, between 2000 and 2300, heart transplants have been performed each year. In the same time, over 3000 patients are listed for heart transplant at year's end. This number peaked at slightly over 4000 in 1999 and 2000. In spite of this, United Network for Organ Sharing data already demonstrate a progressive decrease in waiting time for those in all statuses [65]. It is unlikely that the relatively low number of destination therapy cases had a significant impact on the decreased wait time for heart transplant. Presumably, wait times have shortened because of improved medical therapy, leading to fewer patients being listed and, perhaps, expanded use of nonstandard organs.

Limited impact

The new indication LVADs for destination therapy may not have affected how patients are treated for end-stage CHF. This is likely due to several factors that mitigate physicians and patients choosing them for long-term implantation. Potential reasons for this include competition with established therapy and the various social and financial costs.

The previously established paradigms for treatment of end-stage CHF have established loyalty from physicians. While associated with peri- and postoperative risks as well as limitations of donor availability, cardiac transplantation still presents the best option for long-term survival for patients with end-stage heart failure. Figure 12.5 superimposes the ISHLT reporting 2-year survival curve for heart transplant recipients in the years between 1999 and 2003 with the data presented by Rose et al. comparing LVAD destination therapy with OMM [4,67].

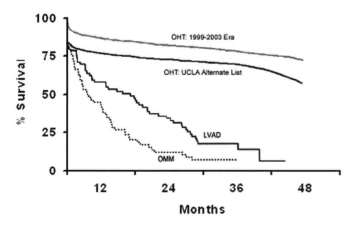

Figure 12.5 Kaplan–Meier actuarial survival curve comparing 4-year survival of advanced heart failure patients receiving optimal medical management (OMM), LVAD destination therapy (LVAD), orthotopic heart transplantation (OHT) utilizing the UCLA alternate list strategy, and ISHLT survival for all heart transplants between 1999 and 2003 (OHT). Graphs are approximate. (Adapted from [66].)

Table 12.2 Patient concerns regarding long-term LVAD therapy.

Specific concerns expressed by LVAD recipient	Percentage of LVAD ($n = 37$) recipients expressing concern
Infection	52
Difficulty sleeping due to the position of the driveline	52
Pain at the driveline exit site	46
Worry about device malfunction	40
Noise	32

LVAD, left ventricle assist device.

There is a clear survival advantage in patients receiving OHT. The second curve from the top represents that of the UCLA (University of California, Los Angeles) alternate list [68,69]. The emergence of alternate list strategies using otherwise unused donor organs has offered another option for those who would otherwise be excluded from heart transplantation. Thus, the aim of alternate list strategies is to provide hearts, which would typically be rejected as donor hearts, to patients who would typically be considered ineligible for transplant, usually due to age [70–72]. Although 90-day survival is somewhat compromised, recent studies have demonstrated similar medium-term (4-year) outcomes when comparing recipients from alternate lists to patients who were listed under more stringent criteria. Longer term survival in these mostly older patients may be compromised due to the effect of immunosuppression on the incidence of malignancies [68]. This collection of survival curves illustrates the fact that future refinements in long-term devices have the potential to offer an alternative to heart transplant in the elderly.

In addition, LVAD implantation may demand financial cost and trade-off some quality of life, which bias physicians and patients to choose OMM. DiGiorgi et al. compared the cost of LVAD therapy to that of OHT. Hospital costs following OHT were significantly less than those for patients receiving LVAD ($197,957 \pm 77,291$, $151,646 \pm 53,909$ ($p = 0.005$), respectively) [73]. In their analysis of the costs associated with the LVAD recipients in the REMATCH trial, Oz et al. calculated the cost for implant survivors to be $159,271 \pm 106,423$ [74]. Their regression analysis determined factors to affect implant cost include "sepsis, pump housing infection, and perioperative bleeding" [74].

Cowper et al. approximated the 5-year cost of medical management of heart failure with β-blockers to be $49,040—including inpatient, outpatient, and medication costs [75]. In a recent cost analysis of cardiac resynchronization therapy (CRT), the best estimate of the cost of CRT implantation was $33,495 [76].

Dew et al. have surveyed the concerns expressed by LVAD recipients [77]. Although the general perceptions of these patients were reported to be positive, many expressed specific concerns reproduced in Table 12.2.

Future directions: smaller continuous flow devices

The most significant impact of the REMATCH trial may have been its role as proof of the LVAD's utility as destination therapy. As a result, there has been a proliferation of academic and industry initiatives to apply novel technologies to this indication. Of particular interest are impellers, or axial flow pumps. These devices are smaller—making them less obtrusive to the patient and easier to implant. It is anticipated that these devices will be less prone to pocket and driveline infections. They generate higher flows at lower pressures, have decreased areas in contact with blood, and do not require valves [78,79].

Continuous flow devices and the artificial heart

Continuous flow assist devices

Continuous flow LVADs have been shown to support myocardial function; however, the systemic effects of continuous flow remain unclear.

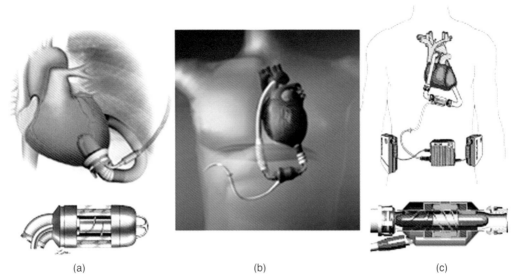

Figure 12.6 Continuous flow devices. (a) The Jarvik 2000 is implanted directly into the left ventricle. The electric motor (orange bar, lower picture) causes the impeller, which contains a magnet, to spin, creating blood flow along the blades. The outflow graft can be sutured to either the descending or ascending thoracic aorta. (b) The HeartMate II, similar to the Jarvik pump, contains blood-immersed bearings. (c) The Incor has a free-floating magnetically suspended impeller that is axially active and radially passive (shown in yellow). The inflow guide vane (shown in blue) allows blood to align itself along the impeller. The outflow guide vane (shown in red) reduces the rotational effects of the blood flow. (Reprinted with permission from the Thoratec, Jarvik Heart, and Berlin Heart Corporations.)

Continuous flow during diastole may be beneficial to end-organ function, or it may be injurious through negative-feedback regulation [80]. Generally, there can be preservation of pulsatile perfusion, as the left ventricle can eject blood through the axial pump, causing an acceleration of flow due to a change in pressure differential across the pump.

Jarvik 2000

The Jarvik 2000, also known as the Flowmaker (Jarvik Heart Inc., New York, NY, USA), provides continuous flow from the left ventricle to the descending or ascending aorta. The former has the advantage of decreased risk of cerebral thromboembolic event, but may cause stasis in the ascending aorta. The device is placed within the left ventricular; thus, no cannula is needed for inflow (Figure 12.6a) [81]. The Jarvik 2000 can provide a flow of 6 L/min [82]. It is 2.5 cm wide × 5.5 cm long and weighs 85 g. An analog controller sets the pump speed that can be changed by patients, on the basis of symptoms and needs. This is a unique biofeedback mechanism. Blood is drawn through the pump by an impeller suspended by ceramic bearings in a titanium housing. The impeller consists of neodymium–iron–boron magnet with two titanium blades. Pump output varies according to a difference in pressure across the pump. Power is supplied via an externalized cable either through the patient's right abdomen or, in cases of destination therapy, at the right mastoid process. Implantation is typically performed with the patient on cardiopulmonary bypass [83]; however, placement without the use of bypass has been reported [84].

Frazier et al. summarized the work of 23 patients who received the Jarvik 2000 device demonstrating an increase in cardiac index and a decrease in systemic vascular resistance and pulmonary capillary wedge pressure [82]. In a study comparing 11 patients receiving HeartMate I devices to 6 patients receiving the Jarvik 2000, Siegenthaler et al. demonstrated a significantly decreased rate of infections in the Jarvik 2000 group (7 patients with infection in the HeartMate group vs 1 in the Jarvik group) [83]. A similar study evaluated the serum creatinine, bilirubin, glutamic-oxaloacetic transaminase, and glutamic–pyruvic transaminase levels in 10 Jarvik 2000 recipients, demonstrating preservation of hepatic and renal function with continuous perfusion [85]. To date, the longest implant is ongoing at over 4 years.

HeartMate II

The HeartMate II is an axial flow pump that weighs 375 g and can provide a maximum flow of 10 L/min [78]. Blood enters the device from the apex of the left ventricle via a valveless sintered cannula (Figure 12.6b). The impeller is spun on a bearing by an electromagnetic motor [80]. The bearing has been tested for a lifespan of >5 years [79]. Exiting blood enters the ascending aorta via a vascular graft. The HeartMate II has a unique control feature that provides a significant advantage by ensuring appropriate ventricle filling and unloading [86]. By measuring afterload as the electrical impedance on the device, the HeartMate II controls its speed to permit pulsatility by the ventricle. The HeartMate II is designed as a modular system to allow for repairs and modifications according to patients' changing needs [79].

The first version of the HeartMate II was tested in Europe with limited results due to thrombus formation [80]. It was improved by adopting a smooth rather than a textured titanium surface of the inflow and outflow stators of impeller [80]. The device has since been approved for investigational purposes in the United States. Pagani et al. reported the outcomes in 25 patients who received the HeartMate II [87]. Complications included 3 incidences of multiple organ failure and 2 with right ventricular dysfunction. There were no embolic events reported. At the time of communication, 15 patients were supported for an average of 99 days while 3 patients were transplanted.

Incor

The Incor LVAD is an impeller device developed by the Berlin Heart Group (Berlin Heart AG, Berlin, Germany) [88]. The pump is 30 mm in diameter and weighs 200 g. Blood enters the device from the left ventricle via a positionable silicone inflow cannula (Figure 12.6c). The flow is driven by an impeller, which does not make contact with other parts of the device. Rather, the impeller is held in suspension by a magnet and can develop a flow of up to 7 L/min [88]. Theoretically, this would prevent wear on the moving impeller, which is in contact only with blood. Blood returns to the ascending aorta via a silicone outflow cannula.

In 2005, Schmid et al. presented the results of the first series of 15 patients receiving the Incor LVAD [88]. Reported complications included systemic emboli and thrombus-related pump dysfunction in 2 and 3 patients, respectively. The device is coated with Carmeda (Carmeda AB, Sweden), a heparin-derived substance that can theoretically be a cause of heparin-induced thrombocytopenia.

Total artificial heart (right and left ventricular replacement)

The quest for a total heart replacement is perhaps the only procedure that has tickled the imagination of humans as much as heart transplantation. The challenge of biventricular replacement lies in positioning two pumps in the abdomen. To date, only the Thoratec implantable VAD has succeeded in this endeavor (Figure 12.7a). This device is pneumatically driven and therefore requires a portable drive console.

Similarly, any artificial heart placed orthotopically must fit into the mediastinal space. Digitalized three-dimensional axial tomography has helped to predict fit. Only the pneumatically driven Cardiowest (originally named Jarvik 7) artificial heart is approved for bridge to transplant in both the United States and Europe (Figure 12.7b). This device consists of two ventricular replacement pumps joined together. The inflow cuffs are sewn onto the annuluses of the tricuspid and mitral valves and the outflow grafts are similarly sewn to the great vessels. It also requires a portable pneumatic driver and has two exiting drivelines. The Abiomed Abiocor total artificial heart is electric and totally implantable with a transcutaneous energy delivery system. (Figure 12.7c). It is still investigational. It has an ingenious design whereby right and left systoles occur in sequence. A single contained pump provides an electrohydraulic energy conversion. The inner hydraulic fluid then shifts via a small set of oscillating windows to alternately compress the right- and left-sided bladders. A compliance chamber on the left accounts for bronchial return.

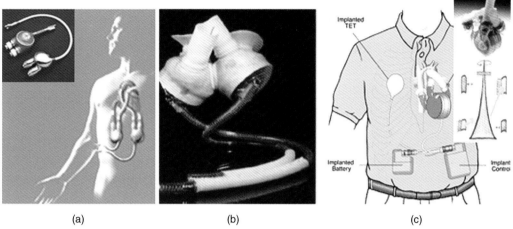

(a)   (b)   (c)

Figure 12.7 Long-term implantable biventricular assist and replacement. (a) The Thoratec implantable ventricular assist device system is a heterotopic long-term system that requires an external pneumatic driver (lower inset). The upper inset shows a comparison to the paracorporeal Thoratec pump. Right and left systoles occur asynchronously. (b) The Cardiowest artificial heart consists of two orthotopically placed ventricles, each requiring a separate pneumatic driveline. (c) The Abiocor electrically powered artificial heart (upper inset) consists of a single pump, which causes sequential right and left systoles. It is designed with a transcutaneous energy transfer system that permits an internal battery to accumulate power as well as a computerized interface with the implantable system controller. The lower part of the inset illustrates the electrohydrolic pumping mechanism. The fluid (shown in blue) shifts to cause compression of a bladder. Polyurethane valves ensure unidirectional flow. (Reprinted with permission from the Thoratec, SynCardia, and ABIOMED Corporations.)

Conclusion

LVADs have proven their ability to support the circulation as a "bridge to transplant." Results of the REMATCH trial demonstrate the expanded role of LVADs in the treatment of heart failure. Destination therapy significantly improved survival for certain subgroups of patients. This was at the cost of the risk of infection and neurological complications. This poses difficult choices for the patients and physicians.

Commensurate with the aging of the overall population, there has been a progressive increase in the number of recipients over the age of 60. As demonstrated in both the REMATCH trial and the MCSD, age is the most common reason for transplant ineligibility. Taken together, these two factors reveal that alternatives to heart transplantation are likely to evolve. The REMATCH trial can be viewed as proof of the concept that LVAD can function as permanent therapy. As a result, it has stimulated the development of newer smaller pumps that are anticipated to continue to improve survival while decreasing complications and burden on the patient's quality of life.

References

1. Farrar DJ, Holman WR, McBride LR, *et al.* Lsong-term follow-up of Thoratec ventricular assist device bridge-to-recovery patients successfully removed from support after recovery of ventricular function. J Heart Lung Transplant 2002;21:516–521.
2. Dandel M, Weng Y, Siniawski H, *et al.* Long-term results in patients with idiopathic dilated cardiomyopathy after weaning from left ventricular assist devices. Circulation 2005;112:I37–145.
3. Stevenson LW, Rose EA. Left ventricular assist devices: bridges to transplantation, recovery, and destination for whom? Circulation 2003;108:3059–3063.
4. Rose EA, Gelijns AC, Moskowitz AJ, *et al.* Long-term use of a left ventricular assist device for end-stage heart failure. N Engl J Med 2001;345:1435–1443.
5. DeBakey ME. Development of mechanical heart devices. Ann Thorac Surg 2005;79:S2228–S2231.
6. Dennis C, Hall DP, Moreno JR, *et al.* Left atrial cannulation without thoracotomy for total left heart bypass. Acta Chir Scand 1962;123:267–279.
7. Debakey M. Left ventricular by-pass pump for cardiac assistance: clinical experience. Am J Cardiol 1971;27:3–11.
8. Cooley DA, Akutsu T, Norman JC, *et al.* Total artificial heart in two-staged cardiac transplantation. Bull Tex Heart Inst 1981;8:305–319.

9. DiGiorgi PL, Rao V, Naka Y, *et al.* Which patient, which pump? J Heart Lung Transplant 2003;22:221–235.

10. Norman J, Brook M, Cooley D, *et al.* Total support of the circulation of a patient with post-cardiotomy stone-heart syndrome by a partial artificial heart (ALVAD) for 5 days followed by heart and kidney transplantation. Lancet 1978;1:1125–1127.

11. Rao V, Oz MC, Flannery MA, *et al.* Revised screening scale to predict survival after insertion of a left ventricular assist device. J Thorac Cardiovasc Surg 2003;125:855–862.

12. Topkara VK, Dang NC, Barili F, *et al.* Predictors and outcomes of continuous veno-venous hemodialysis use after implantation of a left ventricular assist device. J Heart Lung Transplant 2006;25:404–408.

13. Loebe M, Koerner MM, Lafuente JA, *et al.* Patient selection for assist devices: bridge to transplant. Curr Opin Cardiol 2003;18:141–146.

14. Oz MC, Goldstein DJ, Pepino P, *et al.* Screening scale predicts patients successfully receiving long-term implantable left ventricular assist devices. Circulation 1995;92:II169–II173.

15. Aaronson KD, Patel H, Pagani FD. Patient selection for left ventricular assist device therapy. Ann Thorac Surg 2003;75:S29–S35.

16. Miller LW. Patient selection for the use of ventricular assist devices as a bridge to transplantation. Ann Thorac Surg 2003;75:S66–S71.

17. Jessup M, Brozena S. Heart Fail. N Engl J Med 2003;348:2007–2018.

18. Eghtesady P, Nelson D, Schwartz SM, *et al.* Heparin-induced thrombocytopenia complicating support by the Berlin Heart. ASAIO J 2005;51:820–825.

19. Koster A, Sanger S, Hansen R, *et al.* Prevalence and persistence of heparin/platelet factor 4 antibodies in patients with heparin coated and noncoated ventricular assist devices. ASAIO J 2000;46:319–322.

20. Tsukui H, Teuteberg JJ, Murali S, *et al.* Biventricular assist device utilization for patients with morbid congestive heart failure: a justifiable strategy. Circulation 2005;112:I65–I72.

21. Marelli D, Laks H, Fazio D, *et al.* Mechanical assist strategy using the BVS 5000i for patients with heart failure. Ann Thorac Surg 2000;70:59–66.

22. Entwistle JW III, Bolno PB, Holmes E, *et al.* Improved survival with ventricular assist device support in cardiogenic shock after myocardial infarction. Heart Surg Forum 2003;6:316–319.

23. Samuels LE, Holmes EC, Garwood P, *et al.* Initial experience with the Abiomed AB 5000 ventricular assist device system. Ann Thorac Surg 2005;80:309–312.

24. Acker MA. Mechanical circulatory support for patients with acute-fulminant myocarditis. Ann Thorac Surg 2001;71:S73–S76; discussion S82–S85.

25. Furukawa K, Motomura T, Nose Y. Right ventricular failure after left ventricular assist device implantation: the need for an implantable right ventricular assist device. Artif Organs 2005;29:369–377.

26. Booth JV, Schinderle D, Welsby IJ. Pro: vasopressin is the vasoconstrictor of choice after cardiopulmonary bypass. J Cardiothorac Vasc Anesth 2002;16:773–775.

27. Wagner F, Dandel M, Gunther G, *et al.* Nitric oxide inhalation in the treatment of right ventricular dysfunction following left ventricular assist device implantation. Circulation 1997;96:II-291–II-296.

28. Rao V, Slater JP, Edwards NM, *et al.* Surgical management of valvular disease in patients requiring left ventricular assist device support. Ann Thorac Surg 2001;71:1448–1453.

29. Swartz MT, Lowdermilk GA, Moroney DA, *et al.* Ventricular assist device support in patients with mechanical heart valves. Ann Thorac Surg 1999;68:2248–2251.

30. Goldstein DJ, Seldomridge JA, Chen JM, *et al.* Use of aprotinin in LVAD recipients reduces blood loss, blood use, and perioperative mortality. Ann Thorac Surg 1995;59:1063–1067; discussion 1068.

31. Etz C, Welp H, Rothenburger M, *et al.* Analysis of platelet function during left ventricular support with the Incor and Excor system. Heart Surg Forum 2004;7:E423–E427.

32. Strauch JT, Spielvogel D, Haldenwang PL, *et al.* Recent improvements in outcome with the Novacor left ventricular assist device. J Heart Lung Transplant 2003;22:674–680.

33. Deng MC, Edward LB, Hertz MI, *et al.* Mechanical circulatory support device database of the International Society for Heart and Lung Transplantation: Third Annual Report 2005. J Heart Lung Transplant 2005;24:1182–1187.

34. Schenk S, Arusoglu L, Morshuis M, *et al.* Triple bridge-to-transplant in a case of giant cell myocarditis complicated by human leukocyte antigen sensitization and heparin-induced thrombocytopenia type II. Ann Thorac Surg 2006;81:1107–1109.

35. Holman WL, Skinner JL, Waites KB, *et al.* Infection during circulatory support with ventricular assist devices. Ann Thorac Surg 1999;68:711–716.

36. McKellar SH, Allred BD, Marks JD, *et al.* Treatment of infected left ventricular assist device using antibiotic-impregnated beads. Ann Thorac Surg 1999;67:554–555.

37. Itescu S, John R. Interactions between the recipient immune system and the left ventricular assist device surface: immunological and clinical implications. Ann Thorac Surg 2003;75:S58–S65.

38. Ankersmit HJ, Edwards NM, Schuster M, *et al.* Quantitative changes in T-cell populations after left ventricular assist device implantation: relationship to T-cell apoptosis and soluble CD95. Circulation 1999;100:II211–II215.

39. Schuster M, Kocher A, John R, *et al.* B-cell activation and allosensitization after left ventricular assist device implantation is due to T-cell activation and CD40 ligand expression. Hum Immunol 2002;63:211–220.

40. Joyce DL, Southard RE, Torre-Amione G, *et al.* Impact of left ventricular assist device (LVAD)-mediated humoral sensitization on post-transplant outcomes. J Heart Lung Transplant 2005;24:2054–2059.

41. Pamboukian SV, Costanzo MR, Dunlap S, *et al.* Relationship between bridging with ventricular assist device on rejection after heart transplantation. J Heart Lung Transplant 2005;24:310–315.

42. John R, Lietz K, Schuster M, *et al.* Immunologic sensitization in recipients of left ventricular assist devices. J Thorac Cardiovasc Surg 2003;125:578–591.

43. DeRose JJ Jr, Umana JP, Argenziano M, *et al.* Implantable left ventricular assist devices provide an excellent outpatient bridge to transplantation and recovery. J Am Coll Cardiol 1997;30:1773–1777.

44. Ashton RC Jr, Goldstein DJ, Rose EA, *et al.* Duration of left ventricular assist device support affects transplant survival. J Heart Lung Transplant 1996;15:1151–1157.

45. Long JW. Advanced mechanical circulatory support with the HeartMate left ventricular assist device in the year 2000. Ann Thorac Surg 2001;71:S176–S182; discussion S183–S184.

46. Pasque MK, Hanselman T, Shelton K, *et al.* Operative strategies to reduce complications in Novacor left ventricular assist device placement. J Card Surg 2004;19:329–335.

47. Martin J, Siegenthaler MP, Friesewinkel O, *et al.* Implantable left ventricular assist device for treatment of pulmonary hypertension in candidates for orthotopic heart transplantation—a preliminary study. Eur J Cardiothorac Surg 2004;25:971–977.

48. Adamson RM, Dembitsky WP, Jaski BE, *et al.* Left ventricular assist device support of medically unresponsive pulmonary hypertension and aortic insufficiency. ASAIO J 1997;43:365–369.

49. Salzberg SP, Lachat ML, von Harbou K, *et al.* Normalization of high pulmonary vascular resistance with LVAD support in heart transplantation candidates. Eur J Cardiothorac Surg 2005;27:222–225.

50. Vitali E, Colombo T, Bruschi G, *et al.* Different clinical scenarios for circulatory mechanical support in acute and chronic heart failure. Am J Cardiol 2005;96:34L–41L.

51. Moazami N, Pasque MK, Moon MR, *et al.* Mechanical support for isolated right ventricular failure in patients after cardiotomy. J Heart Lung Transplant 2004;23:1371–1375.

52. Goldstein DJ, Oz MC, Rose EA. Implantable left ventricular assist devices. N Engl J Med 1998;339:1522–1533.

53. Mancini DM, Beniaminovitz A, Levin H, *et al.* Low incidence of myocardial recovery after left ventricular assist device implantation in patients with chronic heart failure. Circulation 1998;98:2383–2389.

54. Muller J, Wallukat G, Weng Y-G, *et al.* Weaning from mechanical cardiac support in patients with idiopathic dilated cardiomyopathy. Circulation 1997;96:542–549.

55. Petrou M, Clarke S, Morrison K, *et al.* Clenbuterol increases stroke power and contractile speed of skeletal muscle for cardiac assist. Circulation 1999;99:713–720.

56. Terracciano CMN, Hardy J, Birks EJ, *et al.* Clinical recovery from end-stage heart failure using left-ventricular assist device and pharmacological therapy correlates with increased sarcoplasmic reticulum calcium content but not with regression of cellular hypertrophy. Circulation 2004;109:2263–2265.

57. Bartling B, Milting H, Schumann H, *et al.* Myocardial gene expression of regulators of myocyte apoptosis and myocyte calcium homeostasis during hemodynamic unloading by ventricular assist devices in patients with end-stage heart failure. Circulation 1999;100:216II–223II.

58. Birks EJ, Hall JL, Barton PJR, *et al.* Gene profiling changes in cytoskeletal proteins during clinical recovery after left ventricular-assist device support. Circulation 2005;112:I-57–I-64.

59. Heerdt PM, Holmes JW, Cai B, *et al.* Chronic unloading by left ventricular assist device reverses contractile dysfunction and alters gene expression in end-stage heart failure. Circulation 2000;102:2713–2719.

60. FDA. FDA approves heart assist pump for permanent use. FDA News, 2002.

61. Rose EA, Moskowitz AJ, Packer M, *et al.* The REMATCH trial: rationale, design, and end points. Ann Thorac Surg 1999;67:723–730.

62. Lazar RM, Shapiro PA, Jaski BK, *et al.* Neurological events during long-term mechanical circulatory support for heart failure: the Randomized Evaluation of Mechanical Assistance for the Treatment of Congestive Heart Failure (REMATCH) experience. Circulation 2004;109:2423–2427.

63. Holman WL, Park SJ, Long JW, *et al.* Infection in permanent circulatory support: experience from the REMATCH trial. J Heart Lung Transplant 2004;23:1359–1365.

64. World Heart Corporation. World Heart Corporation Announces Third Quarter 2003 Results. PR Newswire, 5 November 2003.

65. United Network for Organ Sharing. Kaplan-Meier Median Waiting Times for Registrations Listed: Heart. 1997–2002. United Network for Organ Sharing; 2002.

66. Park SJ, Tector A, Piccioni W, *et al*. Left ventricular assist devices as destination therapy: a new look at survival. J Thorac Cardiovasc Surg 2005;129:9–17.

67. Nelson K, Tong K, Ellman A, Long J. Advances in patient and economic outcomes associated with left ventricular assist devices for destination therapy. J Heart Lung Transplant 2005;24:S76–S77.

68. Laks H, Mitropoulos F, Odim J, *et al*. Long-term outcome of alternate list heart transplant patients. International Society for Heart and Lung Transplantation, Twenty-fifth Anniversary Meeting and Scientific Sessions. Philadelphia, PA, 2005; S70.

69. Laks H, Marelli D, Fonarow GC, *et al*. Use of two recipient lists for adults requiring heart transplantation. J Thorac Cardiovasc Surg 2003;125:49–59.

70. Chen JM, Russo MJ, Hammond KM, *et al*. Alternate waiting list strategies for heart transplantation maximize donor organ utilization. Ann Thorac Surg 2005;80:224–228.

71. Felker GM, Milano CA, Yager JE, *et al*. Outcomes with an alternate list strategy for heart transplantation. J Heart Lung Transplant 2005;24:1781–1786.

72. Laks H, Marelli D. The alternate recipient list for heart transplantation: a model for expansion of the donor pool. Adv Card Surg 1999;11:233–244.

73. DiGiorgi PL, Reel MS, Thornton B, *et al*. Heart transplant and left ventricular assist device costs. J Heart Lung Transplant 2005;24:200–204.

74. Oz MCMD, Gelijns ACP, Miller LMD, *et al*. Left ventricular assist devices as permanent heart failure therapy: the price of progress. Ann Surg October 2003; 238(4):577–585.

75. Cowper PA, DeLong ER, Whellan DJ, Allen LaPointe NM, Califf RM. Economic effects of beta-blocker therapy in patients with heart failure. Am J Med 2004;116:135–136.

76. Nichol G, Kaul P, Huszti E, Bridges FP. Cost-effectiveness of cardiac resynchronization therapy in patients with symptomatic heart failure. Ann Intern Med 2004;141:343–351.

77. Dew MA, Kormos RL, Winowich S, et al.. Human factors issues in ventricular assist device recipients and their family caregivers. ASAIO J 2000;46:367–373.

78. Song X, Throckmorton AL, Untaroiu A, *et al*. Axial flow blood pumps. ASAIO J 2003;49:355–364.

79. Burke DJ, Burke E, Parsaie F, *et al*. The HeartMate II: design and development of a fully sealed axial flow left ventricular assist system. Artif Organs 2001;25:380–385.

80. Frazier OH, Delgado RM III, Kar B, *et al*. First clinical use of the redesigned HeartMate II left ventricular assist system in the United States: a case report. Tex Heart Inst J 2004;31:157–159.

81. Frazier OH, Myers TJ, Gregoric ID, *et al*. Initial clinical experience with the Jarvik 2000 implantable axial-flow left ventricular assist system. Circulation 2002;105:2855–2860.

82. Frazier OH, Myers TJ, Westaby S, *et al*. Use of the Jarvik 2000 left ventricular assist system as a bridge to heart transplantation or as destination therapy for patients with chronic heart failure. Ann Surg 2003;237:631–636; discussion 636–637.

83. Siegenthaler MP, Martin J, Pernice K, *et al*. The Jarvik 2000 is associated with less infections than the HeartMate left ventricular assist device. Eur J Cardiothorac Surg 2003;23:748–754; discussion 754–755.

84. Frazier OH. Implantation of the Jarvik 2000 left ventricular assist device without the use of cardiopulmonary bypass. Ann Thorac Surg 2003;75:1028–1030.

85. Letsou GV, Myers TJ, Gregoric ID, *et al*. Continuous axial-flow left ventricular assist device (Jarvik 2000) maintains kidney and liver perfusion for up to 6 months. Ann Thorac Surg 2003;76:1167–1170.

86. Raman J, Jeevanadam V. Destination therapy with ventricular assist devices. Cardiology 2004;101:104–110.

87. Pagani F, Strueber Y, Naka RL, *et al*. Initial multicenter clinical results with the HeartMate II axial flow left ventricular assist device. International Society for Heart and Lung Transplantation, Twenty-fifth Anniversary Meeting and Scientific Sessions. Philadelphia, PA, 2005, p. S74.

88. Schmid C, Tjan TD, Etz C, *et al*. First clinical experience with the Incor left ventricular assist device. J Heart Lung Transplant 2005;24:1188–1194.

CHAPTER 13

The Role of Enhanced External Counterpulsation in Heart Failure Management

Marc A. Silver[1], & William E. Lawson[2]
[1]Advocate Christ Medical Center, Oak Lawn, IL, USA; and University of Illinois, Chicago, IL, USA
[2]SUNY, Stony Brook, Stony Brook, NY, USA

Introduction

Counterpulsation was developed as the prototypical method of circulatory assistance, designed to reduce cardiac workload while preserving cardiac and vital organ perfusion. Currently, counterpulsation is routinely used as the intra-aortic balloon pump, placed during episodes of cardiac decompensation, for acute circulatory support. The intra-aortic balloon pump was first developed in the 1950s and commercially introduced in the 1970s, and has been an essential assist device for cardiac and circulatory support ever since. The development of the invasive, surgically, or percutaneously placed (internal) intra-aortic balloon has, however, been paralleled by the development of a less well-known noninvasive (external) method. Early developmental efforts for both devices targeted acute circulatory decompensation, especially cardiogenic shock, and the first publication comparing both methods appeared in 1973 [1]. Amsterdam et al. in 1980 published the results of the first multicenter trial, demonstrating that external counterpulsation was beneficial in the treatment of acute myocardial infarction complicated by cardiogenic shock [2]. The external counterpulsation used in this and other early studies was a cumbersome hydraulic device, encasing the lower extremities as a single chamber, with residual pressure limiting extremity inflow. These devices were crude, bulky, and less hemodynamically efficient than intra-aortic counterpulsation, hindering their adoption.

In time, major progress was made. First, air replaced water to fill the cuffs, allowing for lighter, faster equipment and allowing elimination of the residual pressure that limited limb inflow. Second, sequential cuff inflation was introduced, significantly increasing the hemodynamic effect. Indeed, the current generation of external counterpulsation devices has greater hemodynamic effects than that of intra-aortic counterpulsation [3].

Simultaneously with investigations into the use of counterpulsation for circulatory support, its use in chronic stable angina was assessed [4]. The results were disappointing, probably due to the brevity (4 × 2 h) of the studied treatment. With a limited clinical application, use in the United States diminished and disappeared from clinical practice. However, Dr Zheng, in China, continued to develop the device and define its clinical applications. After years of work, enhanced external counterpulsation (EECP) (i.e., rapid ECG-gated sequential inflation and simultaneous deflation of cuffs wrapped around the calves, thighs, and buttocks at suprasystolic pressures during diastole) was reintroduced into the United States in the late 1980s by Drs Soroff and Hui. An initial series of small research studies of chronic, stable angina patients, utilizing 35–36 hours of treatment over 4–7 weeks, at Stony Brook

Heart Failure: Device Management. Edited by Arthur Feldman.
© 2010 Blackwell Publishing.

University (New York), confirmed the benefits of treating this population. A pivotal, prospective, multicenter, randomized, blinded, sham-controlled trial was performed (MUST-EECP, Vasomedical, Westbury, NY, USA) demonstrating an increase in time to exercise induced ST-segment depression and a reduction in anginal episodes with treatment. EECP clearly improved the functional and clinical status of patients with chronic stable angina pectoris. Subsequent reports have validated these trial results and demonstrated both long-term symptom relief [5] and sustained improvement in the quality of life [6,7]. Reimbursement coverage by the Centers for Medicare & Medicaid Services began in 1999; today, there are more than 1000 EECP centers worldwide, treating 30,000 patients annually [8].

Mechanisms of action (see Table 13.1)

An initial, overly simplistic, mechanistic model considered only the acute hemodynamic effects of counterpulsation. Led by the evidence of sustained clinical effects, research has focused on the clarification of mechanisms that could lead to sustained effects. While initial efforts to understand the mechanism of action of EECP focused on angiogenesis, emerging evidence suggests a broader role in endovascular health and neurohumoral passivation mediated primarily by shear stress. EECP appears to produce a complex ensemble of effects that supports the overall benefits of treatment.

Michaels et al. studied a portable EECP device in patients invasively assessed with pressure and flow wires in the cardiac catheterization laboratory, showing that EECP produces marked diastolic augmentation of pressure and flow in the coronary arteries [3]. Taguchi extended the hemodynamic understanding of EECP, demonstrating that the increase in venous return with EECP is largely responsible for the significant increase in cardiac output compared to IABP, presumably through the Starling mechanism, with similar effects on ventricular unloading [9]. Confirming evidence of increased venous return is the parallel acute increase in atrial natriuretic peptide (ANP), an indicator of left ventricular filling [10]. By improving cardiac output, EECP acutely provides circulatory support and improved perfusion to the body's organ systems. Studies of EECP have demonstrated improved perfusion

of the heart [3], the eye [11], the brain [12], the skin [13], and the kidney [14].

Interestingly, EECP increased flow velocity in the eye only in areas of decreased perfusion or when atherosclerosis was present, suggesting that local autoregulation may be dependent on local endovascular function [10]. A unifying hypothesis for a mechanism of action arises from our understanding of the acute hemodynamic effects of EECP. EECP increases venous return, produces diastolic augmentation, and increases cardiac output as well as coronary flow, all factors increasing intravascular shear stress. Increased shear stress is known to trigger angiogenesis and to improve vascular function through the modulation of vasoactive factors. In the dog model of acute infarction, Wu et al. demonstrated that EECP produced coronary collaterals, confirming findings of angiogenesis noted in a much earlier study [15,16]. While this model may not directly apply to man, the extensive literature supporting improvement in myocardial perfusion after EECP is indirect evidence of improved vascularity. Recent evidence has shown that EECP dramatically increased levels of serum vascular endothelial growth factor [17] and other, similarly active factors in patients [18]. More direct evidence is provided in an elegant study by Werner et al. using assessments of changes in ocular blood flow after a short course of EECP [19]. A recent randomized trial of EECP in chronic stable angina patients by Barsheshet et al. demonstrated that EECP significantly increased circulating endothelial progenitor cells positive for CD34 measured by flow cytometry and kinase insert domain receptor measured by the number of colony-forming units, suggesting a potential role for EECP in vasculogenesis and endovascular repair [20].

The positive role of EECP-mediated shear stress in maintenance of endovascular health has been further demonstrated by Zhang et al. in high–cholesterol-diet pigs randomized to EECP. EECP increased peak diastolic arterial wall shear stress and reduced intima-to-media area ratio by 42% compared with high-cholesterol group. EECP treatment increased the protein expression of endothelial nitric oxide synthase and suppressed phosphorylation of extracellular signal-regulated kinases [21].

EECP has also been demonstrated to suppress pro-inflammatory markers, often associated with

Table 13.1 Mechanism of action.

Reference	Inventor	Year	N	Population	Design	Effects
14	Jacobey	1963	21	Dogs	Two groups: Acute coronary occlusion with and without EECP	After acute coronary occlusion, mortality of 54% in control group vs 11% in EECP group
					Additional testing of EECP on normal dogs and dogs with chronic ischemia	EECP (×2 h) opened dormant coronary collaterals in dogs with conditions of ischemia (acute or chronic) but not in normal dogs
59	Lawson	1996	27	CAD	Single group; RNGXT pre and post 35 h EECP	81% improved exercise tolerance, 78% improved radionuclide stress perfusion images. Attenuation of blood pressure rise with exercise suggested a peripheral "training" effect. Increased post-EECP exercise tolerance may relate to improved myocardial perfusion and a decrease in cardiac workload
12	Applebaum	1997	35 18	CAD	Single group: two subgroups (carotid and renal blood flow)	Significantly increased carotid and renal blood flow in all subjects studied (35 and 18, respectively)
9	Taguchi	2000	23 12	AMI	Two groups EECP (1 h) vs IABP	Similar diastolic augmentation in the two groups. Increased right atrial pressure, pulmonary capillary wedge pressure, and cardiac index in the EECP group only
18	Masuda	2001	11	Chronic stable angina	Single group EECP 35 (1 h) sessions	Promoted release of angiogenesis factors, especially HGF, through increased shear stress, and resulted in increased functional collateral vessels
19	Werner	2001	12 12	Healthy CAD	Two groups: healthy vs CAD Blood flow velocity measured during first minute of EECP application	Significantly increased blood flow velocity in the ophthalmic artery of CAD subjects by 11.4%, but not in healthy subjects
27	Urano	2001	12	Stable Angina	Single group EECP 35 (1 h) sessions	Improved LV diastolic filling and reduced myocardial ischemia as measured by thallium scintigraphy
28	Masuda	2001	11	Stable Angina	Single group EECP 18–35 (1 h) sessions	Improved myocardial perfusion measured at stress by N-ammonia PET scan, at the same cardiac workload, follow-up vs baseline
3	Michaels	2002	10	Diagnostic Cath	Single group EECP (300 mmHg)	Acutely increased coronary artery pressure and flow velocity following significant increase in diastolic pressure in the central aorta

(Cont.)

Table 13.1 (*Continued*)

Reference	Inventor	Year	N	Population	Design	Effects
30	Stys	2002	175	Stable Angina	Single group EECP 35 (1 h) sessions	Improved myocardial perfusion measured at stress by radionuclide scan, at the same cardiac workload, follow-up vs baseline
23	Bonetti	2003	23	CAD	Single group EECP 35 (1 h) sessions	Improved endothelial function as shown by increased reactive hyperemia index
29	Tartaglia	2003	25	Stable Angina	Single group EECP 35 (1 h) sessions	Improved myocardial perfusion measured at stress by SPECT and maximal exercise (different workloads at baseline follow-up)
36	Levenson	2003	55	30 subjects with chronic, stable CAD, 25 with high CV risk factors	Randomized, Sham controlled EECP vs Sham EECP, single (1 h) session	Significantly increased plasma cGMP concentration and platelet content; inhibition reduced and stimulation increased cGMP, suggesting activation of nitric oxide pathway
10	Taguchi	2004	24	AMI	Single group EECP (1 h)	Increased CI and ANP, but not BNP (increase in BNP being associated with worsening of cardiac function)
11	Werner	2004	20	Central or branch retinal artery occlusion	Two groups: hemodilution and EECP (2 h) vs hemodilution alone	Immediately increased perfusion in ischemic retinal areas in EECP group. Increase in perfusion in both groups, with no difference between groups 48 h later
60	Bagger	2004	23	Stable angina + dobutamine stress echo	Single group EECP 35 (1 h) sessions	Stress-induced wall motion score (WMS) improved by ≥ 2 grades in 43% of the patients and exercise capacity increased by 73 s in the 18 patients who were able to exercise
5	Michaels	2004	34	Stable angina	Single group EECP 35 (1 h) sessions	No change in myocardial perfusion measured at stress by radionuclide, at same cardiac workload at baseline and follow-up. Clinical and exercise capacity improvements following EECP attributed to peripheral training effect
16	Wu	2005	12	Dogs	Randomized controlled Acute coronary occlusion with and without EECP	Significantly increased density of microvessels in infarcted regions of EECP group compared to controls Improved myocardial perfusion as assessed by SPECT
39	Grayson	2004	20	Chronic, stable CAD and healthy, sedentary volunteers	Two groups, CAD (10) and healthy, sedentary volunteers (10) Single (1 h) EECP session	Increased oxygen uptake (VO_2) during active EECP in both groups

Table 13.1 (*Continued*)

Reference	Inventor	Year	N	Population	Design	Effects
40	Ochoa	2006	20	Chronic, stable CAD and healthy, sedentary volunteers	Two groups, CAD (10) and healthy, sedentary volunteers (10) Single (30 min) EECP session	Increased oxygen uptake (VO_2) during active EECP in both groups
25	Nichols	2006	20	Chronic, stable angina	Single group 34 (1 h) sessions	Significant decrease in augmentation index and increase in reflected wave travel time consistent with reduced arterial stiffness. Decreases left ventricular afterload, myocardial oxygen demand, improves CCS class
37	Levenson	2006	55	30 CAD and 25 controls with cardiac risk factors	Two groups, CAD and controls with cardiac risk factors randomized to Sham or (1 h) EECP session	EECP increased cGMP plasma concentration and platelet content, suggesting nitric oxide synthase activation
26	Levenson	2007	30	Chronic, stable CAD	Randomized, sham controlled EECP vs Sham EECP, 35 (1 h) sessions	Significantly decreased carotid artery wall stiffness and vascular resistance, EECP vs Sham EECP
21	Zhang	2007	35	Male swine	Randomized, control, high cholesterol diet $\pm$ EECP	EECP increased peak diastolic arterial wall shear stress and reduced intima-to-media area ratio by 42% compared with high-cholesterol group. EECP treatment increased the protein expression of endothelial nitric oxide synthase and suppressed phosphorylation of extracellular signal-regulated kinases.
49	Estahbanaty	2007	25	Chronic, stable angina	Single group 35 h EECP	EECP significantly reduced systolic and diastolic volumes and increased ejection fraction in patients with baseline LVEF $\leq$ 50%, E/Ea $\geq$ 14, grade II or III diastolic dysfunction (decreased compliance), Ea < 7 cm/s and baseline Sm < 7 cm/s, but not in patients without these findings
61	Michaels	2007	27	Chronic, stable angina	Single group 35 h EECP	48-h Holter showed no significant changes in the time- or frequency-domain HR. Variability measures after EECP. Diabetics increased low-frequency HRV, which has been associated with reduced mortality

(*Cont.*)

Table 13.1 (*Continued*)

Reference	Inventor	Year	N	Population	Design	Effects
20	Barsheshet	2008	25	Chronic, stable angina	Randomized (15 EECP; 10 control)	Circulating endothelial progenitor cells positive for CD34 measured by flow cytometry and kinase insert domain receptor measured by the number of colony-forming units. Significant increase in EECP group; no significant change in Sham group
22	Casey	2008	21	Chronic, stable angina	Randomized, sham controlled (12 EECP; 9 Sham)	Tumor necrosis factor was reduced by 29% and monocyte chemoattractant protein-1 by 19% in EECP group; no significant change in Sham group
62	Hashemi	2008	15	Ischemic cardiomyopathy	Single group EECP 35 (1 h) sessions	EECP improved endothelium-dependent, but not - independent relaxation. However, endothelium-dependent vasorelaxation returned to baseline by 1-mo post-EECP

AMI, acute myocardial infarction; ANP, atrial natriuretic peptide; BNP, brain natriuretic peptide; CAD, coronary artery disease; CCS, Canadian Cardiovascular Society; cGMP, cyclic guanosine monophosphate; CI, cardiac index; EECP, enhanced external counterpulsation; HGF, human growth factor; HR, heart rate; HRV, heart rate variability; IABP, intra-aortic balloon pump; LV, left ventricular; LVEF, left ventricular ejection fraction; RNGXT, radionucleotide-graded exercise test; SPECT, single photon emission computed tomography.

an increased risk of cardiac events. In a randomized study of EECP in patients with chronic, stable angina, Casey et al. demonstrated a 29% reduction in tumor necrosis factor and a 19% reduction in monocyte chemoattractant protein-1 in the EECP group [22].

In sum, the preponderance of evidence suggests that EECP positively effects endovascular structure and function. The effect on vascular health is not confined to the heart but includes all vessels. Well-controlled investigations have demonstrated that EECP improves brachial vasoreactivity [23], arterial compliance [24], and vascular resistance [25,26].

While inferential as to mechanism, most studies of EECP have demonstrated improved myocardial perfusion [27–30], though one study, while failing to show increased perfusion, still confirmed the clinical benefits of EECP [31]. Further substantiation for the endovascular "health" benefits of EECP are illustrated by a case of coronary vascular dysfunction reported by the Mayo Clinic [32] and a case series of 30 patients with cardiac syndrome X, also known as microvascular angina, in which EECP treatment resulted in improvement in angina, sustained at 1 year in 87% (and resolution of exercise-induced wall motion abnormalities) [33].

EECP alters endovascular tone, changing the local milieu and balance of vasodilators and vasoconstrictors. Treatment is associated with a marked decrease in the potent vasoconstrictor, endothelin, with a gradual return to baseline after stopping the treatment [34]. Similarly, nitric oxide, a potent vasodilator, increased during treatment with EECP, with elevated, though diminishing levels over the 3 months following treatment [35]. Corroborating this evidence, Levenson et al. demonstrated that a single hour of EECP increases cGMP in plasma and platelets, consistent with activation of the nitric oxide pathway [36,37].

Other authors have found that ANP tends to decrease following the application of EECP [12,22]. In addition, these authors showed that BNP, which was significantly elevated prior to treatment, was markedly lowered upon treatment initiation and continued to decrease thereafter.

In summary, these data suggest that EECP favorably affects perfusion by favoring angiogenesis and improving vascular function. These effects seem to benefit all organs and appear dose dependent, as changes occur immediately upon treatment initiation, increase with the number of treatment sessions, and most often are maintained well beyond the end of therapy.

There have been studies to suggest that EECP effects cellular energetics and metabolism, but the picture is incomplete. Masuda et al. found that EECP has a favorable effect on regional myocardial oxygen metabolism in ischemic regions, as indicated by others [38]. By contrast, nonischemic regions were unchanged, suggesting that EECP primarily affects areas where vascular or metabolic abnormalities are present. In studies of EECP in patients with heart failure, exploratory results indicated that the etiology of heart failure did not significantly impact the effectiveness of the device, suggesting that EECP may directly affect contractility [36]. During the application of EECP to coronary artery disease patients and healthy volunteers, oxygen uptake increased [39,40].

Likewise, no difference was observed in the benefit derived in large cohorts of stable angina patients with heart failure irrespective of whether the etiology was systolic or diastolic dysfunction [41]. In studies in the dog model of acute myocardial infarction, the acute hemodynamic effects of EECP also produce significant downregulation of tissue and circulating levels of components of the renin–angiotensin system, potentially benefiting cardiovascular remodeling and function [42].

Taken together, these data suggest that EECP may affect the myocardium in ways other than vascular, i.e., at the level of cellular metabolism or by modification of neurohumoral activation.

While the acute mechanistic effects of EECP are readily apparent, the means by which the immediate hemodynamic effects translate into the observed long-term clinical benefit is less clear. Working hypotheses embrace neurohumoral, structural, and endovascular effects. Given that the benefit of EECP appears to be time and/or dose dependent, it is likely that the benefit is related to cumulative effects occurring at the vascular and possibly cellular levels.

EECP in heart failure: evidence (see Table 13.2)

The initial studies of the safety and benefit of EECP in patients with left ventricular dysfunction and heart failure were performed in a large prospective registry (International EECP Patient Registry, IEPR) coordinated by the University of Pittsburgh. The IEPR tracked immediate and up to 3-year outcomes in sequentially enrolled patients from numerous centers. While the bulk of the patients had angina refractory to medical or revascularization therapy, a large proportion (about 22%) of the patients treated for stable angina pectoris also had systolic dysfunction or symptoms of heart failure. The initial report from the IEPR showed the heart failure patients to be sicker, less likely to complete EECP, and more likely to have exacerbation of heart failure during treatment; overall major adverse cardiac events (death, myocardial infarction, revascularization) were similar to the patients without heart failure. Angina class improved in 68% of heart failure patients, with comparable quality of life benefit. At 6 months, patients with heart failure maintained their reduction in angina but were significantly more likely to have experienced a major adverse clinical event (MACE) endpoint than did patients without heart failure [43].

Soran et al. [44] published results comparing subgroups with preserved and compromised systolic function, reporting that the cohort of patients with systolic dysfunction had more severe background disease compared to patients with normal ventricular function. However, both populations showed significant benefits in terms of symptom relief (67.8% vs 76.2% improved by one or more CCS classes, $p < 0.01$) and quality of life immediately after treatment with EECP as well as 6 months thereafter. MACEs (death, myocardial infarction, coronary artery bypass grafting, percutaneous coronary intervention) were similar during treatment, but exacerbation of heart failure (5.4% vs 1.0%, $p < 0.001$) and unstable angina (4.2% vs 2.0%, $p < 0.05$) were higher in patients with left ventricular dysfunction. Subsequently, these authors reported that such benefits were sustained at 2 years in the majority of patients, with a 2-year survival of 83% and a major cardiovascular event-free survival rate of 70% [45].

Table 13.2 Evidence in heart failure.

Reference	Inventor	Year	N	Population	Design	Results
43	Lawson	2001	1957	CAD ± HF	Observational (EECP registry) two groups CAD (1409) CAD + HF (548)	HF group was sicker, less likely to complete EECP, and more likely to have exacerbation of HF; overall major adverse cardiac events (death, myocardial infarction, revascularization) were similar. Angina class improved in 68%, with comparable quality of life benefit. At 6 mo, patients with HF maintained their reduction in angina but were significantly more likely to have experienced an MACE endpoint.
44	Soran	2002	1402	Chronic stable angina	Observational (EECP registry) two groups LVEF > 35% (1090) LVEF ≤ 35% (312)	Patients with LVD had improved anginal status similar to patients without LVD immediately post-EECP and 6-mo after EECP, despite more history of MI and CHF, longer duration of CAD, and more severe CCS class at baseline. Patients with LVD experienced more AEs during EECP treatment and at 6-mo follow-up. A significantly higher proportion of patients in the LVD group had CV outcomes (15.4% vs 8.3%)
46	Soran	2002	32 enrolled 26 treated 23 with FU 19 completed study	Chronic stable HF LVEF ≤ 35% NYHA II–III	Open, single group EECP 35 (1 h) sessions 6-mo follow-up	6-mo follow-up • NYHA (N = 23): 12 maintained improvement, 5 had no change, and 4 worsen • Exercise duration: 15.6% increase (N = 19) • Peak VO$_2$: 27% increase (N = 19) • Quality of life: improvement maintained (N = 19) • Echo substudy: significant increase in PAMP was observed after EECP therapy from 4.2 ± 2.0 to 5.4 ± 2.0 mW/cm^4; p < 0.05 vs baseline in 8 subjects participating in the substudy
52	Feldman	2005	187 randomized 178 treated 164 with FU	Chronic stable HF LVEF ≤ 35% NYHA II–III Optimal care	Controlled, single blind EECP 35 (1 h) sessions 6-mo follow-up	6-mo follow-up: 164 subjects • Ex duration: increase ≥ 60 s in 35% (EECP) vs 25% (control); p = 0.016 • Peak VO$_2$: no difference between groups in % subjects who improved by 1.5 mL/kg/min or more; peak VO$_2$ increased at 1-wk posttreatment overall (strong trend) and in ischemic heart disease subgroup (p < 0.05). EECP group on average tended to maintain improvement, while control group showed a progressive deterioration of peak VO$_2$ over time • NYHA: shift in NYHA class significantly better in EECP group • Quality of life: significantly greater improvement from baseline as measured by MLHQ physical and emotional scores. A significantly higher proportion of subjects in EECP group reported improvement in their health as compared to 1 yr ago (SF-36)

	Author	Year	Population	Study type	Results
48	Arora	2005	Chronic stable refractory angina CCS I–III	Single group EECP 35 (1 h) sessions	Improved systolic function as measured by increase of LVEF at rest and at stress using echocardiography in subjects with normal and mild systolic dysfunction
51	Lawson	2005	Chronic stable angina with CCS III (90%) IV (10%) History of HF	Observational (EECP registry) two groups LVEF > 35% (391 S) LVEF ≤ 35% (355 D)	Post-EECP (32 h) • Angina reduced by ≥1 class in 72% in both groups 1-yr follow-up • Angina: less than pre-EECP in 78% (D) vs 76% (S) • MACE: 24.3% (D) vs 23.8% (S)
53	Feldman	2006	NYHA class II–III	Prospective, randomized (PEECH trial)	35% EECP and 25% of controls increased exercise time $\geq$ 60 s ($p = 0.016$) at 6 mo. No difference in the percentage with $\geq$1.25 mL/kg/min increase in MVO_2. NYHA improved in with EECP at 1-wk ($p < 0.01$), 3 mo ($p < 0.02$), and 6 mo ($p < 0.01$) posttreatment. The Minnesota Living with Heart Failure score also improved significantly in the treated group at 1 wk ($p < 0.002$) and 3 mo ($p = 0.01$) after treatment versus no significant changes in the controls
63	Abbottsmith	2006	NYHA class II–III	Prespecified subgroup ($\geq$65 yr) of PEECH trial	At 6 mo, 35.1% EECP vs 25.0% controls increased exercise time $\geq$ 60 s ($p = 0.008$) and 29.7% EECP vs 11.4% controls increased MVO_2 > 1.25 mL/kg/min ($p = 0.017$). The mean changes in exercise duration and MVO_2 from baseline were significantly increased compared with the controls at 1 wk, 3 mo, and 6 mo
45	Soran	2006	Refractory angina and LVEF ≤ 35%	Observational (IEPR-EECP registry)	EECP resulted in improved angina, and quality of life, maintained at 2 yr
64	Soran	2007		Observational (IEPR-EECP registry)	ER visits and hospitalizations decreased significantly ($p < 0.001$) in the 6-mo post-EECP, realizing an estimated cost savings of $10,000/patient
57	Cohen	2007	Acute coronary syndrome and/or heart failure	Observational (2–4 h EECP)	EECP was safe and effective in treating acute coronary syndrome alone ($n = 4$), cardiogenic shock alone ($n = 3$), or both ($n = 3$) in patients who were not candidates for IABP support

AE, adverse events; CAD, coronary artery disease; CCS, Canadian Cardiovascular Society; CHF, congestive heart failure; EECP, enhanced external counterpulsation; HF, heart failure; LVD, left ventricular dysfunction; LVEF, left ventricular ejection fraction; MI, myocardial infarction; MACE, major adverse clinical event; NYHA, New York Heart Association; PAMP, pulmonary artery mean pressure; MLHQ, Minnesota Living with Heart Failure Questionnaire.

The registry data from the IEPR demonstrated that EECP could be used safely in patients with a history of systolic or diastolic heart failure and with persistent left ventricular dysfunction. Anginal symptoms improved and the improvements in angina and quality of life were maintained. However, the obvious questions of whether EECP was effective in patients with the primary diagnosis of heart failure and at what stage of decompensation remained unanswered.

To provide an estimate of the number needed for a pivotal trial of effectiveness, a pilot safety trial was performed in patients with the primary diagnosis of heart failure [46].

Heart failure patients were carefully selected to include only patients in stable clinical condition and without any overt fluid overload (rales or peripheral edema). In this single group, feasibility study, EECP (35 1-h sessions) proved to be safe, with preliminary indications of effectiveness. Peak oxygen uptake (+27.1%) and exercise duration (+15.6%) were increased at 6 months, as were symptoms and quality of life measures. The benefits in ischemic and idiopathic heart failure cohorts were similar, with echocardiography suggesting an improvement in ventricular function that was sustained over the follow-up period [47].

In small, prospective or retrospective, single-group studies, EECP effected on increase in left ventricular ejection fraction (LVEF) in groups of patients with normal or mildly depressed left ventricular function, while no changes in diastolic function were found [48]. A similar echocardiographic study demonstrated that EECP significantly reduced systolic and diastolic volumes and increased ejection fraction in patients with baseline LVEF $\leq$ 50%, E/Ea $\geq$ 14, grade II or III diastolic dysfunction (decreased compliance), Ea < 7 cm/s and baseline Sm < 7 cm/s, but not in patients without these findings [49].

In the IEPR, EECP was shown to improve functional capacity in patients with left ventricular dysfunction as assessed by the Duke Activity Status Index, a questionnaire that correlates well with peak oxygen uptake [50]. Other data from the same registry showed that in patients with angina pectoris and a history of congestive heart failure, the effects of EECP were similar when systolic function was preserved (diastolic heart failure) or depressed [51].

Symptoms, functional status, frequency of anginal episodes, and use of on-demand nitroglycerin improved to a similar degree, while MACEs were also similar in both groups. EECP resulted in improved angina and quality of life maintained at 2 years [45].

On the basis of the favorable pilot trial results, a controlled, multicenter, prospective, and randomized trial, the Prospective Evaluation of EECP® in Congestive Heart Failure (PEECH) trial, was performed to definitively evaluate the role of EECP in heart failure patients [52]. The PEECH trial enrolled heart failure patients (ischemic or idiopathic; LVEF $\leq$ 35%, NYHA class II/III) receiving optimal medical therapy. After a 2-week baseline period, subjects were randomized to either optimal medical therapy alone or optimal care plus EECP. The EECP cohort received 35 hours of EECP as 1-hour sessions spaced over 7 weeks. Both groups were followed for an additional 6 months with blinded evaluations (core laboratory and site investigators) at 1 week, 3 months, and 6 months. Two primary endpoints were defined measuring changes in exercise capacity, the percentage of subjects who increased exercise duration by 60 seconds or more, and the percentage of subjects who increased peak oxygen uptake by 1.5 mL/kg/min or more. Both thresholds were selected to be above any effect observed in the placebo groups or inactive drug groups of prior trials in similar populations.

Results at 6 months showed that exercise duration increased by 60 seconds or more in a 35.4% of subjects receiving EECP compared to 25.3% of controls at 6 months ($p = 0.016$). Mean exercise duration (a secondary endpoint) was also significantly increased at 1 week, 3 months, and 6 months (21.7 vs −9.9 s at 6 mo, $p = 0.01$) in the EECP compared to the control cohort. By contrast, peak oxygen uptake increased at 1 week, but not at later time points. The secondary endpoint of improved NYHA significantly favored EECP at all time points (31.3% vs 14.3% at 6 mo, $p < 0.01$). Quality of life, as assessed by the Minnesota Living with Heart Failure score, increased significantly in EECP-treated patients compared to controls at 1 week and 3 months posttreatment, but was not significantly different at 6 months. Thus, results showed that in optimally treated patients with mild-to-moderate heart failure, EECP provided benefits in only select outcome markers [53]. These results were not convincing to individuals or the CMS panel and therefore Medicare will not reimburse for EECP where the indication is heart failure.

When to recommend EECP for patients with heart failure

Indications for use of EECP therapy approved by Food and Drug Administration include stable and unstable angina, congestive heart failure, acute myocardial infarction, and cardiogenic shock. Use in acute conditions has been scarce to date. Large registry studies suggest that EECP provides consistent benefits in patients regardless of age, ventricular function, prior diagnosis of heart failure, or gender [43,54,55,44]. Furthermore, EECP is effective in the presence of diabetes mellitus [56]. This experience is important as about 25% of patients treated for symptoms of stable angina pectoris have a concomitant diagnosis of heart failure and experience similar benefit, though, as expected, they incur a slightly higher rate of clinical events. As in most clinical trials some but not all endpoints were attained in heart failure patients, leading CMS to deny funding approval. In addition, routine use is not recommended by the American Heart Association/American College of Cardiology Heart Failure Guidelines Committee. Furthermore, patients in the PEECH trial were clinically stable, essentially free of edema (trace ankle edema only), and treated with guideline-recommended medications (angiotensin converting enzyme inhibitor or angiotensin receptor blocker and beta-blocker) titrated to appropriate doses at baseline.

The population observed in the registries was quite different from the PEECH trial population in that when present, heart failure is not the primary indication for EECP. Rather, the indications for EECP were anginas. The registries showed EECP to be well tolerated and able to provide benefits equally in patients with or without heart failure. Thus EECP may provide a useful therapeutic tool in patients with angina and mild-to-moderate heart failure.

While the safety of EECP in patients without significant fluid overload has been demonstrated, there exist little data to guide the use of EECP in patients with more severe fluid overload or acute decompensated heart failure. Further experience and

investigation is clearly needed in this area. Experience from spontaneous adverse event reports and studies show that when applied at lower pressure to patients with unsatisfactory fluid balance, EECP can precipitate pulmonary edema. This is consistent with data discussed earlier, showing that EECP increases venous return and transiently increases pulmonary capillary wedge pressure [57].

Also, experience gathered from various studies, in particular the PEECH trial and the IEPR, shows that there is little or no reason for concern treating patients with pacemakers, including biventricular devices [58].

Conclusions

In conclusion, EECP can benefit patients with anginas and left ventricular dysfunction who already receive optimal medical care without having achieved the degree of functional benefit they desire. The available data are consistent across several studies and the results of the PEECH trial provide the best available basis to date to assess the safety of this therapy. It can be argued that EECP may well be the intervention of choice in patients with coronary artery disease not remediable by surgery or percutaneous coronary intervention and congestive heart failure, provided that medical therapy is optimal and edema is very limited or absent. Certainly its impact on residual ischemic burden will play a role in patient outcomes. When one considers its noninvasive approach and the wealth of data supporting its safety and improved outcomes, it is possible that EECP therapy will gain an important role in the treatments for symptomatic coronary artery disease complicated by heart failure.

More research will help to define the effectiveness of EECP and establish the cost-effectiveness of this therapeutic approach in patients with heart failure but not angina. It may be of value to evaluate different treatment courses in the heart failure patient. Perhaps a chronic maintenance schedule more akin to the treatment of end-stage renal disease might be more effective than a single 35-hour course of therapy. Work is currently in progress to evaluate whether variations in the placement of EECP cuffs may allow manipulation in the degree of venous return versus afterload reduction, potentially increasing the spectrum of heart failure patients amenable to therapy. In addition to clarifying the role of EECP in the treatment of chronic heart failure, exciting new frontiers for the application of EECP include the potential for treating the diuretic-resistant patient and the patient with acute decompensated heart failure.

References

1. Beckman CB, Romero LH, Shatney CH, et al. Clinical comparison of the intra-aortic balloon pump and external counterpulsation for cardiogenic shock. Trans Am Soc Artif Intern Organs 1973;19:414–418.

2. Amsterdam EA, Banas J, Criley JM, et al. Clinical assessment of external pressure circulatory assistance in acute myocardial infarction: report of a cooperative clinical trial. Am J Cardiol February 1980;45(2):349–356.

3. Michaels AD, Accad M, Ports TA, Grossman W. Left ventricular systolic unloading and augmentation of intracoronary pressure and Doppler flow during enhanced external counterpulsation. Circulation 3 September 2002;106(10):1237–1242.

4. Solignac A, Ferguson RJ, Bourassa MG. External counterpulsation: coronary hemodynamics and use in treatment of patients with stable angina pectoris. Cathet Cardiovasc Diagn 1977;3(1):37–45.

5. Michaels AD, Linnemeier G, Soran O, et al. Two-year outcomes after enhanced external counterpulsation for stable angina pectoris (from the International Patient Registry [IEPR]). Am J Cardiol 15 February 2004;93(4):461–464.

6. Arora RR, Chou TM, Jain D, et al. Effects of enhanced external counterpulsation on health-related quality of life continue 12 months after treatment: a substudy of the multicenter study of enhanced external counterpulsation. J Investig Med January 2002;50(1):25–32.

7. Loh PH, Cleland JG, Louis AA, et al. Enhanced external counterpulsation in the treatment of chronic refractory angina: a long-term follow-up outcome from the International Enhanced External Counterpulsation Patient Registry. Clin Cardiol 2008;31(4):159–164.

8. Data on file, Vasomedical, Inc., Westbury, NY, USA.

9. Taguchi I, Ogawa K, Oida A, et al. Comparison of hemodynamic effects of enhanced external counterpulsation and intra-aortic balloon pumping in patients with acute myocardial infarction. Am J Cardiol 15 November 2000;86(10):1139–1141.

10. Taguchi I, Ogawa K, Kanaya T, et al. Effects of enhanced external counterpulsation on hemodynamics and its mechanism. Circ J November 2004;68(11):1030–1034.

11. Werner D, Michalk F, Harazny J, et al. Accelerated reperfusion of poorly perfused retinal areas in central retinal

12. Applebaum RM, Kasliwal R, Tunik PA, et al. Sequential external counterpulsation increases cerebral and renal blood flow. Am Heart J 1997;133:611–615.

13. Hilz MJ, Werner D, Marthol H, et al. Enhanced external counterpulsation improves skin oxygenation and perfusion. Eur J Clin Invest June 2004;34(6):385–391.

14. Werner D, Trägner P, Wawer A, et al. Enhanced external counterpulsation: a new technique to augment renal function in liver cirrhosis. Nephrol Dial Transplant 23 March 2005;20:920–926.

15. Jacobey JA, Taylor WJm, Snith GP, et al. A new therapeutic approach to acute coronary occlusion. Am J Cardiol 1963;11(2):218–227.

16. Wu GF, Du ZM, Hu CH, et al. Microvessel angiogenesis: a possible cardioprotective mechanism of external counterpulsation for canine myocardial infarction. Chin Med J (Engl) 20 July 2005;118(14):1182–1189.

17. Kho S, Liuzzo J, Suresh K, et al. Vascular endothelial growth factor and atrial natriuretic peptide in enhance counterpulsation. Program and Abstract of the 82nd Annual Meeting of the Endocrine Society, Toronto, Ontario, Canada, 21–24 June 2000 (abstract 561).

18. Masuda D, Nohara R, Kataoka K, et al. Enhanced external counterpulsation promotes angiogenesis factors in patients with chronic stable angina. Circulation 23 October 2001;104(17, Suppl II):445.

19. Werner D, Michelson G, Harazny J, et al. Changes in ocular blood flow velocities during external counterpulsation in healthy volunteers and patients with atherosclerosis. Graefes Arch Clin Exp Ophthalmol August 2001;239(8):599–602.

20. Barsheshet A, Hod H, Shechter M, et al. The effect of external counter pulsation therapy on circulating endothelial progenitor cells in patients with angina pectoris. Cardiology 2008;110(3):160–166.

21. Zhang Y, He X, Chen X, et al. Enhanced external counterpulsation inhibits intimal hyperplasia by modifying shear stress responsive gene expression in hypercholesterolemic pigs. Circulation 31 July 2007;116(5):526–534.

22. Casey DP, Conti CR, Nichols WW, Choi CY, Khuddus MA, Braith RW. Effect of enhanced external counterpulsation on inflammatory cytokines and adhesion molecules in patients with angina pectoris and angiographic coronary artery disease. Am J Cardiol 2008;101(3):300–302.

23. Bonetti PO, Barsness GW, Keelan PC, et al. Enhanced external counterpulsation improves endothelial function in patients with symptomatic coronary artery disease. J Am Coll Cardiol 21 May 2003;41(10):1761–1768.

24. Nichols WW, Braith RW, Aggarwal R, *et al.* Enhanced external counterpulsation decreases wave reflection amplitude and reduces left ventricular afterload and systolic stress in patients with refractory angina. J Am Coll Cardiol 3 March 2004;43(5, Suppl A):307A.

25. Nichols WW, Estrada JC, Braith RW, Owens K, Conti CR. Enhanced external counterpulsation treatment improves arterial wall properties and wave reflection characteristics in patients with refractory angina. J Am Coll Cardiol 2006;48(6):1209–1215.

26. Levenson J, Simon A, Megnien JL, *et al.* Effects of enhanced external counterpulsation on carotid circulation in patients with coronary artery disease. Cardiology 2007;108(2):104–110.

27. Urano H, Ikeda H, Ueno T, *et al.* Enhanced external counterpulsation improves exercise tolerance, reduces exercise-induced myocardial ischemia and improves left ventricular diastolic filling in patients with coronary artery disease. J Am Coll Cardiol January 2001;37(1):93–99.

28. Masuda D, Nohara R, Hirai T, *et al.* Enhanced external counterpulsation improved myocardial perfusion and coronary flow reserve in patients with chronic stable angina: evaluation by ^{13}N-ammonia positron emission tomography. Eur Heart J August 2001;22(16):1451–1458.

29. Tartaglia J, Stenerson J Jr, Charney R. Exercise capability and myocardial perfusion in chronic angina patients treated with enhanced external counterpulsation. Clin Cardiol June 2003;(26):287–290.

30. Stys TP, Lawson WE, Hui JCK, *et al.* Effects of enhanced external counterpulsation on stress radionuclide coronary perfusion and exercise capacity in chronic stable angina pectoris. Am J Cardiol 1 April 2002;89(7):822–824.

31. Michaels AD, Raisinghani A, Soran O, *et al.* The effects of enhanced external counterpulsation on myocardial perfusion in patients with stable angina: a single blind multicenter pilot study. J Am Coll Cardiol 3 March 2004;43(5, Suppl A):308A.

32. Bonetti PO, Gadasalli SN, Lerman A, *et al.* Successful treatment of symptomatic coronary endothelial dysfunction with enhanced external counterpulsation. Mayo Clin Proc May 2004;79(5):690–692.

33. Kronhaus K, Lawson WE. Enhanced external counterpulsation is an effective treatment for syndrome X. Int J Cardiol 2008;135:256–257.

34. Wu GF, Qiang SZ, Zheng ZS, *et al.* A neurohormonal mechanism for the effectiveness of enhanced external counterpulsation. Circulation 1999;100(18):I-832.

35. Qian X, Wu W, Zheng ZS, *et al.* Effect of enhanced external counterpulsation on nitric oxide production in coronary disease. J Heart Dis May 1999;1(1):193.

36. Levenson J, Pernollet MG, Iliou MC, *et al.* Enhanced external counterpulsation acutely increases blood and platelet cGMP. Circulation 28 October 2003;108(17, Suppl IV):589–590.

37. Levenson J, Pernollet MG, Iliou MC, Devynck MA, Simon A. Cyclic GMP release by acute enhanced external counterpulsation. Am J Hypertens 2006;19(8):867–872.

38. Masuda D, Fujita M, Nohara R, *et al.* Improvement of oxygen metabolism in ischemic myocardium as a result of enhanced external counterpulsation with heparin pretreatment for patients with stable. Heart Vessels March 2004;19(2):59–62.

39. Grayson D, de Jong A, Ochoa A, *et al.* Oxygen consumption changes during EECP treatment in patients with and without coronary artery disease. Med Sci Sports Exerc May 2004;36(5, Suppl):S214.

40. Ochoa AB, deJong A, Grayson D, Franklin B, McCullough P. Effect of enhanced external counterpulsation on resting oxygen uptake in patients having previous coronary revascularization and in healthy volunteers. Am J Cardiol 2006;98(5):613–615.

41. Lawson WE, Silver MA, Kennard L, *et al.* Angina patients with diastolic or systolic heart failure demonstrate comparable immediate and one year benefit from enhanced external counterpulsation. J Card Fail October 2003;9(5):107.

42. Lu L, Zheng ZS, Wu WK, Lawson W, Hui JCK. Effects of enhanced external counterpulsation on renin–angiotensin system in experimental AMI. In: Kimchi A, editor. Heart Disease: New Trends in Research, Diagnosis and Treatment. Engelwood, NJ: Medimond Medical Publications; 2001: 275–279.

43. Lawson WE, Kennard ED, Holubkov R, et al; IEPR Investigators. Benefit and safety of enhanced external counterpulsation in treating coronary artery disease patients with a history of congestive heart failure. Cardiology 2001;96(2):78–84.

44. Soran O, Kennard ED, Kelsey S, *et al.* Enhanced external counterpulsation as treatment for chronic angina in patients with left ventricular dysfunction: a report from the International EECP Patient Registry (IEPR). Congest Heart Fail 2002 8(6):297–302.

45. Soran O, Kennard ED, Kfoury B, et al; IEPR Investigators. Two year clinical outcomes, after enhanced external counterpulsation (EECP) therapy in patients with refractory angina pectoris and left ventricular dysfunction: (report from the International EECP Patient Registry. Am J Cardiol 2006;97(1):17–20.

46. Soran O, Fleishman B, Demarco T, *et al.* Enhanced external counterpulsation in patients with heart failure: a multicenter feasibility study. Congest Heart Fail July–August 2002;8(4):204–208, 227.

47. Gorscan J III Crawford L, Soran O, et al. Improvement in left ventricular performance by enhanced external counterpulsation in patients with heart failure. J Am Coll Cardiol February 2000;35(2, Suppl A):230.

48. Arora RR, Lopez S, Saric M. Enhanced external counterpulsation improves systolic function by echocardiography in patients with coronary artery disease. Heart Lung March–April 2005;34(2):122–125.

49. Estahbanaty G, Samiei N, Maleki M, et al. Echocardiographic characteristics including tissue Doppler imaging after enhanced external counterpulsation therapy. Am Heart Hosp J 2007;5(4):241–246.

50. Linnemeier GC, Kennard ED, Soran O, et al. Enhanced external counterpulsation improves functional capacity in patients with left ventricular dysfunction as assessed by the Duke activity status index—a questionnaire correlated with peak oxygen uptake. J Card Fail 2003;9(5, Suppl):S107.

51. Lawson WE, Silver MA, Hui JCK. Angina patients with diastolic versus systolic heart failure demonstrate comparable immediate and one-year benefit from enhanced external counterpulsation. J Card Fail February 2005;11(1):61–66.

52. Feldman AM, Silver AM, Francis GS, et al. Treating heart failure with enhanced external counterpulsation (EECP): design of the prospective evaluation of EECP in heart failure (PEECH) trial. J Card Fail April 2005;11(3):240–245.

53. Feldman AM, Silver MA, Francis GS, et al; for the PEECH Investigators. Enhanced external counterpulsation improves exercise tolerance in patients with chronic heart failure. J Am Coll Cardiol 2006;48(6):1199–1206.

54. Lawson WE, Hui JC, Kennard ED, et al. Benefit and safety of enhanced external counterpulsation in the treatment of ischemic heart disease with history of congestive heart failure. J Card Fail September 2000;6(3):84.

55. Linnemeier G, Michaels AD, Soran O, et al. Enhanced external counterpulsation in the management of angina in the elderly. Am J Geriatr Cardiol March–April 2003;12(2):90–96.

56. Linnemeier G, Rutter MK, Barsness G, et al. Enhanced external counterpulsation for the relief of angina in patients with diabetes: safety, efficacy and 1-year clinical outcomes. Am Heart J September 2003;146(3):453–458.

57. Cohen J, Grossman W, Michaels AD. Portable enhanced external counterpulsation for acute coronary syndrome and cardiogenic shock: a pilot study. Clin Cardiol 2007;30(5):223–228.

58. Tartaglia J, Stenerson J Jr, Ramasamy S, et al. Safety and efficacy of enhanced external counterpulsation in patients with permanent pacemakers in the treatment of chronic heart angina. J Investig Med March 2005;53(2):402.

59. Lawson WE, Hui JC, Zheng ZS, et al. Improved exercise tolerance following enhanced external counterpulsation: cardiac or peripheral effect? Cardiology 1996;87(4):271–275.

60. Bagger JP, Hall RJ, Koutroulis G, Nihoyannopoulos P. Effect of enhanced external counterpulsation on dobutamine-induced left ventricular wall motion abnormalities in severe chronic angina pectoris. Am J Cardiol 2004;93(4):465–467.

61. Michaels AD, Bart BA, Pinto T, Lafferty J, Fung G, Kennard ED. The effects of enhanced external counterpulsation on time- and frequency-domain measures of heart rate variability. J Electrocardiol 2007;40(6):515–521.

62. Hashemi M, Hoseinbalam M, Khazaei M. Long-term effect of enhanced external counterpulsation on endothelial function in the patients with intractable angina. Heart Lung Circ. 2008;17(5):383–387.

63. Abbottsmith CW, Chung ES, Varricchione T, et al. Prospective Evaluation of EECP in Congestive Heart Failure (PEECH) Investigators. Enhanced external counterpulsation improves exercise duration and peak oxygen consumption in older patients with heart failure: a subgroup analysis of the PEECH trial. Congest Heart Fail 2006;12(6):307–311.

64. Soran O, Kennard ED, Bart BA, Kelsey SF. Impact of external counterpulsation treatment on emergency department visits and hospitalizations in refractory angina patients with left ventricular dysfunction. Congest Heart Fail 2007;13(1):36–40.

CHAPTER 14

Ultrafiltration in the Management of Heart Failure

Maria Rosa Costanzo
Edward Heart Hospital, Naperville, IL, USA

In the United States, 90% of 1 million annual hospitalizations for heart failure (HF) are due to volume overload [1,2]. Hypervolemia contributes to HF progression and mortality. Guidelines recommend that therapy for HF patients be aimed at achieving euvolemia. Intravenous loop diuretics induce rapid diuresis that reduces lung congestion and dyspnea. However, loop diuretics' effectiveness declines with repeated exposure [3]. Unresolved congestion may contribute to high rehospitalization rates. Furthermore, loop diuretics may be associated with increased morbidity and mortality due to deleterious effects on neurohormonal activation, electrolyte balance, and cardiac and renal function [3–7]. Ultrafiltration is an alternative method of sodium and water removal, which safely improves hemodynamics in HF patients [8]. Application of this technology has been limited by the need for high flow rates, large extracorporeal blood volumes, and large-bore central venous catheters. A modified ultrafiltration device has overcome these limitations.

The process

Ultrafiltration is the production of plasma water from whole blood across a semipermeable membrane (hemofilter) in response to a transmembrane pressure gradient generated by the hydrostatic pressures in the blood and in the filtrate compartments and by the oncotic pressure produced by plasma proteins [8]. Hydrostatic pressure is determined by

the blood pressure in the filtering device, generated either by the patient's blood pressure or by an extracorporeal pump plus the suction occurring in the ultrafiltrate compartment [8]. With isolated ultrafiltration, the solute is passively removed by accompanying the solvent flow (convective transport): the sodium concentration in the ultrafiltrate is equal to that in the water component of the plasma [8]. After cannulation of an artery or vein, ultrafiltration is performed on blood extracted from and then returned to the patient via a separate access to the venous circulation [8]. Ultrafiltration can be isolated, intermittent, or continuous. With appropriate ultrafiltration rates, the extracellular fluid gradually refills the intravascular space and blood volume is maintained. If the ultrafiltration rate is too high, blood volume may decrease because intravascular volume depletion exceeds reabsorption of fluid from the interstitium into the vascular space. Accurate determination of the amount of fluid to be removed, optimization of fluid removal rate, and maintenance of circulating blood volume are critically important [8].

The fluid removed with diuretics is hypotonic. In contrast, the ultrafiltrate is essentially isosmotic and isonatric compared with plasma. Therefore, for any amount of fluid withdrawn, more sodium is removed with ultrafiltration than with diuretics [8]. With diuretics, intravascular hypovolemia is prolonged and inhibition of sodium chloride uptake in the macula densa enhances renal renin secretion [8]. The augmented neurohormonal activation, in turn, promotes sodium and water retention, ultimately reducing the diuretics' ability to relieve circulatory congestion [3]. Ultrafiltration does not

Heart Failure: Device Management. Edited by Arthur Feldman.
© 2010 Blackwell Publishing.

stimulate macula densa-mediated neurohormonal activation and it does not produce prolonged intravascular hypovolemia because ultrafiltration removes fluid from the blood at the same rate at which fluid is reabsorbed from the edematous interstitium [9].

Use of ultrafiltration in HF

Ultrafiltration improves congestion, lowers right atrial and pulmonary arterial wedge pressures, improves cardiac output, decreases neurohormone levels, corrects hyponatremia, restores diuresis, and reduces diuretic requirements [10].

Use of ultrafiltration in patients with moderate HF has shed light on the mechanisms of ultrafiltration's benefit [11]. Sixteen patients with NYHA (New York Heart Association) class II and III HF were randomly allocated to receive either a single ultrafiltration treatment ($n = 8$) or intravenous furosemide ($n = 8$, mean dose = 248 mg) to remove 1600 mL of fluid [11]. Soon after fluid withdrawal by either method, biventricular filling pressures and body weight were reduced and plasma renin, norepinephrine, and aldosterone levels were increased. After furosemide, neurohormone levels remained elevated over 4 days and during this period patients had positive water balance, recurrent elevation of filling pressures, and lung congestion without improvement of VO_{2max}. After ultrafiltration, neurohormone levels fell below baseline within 48 hours, whereas water metabolism was equilibrated at a new set point (less fluid intake and diuresis without weight gain). Improvement was sustained at 3 months after ultrafiltration [11]. Although ultrafiltration and furosemide are equally effective in terms of acute volume of fluid removed and resolution of congestive symptoms, their long-term effects are different. The effects of ultrafiltration on pulmonary water metabolism and neurohormone levels may be due to mechanisms not occurring with diuretics. The ultrafiltrate has different sodium content compared to the fluid removed with diuretics. Ultrafiltration removes fluid with a sodium concentration similar to that of plasma, so that approximately 150 mmol of sodium is withdrawn with each liter of ultrafiltrate. In contrast, the urine of HF patients is hypotonic compared with plasma and the 50 mmol of sodium usually present in 1 L of urine

increases to only 100 mmol with furosemide administration [12]. The different amounts of sodium removed with similar amounts of fluid account for the differential effects of ultrafiltration and diuretics on neurohormonal responses, which in turn will result in different renal sodium and water reabsorption.

Among 32 NYHA class II to IV hypervolemic HF patients the baseline 24-hour diuresis and natriuresis were inversely correlated with neurohormone levels and renal perfusion pressure [13]. The response to ultrafiltration ranged from neurohormonal activation and reduction of diuresis in patients with the mildest hypovolemia and urine output greater than 1000 mL/24 h to neurohormonal inhibition and enhanced diuresis and natriuresis in those with the most severe volume overload and urine output less than 1000 mL/24 h [13]. Decreases in norepinephrine level were proportional to enhancement of diuresis. Thus subtraction of total body water uncovers enough cardiac reserve to increase cardiac output and attenuate neurohormonal activation. Benefits are then maintained because the enhanced diuresis improves norepinephrine clearance from the circulation [11]. The earliest effect of ultrafiltration may be the reduction of the extravascular pulmonary fluid, with a subsequent decrease in pulmonary extravascular resistance, improvement of ventilation and gas exchange, and a decrease in hypoxia-induced vasoconstriction. Ultrafiltration itself, via baroreceptor-mediated reflexes, may reset neurohormonal activation, which in turn may explain the intermediate- and long-term benefits observed after ultrafiltration [11]. The removal of myocardial depressant factors may also occur [14]. In 36 patients with acutely decompensated HF, ultrafiltration was associated with increased cardiac index and oxygenation status, decreased pulmonary artery pressure and vascular resistance, as well as reduced requirement for inotropes [15].

It is unknown if the clinical benefits of ultrafiltration translate into improved survival. In decompensated HF patients, ultrafiltration has been used predominantly after diuretics have failed or in the presence of acute renal failure. Earlier utilization of ultrafiltration can expedite and maintain compensation of acute HF by simultaneously reducing volume overload without causing intravascular volume depletion and reestablishing acid–base and electrolyte balance. However, overly aggressive ultrafiltration in patients with decompensated HF can convert nonoliguric renal dysfunction into oliguric renal failure by increasing neurohormonal activation and decreasing renal perfusion pressure, with minimal opportunity of recovery of renal function.

Ultrafiltration therapies

The continuous ultrafiltration techniques include continuous hemofiltration in the arterial–venous (CAVH) or veno-venous mode (CVVH) and slow continuous ultrafiltration (SCUF) in arterial–venous or veno-venous modes [16]. Using a large-bore catheter inserted into the femoral artery and the patients' own blood pressure, arterial blood is delivered to a hemofilter. Systemic blood pressure provides the driving force to achieve sufficient blood flow. When hydrostatic pressure exceeds oncotic pressure, ultrafiltrate is generated. Ultrafiltrate drains by gravity through tubing into a collection bag, creating mild negative pressure in the filter's blood chamber, favoring further ultrafiltration [16]. With SCUF, replacement volumes are much lower than with CAVH. Recently extracorporeal blood pumps have been reintroduced to eliminate the need for an arterial–venous pressure gradient and permit veno-venous vascular access [17]. Until the introduction of simplified intermittent peripheral veno-venous ultrafiltration techniques, CVVH and SCUF were the recommended therapies for the more critically ill, hypotensive HF patients [17]. Because CVVH requires an extracorporeal blood pump, air embolism and blood loss can occur. With SCUF, air embolism is uncommon and blood loss is self-limited. Extracorporeal blood pumps, by producing a constant blood flow, can provide ultrafiltration rates not achievable with SCUF. All continuous therapies require anticoagulation. Hypovolemia can be avoided by careful clinical management. Complication rates are acceptable [18]. With SCUF, ultrafiltration rate can vary from 0 to 20 mL/min, with a goal of approximately 5 mL/min. Clinical urgency will dictate the ultrafiltration rate, which can easily be adjusted. For CVVH, an ultrafiltration rate of 40 mL/min is achievable. Without an extracorporeal blood

pump, vascular access must guarantee an adequate arterial–venous gradient. Placement of large-bore catheters requires specific technical skills. In CVVH the extracorporeal blood pump produces flow rates of 100–150 mL/min. The veno-venous double lumen catheters can be placed in the internal jugular, subclavian, or femoral veins. The extracorporeal blood pump includes a roller pump, arterial pressure sensor, air detector, and venous pressure alarms. Use of this equipment requires trained hemodialysis personnel. Ultrafiltration rate can be controlled directly by a pump on the ultrafiltration line or indirectly by altering blood flow. Alternatively, venous pressure can be raised by placing a screw clamp on the venous bloodline or negative pressure can be applied by suction to the ultrafiltrate compartment.

With intermittent isolated ultrafiltration, the blood is pumped through a filter by an extracorporeal blood pump aided either by suction applied to the ultrafiltrate compartment (negative pressure) or from resistance induced in the venous line (positive pressure). Because of the pump, a dual lumen veno-venous catheter will generate a blood flow of 500–1000 mL/h. Slower rates over longer periods of time improve hemodynamic tolerance [19]. Intermittent isolated ultrafiltration is effective in removing salt and water in hypervolemic patients with moderate and severe HF [19]. Many patients regain responsiveness to diuretics after one or more ultrafiltration treatments, suggesting that untapped cardiac functional reserve is recruited by ultrafiltration [19]. Ascites, edema, dyspnea, and hyponatremia may improve. Plasma volume falls and oncotic pressure rises [19]. Ultrafiltration increases plasma colloid osmotic pressure and transcapillary gradient [8]. This increase is maximal in the first 60 minutes of ultrafiltration and then levels off as refilling occurs. After ultrafiltration, the decreased venous pressure further enhances the net transcapillary pressure gradient change, favoring interstitial fluid reabsorption.

If the ultrafiltration rate is limited to 500–1000 mL/h for only a few hours, heart rate, blood pressure, and systemic vascular resistance remain unchanged [10]. Cardiac output either rises or is stable. Pulmonary capillary wedge pressure is unchanged or decreased. Right atrial pressure and pulmonary vascular resistance fall. An improved ejection fraction and a decreased radiographic cardiothoracic ratio have also been described [10]. Advantages of intermittent isolated ultrafiltration include the avoidance of an arterial puncture and the short exposure to systemic anticoagulation. Disadvantages include the need for dialysis equipment and personnel, and the removal of large amounts of fluid in a short time period. Hemorrhage from anticoagulation and extracorporeal blood pump complications, such as air embolism, can occur.

Intermittent isolated ultrafiltration has been described in more than 100 patients with NYHA class IV refractory HF [20]. Of 52 such patients treated with slow isolated ultrafiltration, 13 died in less than 1 month during treatment (nonresponders), 24 had both cardiac and renal improvement (responders) for either less than 3 ($n = 6$) or for greater than 3 months ($n = 18$), and 15 (partial responders) had hemodynamic improvement but worsening renal function requiring either long-term weekly ultrafiltration ($n = 8$), continuous ambulatory peritoneal dialysis ($n = 1$), or intermittent renal replacement therapy ($n = 6$). Adequate diuresis was restored in 1 month in 24 of the 39 responders and partial responders. Four of the 15 partial responders had sufficient recovery of renal function to undergo heart transplantation within 3–9 months. Thus, intermittent ultrafiltration can be used to treat HF refractory to maximally tolerated medical therapy. Restoration of diuresis and natriuresis after intermittent ultrafiltration identified patients with recoverable cardiac functional reserve. Intermittent isolated ultrafiltration is valuable in partial responders because it improves quality of life and may be used as a bridge to heart transplantation. The high short-term mortality is consistent with the poor prognosis of advanced HF.

A new device (Aquadex System 100, CHF Solutions, Minneapolis, MN, USA) permits both withdrawal of fluid and blood return through peripheral veins (Figure 14.1). However, central venous access remains an option. Fluid removal can range from 10 to 500 mL/h; blood flow can be set at 10–40 mL/min, and total extracorporeal blood volume is only 33 mL. The device consists of a console, an extracorporeal blood pump, and venous catheters. The console controls blood removal rates and extracts ultrafiltrate at a user-set maximum rate. The device is

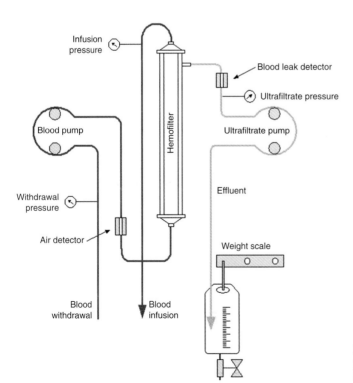

Figure 14.1 The Aquadex System 100 peripheral veno-venous system (CHF Solutions, Minneapolis, MN, USA).

designed to monitor the extracorporeal blood circuit and to alert the user to abnormal conditions. Ultrafiltrate drains into a bag. Blood is withdrawn from a vein through the withdrawal catheter. Tubing connects the withdrawal catheter to the blood pump. Blood passes through the withdrawal pressure sensor just before it enters the blood pump tubing loop. During operation, the pump loop is compressed by rotating rollers that propel the blood through the tubing. After exiting the blood pump, blood passes through the air detector and enters the hemofilter. The hemofilter is bonded to a clip-on cartridge that mounts onto the ultrafiltrate pump raceway on the side of the console. Blood enters the filter through a port on the bottom, exits through the port at the top of the filter, and passes through the infusion pressure sensor before returning to the patient. Inside the hemofilter, there is a bundle of hollow fibers. The ultrafiltrate passes through the fiber walls, fills the space between these fibers, and exits through a port near the top of the filter case. Ultrafiltrate then passes through a blood leak detector. Ultrafiltrate sequentially passes through the ultrafiltrate pressure sensor, the ultrafiltrate pump, and the collecting bag that is suspended from the weight scale. Treatment can be performed by any nurse trained in the use of the device.

Three pilot trials of intermittent peripheral veno-venous ultrafiltration have been published. In the first study, in 21 fluid-overloaded patients, removal of an average of 2611 ± 1002 mL over 6.4 ± 1.5 hours reduced weight from 92 ± 17 to 89 ± 17 kg ($p < 0.0001$) and congestion without changes in heart rate, blood pressure, electrolytes, or hematocrit [21]. The aim of the second study was to determine if ultrafiltration with the Aquadex System 100 before intravenous diuretics in patients with decompensated HF and diuretic resistance resulted in euvolemia and hospital discharge in 3 days, without hypotension or worsening renal function. Ultrafiltration was initiated within 4.7 ± 3.5 hours of hospitalization and before intravenous diuretics in 20 HF patients with volume overload and diuretic resistance (age 74.5 ± 8.2 yr, 75% ischemic disease, ejection fraction $3 \pm 15\%$), and continued until euvolemia. An average of 8654 ± 4205 mL was removed with 2.6 ± 1.2 8 hours of ultrafiltration courses (8 h each). Twelve patients (60%) were discharged in 3 days. One patient was readmitted in 30 days and 2 patients in 90 days for reasons unrelated to recurrent volume overload. Weight ($p = 0.006$), Minnesota Living with Heart Failure scores ($p = 0.003$), and global assessment ($p = 0.00,003$) were improved after ultrafiltration at 30 and 90 days. B-type natriuretic peptide levels were decreased after ultrafiltration (from 1236 ± 747 to 988 ± 847 pg/mL) and at 30 days (816 ± 494 pg/mL, $p = 0.03$). Blood pressure, renal function, and medications were unchanged. Thus in HF patients with volume overload and diuretic resistance, early ultrafiltration before intravenous diuretics effectively and safely decreases length of stay and readmissions. Benefits persisted at 3 months after treatment [22]. The aim of the third study was to compare the safety and efficacy of ultrafiltration with the Aquadex System 100 device versus those of intravenous diuretics in decompensated HF patients. Compared to the 20 diuretic-treated patients, the 20 patients randomized to a single, 8-hour ultrafiltration session had greater median fluid removal (2838 vs 4650 mL, $p = 0.001$) and weight loss (1.86 vs 2.5 kg, $p = 0.24$). Ultrafiltration was well tolerated and not associated with adverse hemodynamic or renal effects. Thus early ultrafiltration in decompensated HF patients results in greater fluid removal and improvement of congestion than those achieved with intravenous diuretics [23]. The findings of these studies stimulated the design and implementation of the Ultrafiltration Versus Intravenous Diuretics for Patients Hospitalized for Acute Decompensated Heart Failure (UNLOAD) trial [24]. This study was designed to compare the safety and efficacy of venovenous ultrafiltration and standard intravenous diuretic therapy for hospitalized HF patients with two or more than two signs of hypervolemia. Two hundred patients (63 ± 15 yr, 69% men, 71% had ejection fraction $\leq 40\%$) were randomized to ultrafiltration or intravenous diuretics. At 48 hours, weight (5.0 ± 3.1 vs 3.1 ± 3.5 kg, $p = 0.001$) and net fluid loss (4.6 vs 3.3 L, $p = 0.001$) were greater in the ultrafiltration group. Dyspnea scores were similar. At 90 days, the ultrafiltration group had fewer patients rehospitalized for HF (16 of 89 [18%] vs 28 of 87 [32%], $p = 0.037$), HF rehospitalizations (0.22 ± 0.54 vs 0.46 ± 0.76, $p = 0.022$), rehospitalization days (1.4 ± 4.2 vs 3.8 ± 8.5, $p = 0.022$) per patient, and unscheduled visits (14 of 65 [21%] vs 29 of 66 [44%], $p = 0.009$). Changes in serum creatinine were similar in the two groups through-out the study. The percentage of patients with rises in serum creatinine levels > 0.3 mg/dL was similar in the ultrafiltration and standard care group at 24 hours (13/90 [14.4%] vs 7/91 [7.7%], $p = 0.528$), at 48 hours (18/68 [26.5%] vs 15/74 [20.3%], $p = 0.430$), and at discharge (19/84 [22.6%] vs 17/86 [19.8%], $p = 0.709$). There was no correlation be-tween net fluid removed and changes in serum crea-tinine in the ultrafiltration ($r = -0.050$, $p = 0.695$) or in the intravenous diuretics group ($r = 0.028$, $p = 0.820$). No clinically significant changes in serum blood urea nitrogen, sodium, chloride, and bicar-bonate occurred in either group. Serum potassium < 3.5 mEq/L occurred in 1/77 (1%) patient in the ultrafiltration and in 9/75 (12%) patients in the di-uretics group ($p = 0.018$). Episodes of hypotension during 48 hours after randomization were similar (4/100 [4%] vs 3/100 [3%]). Thus the UNLOAD trial demonstrated that in decompensated HF, ul-trafiltration safely produces greater weight and fluid loss than intravenous diuretics, reduces 90-day re-source utilization for HF, and is an effective alterna-tive therapy [24]. It is also important to recognize the limitations of the UNLOAD trial. The treat-ment targets for both diuretics and ultrafiltration were not prespecified. Although treatment was not blinded, it is unlikely that a placebo effect influenced either weight loss or the improved 90-day outcomes associated with ultrafiltration. The possibility that standard care patients were inadequately treated is diminished by the observation that improvements in symptoms of HF, biomarkers, and quality of life were similar in the two treatment groups through-out the study. Furthermore, 43% of patients in the standard care group lost at least 4.5 kg during hospi-talization, a weight loss greater than that observed in 75% of patients enrolled in the Acute Decom-pensated Heart Failure National Registry [2].

Although the study did not include measure-ments of blood volume, plasma refill rate, intersti-tial salt and water, cardiac performance, or hemo-dynamics, ultrafiltration was not associated with excessive hypotension or renal or electrolyte abnor-malities.

The economic impact of ultrafiltration as an ini-tial strategy for decompensated HF was also not addressed in this trial. While the costs associated with ultrafiltration during the index hospitalization may exceed those of intravenous diuretics, total cost over time may be lower due to decreased resource utilization for HF.

Conclusion

Of the ultrafiltration approaches described, the most practical are veno-venous ultrafiltration tech-niques in which isotonic plasma is propelled through the filter by an extracorporeal pump. These approaches avoid an arterial puncture, remove a predictable amount of fluid, are not associated with significant hemodynamic instability, and, in the case of peripheral veno-venous ultrafiltration, do not require specialized dialysis personnel. Ultrafil-tration has been used in patients with decompen-sated HF and volume overload refractory to diuret-ics. These patients generally have preexisting renal insufficiency and, despite daily oral diuretic doses, develop signs of pulmonary and peripheral conges-tion. Ultrafiltration and diuretic holiday may re-store diuresis and natriuresis. Some patients with volume overload refractory to all available intra-venous vasoactive therapies have had significant improvements of symptoms, hemodynamics, and renal function following ultrafiltration. A strategy of *early* ultrafiltration and diuretic holiday can re-sult in more effective weight reduction and can shorten hospitalization. Patients should not be con-sidered for ultrafiltration if the following conditions exist: venous access cannot be obtained; there is a hypercoagulable state; systolic blood pressure is <85 mmHg or there are signs or symptoms of car-diogenic shock; patients require intravenous pres-sors to maintain an adequate blood pressure; or there is end-stage renal disease, as documented by a requirement for dialysis approaches. Ultrafiltra-tion can be carried out in patients with hematocrit >40% only if it can be proven that hypovolemia is absent.

Many questions regarding the use of ultrafiltra-tion in HF patients remain unanswered and must be addressed in future studies. These include op-timal fluid removal rates in individual patients, effects of ultrafiltration on cardiac remodeling, in-fluence of a low oncotic pressure occurring in pa-tients with cardiac cachexia on plasma refill rates, and the economic impact of ultrafiltration to de-termine if the expense of disposable filters is offset by the cost savings due to reduced rehospitalization rates.

References

1. Thom T, Haase N, Rosamond W, *et al.* Heart disease and stroke statistics—2006 update. A report from the American Heart Association Statistics Committee and the Stroke Statistics Subcommittee. Circulation 2006;113:e85–e151.

2. Adams KF, Fonarow GC, Emerman CL, *et al.* Characteristics and outcomes of patients hospitalized for heart failure in the United States: rationale, design, and preliminary observations from the first 100000 cases in the Acute Decompensated Heart Failure National Registry (ADHERE). Am Heart J 2005;149:209–216.

3. Ellison DH. Diuretic therapy and resistance in congestive heart failure. Cardiology 2001;96:132–143.

4. Philbin EF, Cotto M, Rocco TA Jr, Jenkins PL. Association between diuretic use, clinical response and death in acute heart failure. Am J Cardiol 1997;80:519–522.

5. Butler J, Forman DE, Abraham WT, *et al.* Relationship between heart failure treatment and development of worsening renal function among hospitalized patients. Am Heart J 2004;147:331–338.

6. Francis GS, Benedict C, Johnstone DE, *et al.* Comparison of neuroendocrine activation in patients with left ventricular dysfunction with and without congestive heart failure: a substudy of the Studies Of Left ventricular Dysfunction (SOLVD). Circulation 1990;82:1724–1729.

7. Gottlieb SS, Brater DC, Thomas I, *et al.* BG9719 (CVT-124), an A1 adenosine receptor antagonist, protects against the decline in renal function observed with diuretic therapy. Circulation 2002;105:1348–1353.

8. Ronco C, Ricci Z, Bellomo R, Bedogni F. Extracorporeal ultrafiltration for the treatment of overhydration and congestive heart failure. Cardiology 2001;96:155–168.

9. Marenzi GC, Lauri G, Grazi M, *et al.* Circulatory response to fluid overload removal by extracorporeal ultrafiltration in refractory congestive heart failure. J Am Coll Cardiol 2001;38:963–968.

10. Marenzi G, Grazi S, Lauri G, *et al.* Interrelation of humoral factors, hemodynamics and fluid and salt metabolism in congestive heart failure: effects of extracorporeal ultrafiltration. Am J Med 1993;94:49–56.

11. Agostoni PG, Marenzi GC, Lauri G, *et al.* Sustained improvement in functional capacity after removal of body fluid with isolated ultrafiltration in chronic cardiac insufficiency: failure of furosemide to provide the same result. Am J Med 1994;96:191–199.

12. Canaud B, Leray-Moragues H, Garred LJ, *et al.* Slow isolated ultrafiltration for the treatment of congestive heart failure. Am J Kidney Dis 1996;28(Suppl 3):S67–S73.

13. Cipolla CM, Grazi S, Rimondini A, *et al.* Changes in circulating norepinephrine with hemofiltration in advanced congestive heart failure. Am J Cardiol 1990;66: 987–994.

14. Blake P, Hasewaga Y, Khosla MC, *et al.* Isolation of "myocardial depressant factor(s)" from the ultrafiltrate of heart failure patients with acute renal failure. ASAIO J 1996;42:M911–M915.

15. Coraim FI, Wolner E. Continuous hemofiltration for the failing heart. New Horiz 1995;3:725–731.

16. Burchardi H. History and development of continuous renal replacement techniques. Kidney Int 1998;66(Suppl):S120–S124.

17. Canaud B, Cristol JP, Klouche K, *et al.* Slow continuous ultrafiltration: a means of unmasking myocardial functional reserve in end stage cardiac disease. Contrib Nephrol 1991;93:79–85.

18. Grone HJ, Kramer P. Puncture and long-term cannulation of the femoral artery and vein in adults. In: Kramer P, editor. Arteriovenous Hemofiltration. Berlin: Springer-Verlag; 1985:35–47.

19. Dileo M, Pacitti A, Bergerone S, *et al.* Ultrafiltration in the treatment of refractory heart failure. Clin Cardiol 1988;11:449–459.

20. Silverstein ME, Ford CA, Lysaght MJ, *et al.* Treatment of severe volume overload by ultrafiltration. N Engl J Med 1974;291:747–751.

21. Jaski BE, Ha J, Denys BG, *et al.* Peripherally inserted veno-venous ultrafiltration for rapid treatment of volume overloaded patients. J Card Fail 2003;9:227–231.

22. Costanzo MR, Saltzberg MT, O'Sullivan JE, *et al.* Early ultrafiltration in patients with decompensated heart failure and diuretic resistance. J Am Coll Cardiol 2005;46:2043–2051.

23. Bart BA, Boyle A, Bank AJ, *et al.* Randomized controlled trial of ultrafiltration versus usual care for hospitalized patients with heart failure: relief for acutely fluid overloaded patients with decompensated congestive heart failure. J Am Coll Cardiol 2005;46:2043–2046.

24. Costanzo MR, Guglin ME, Saltzberg MT, *et al.* Ultrafiltration versus intravenous diuretics for patients hospitalized for acute decompensated heart failure. J Am Coll Cardiol 2007;49:675–683.

Conclusion: Finding the Right Device or the Right Patient

As was pointed out in the introduction and has been discussed throughout the various chapters, one of the challenges in choosing a therapeutic or diagnostic device for the treatment of a patient with heart failure is not as straightforward as deciding what drugs should be routinely used in the care of this patient population. We have seen that two devices carry substantive recommendations from leading panels of experts: the use of an implantable cardioverter-defibrillator (ICD) and the use of resynchronization devices – cardiac resynchronization therapy (CRT) – with or without an ICD. However, even with these devices, both of which have been shown to improve survival and to decrease hospitalizations in patients with heart failure, a physician must carefully evaluate each patient before initiating therapy. For example, all heart failure patients must undergo treatment with routine pharmacologic agents including a *ubeta*-blocker and an angiotensin-converting enzyme inhibitor before beginning device therapy. In addition, patients with end-stage heart failure might benefit from a resynchronization device to improve symptoms but may not want to receive an ICD. This is particularly true in patients with a short life expectancy due to severe heart failure or a concomitant disease. In addition, some patients might not want to increase their life expectancy if it means that they will have an extensive number of shocks but may decide to have a resynchronization device implanted with the hope that it will improve their symptoms.

Far less is known about which patient will benefit from other devices that, at least in preliminary studies, appear to enhance cardiac performance. For example, the use of electrical signals applied during absolute refractory period as a means to enhance cardiac performance has shown interesting effects in patients with left ventricular dysfunction. Sim-ilarly, the application of cardiac restraint devices may benefit selective patient populations. Both of these novel devices will require additional clinical trials before they receive Food and Drug Administration approval and before physicians can fully understand the risk/benefit ratio associated with their use as well as to define the patient population in which they are most effective.

The role of invasive monitoring in patients with heart failure has also been controversial and requires a careful analysis before electing to utilize one of the many new technologies that are available in a given patient. Until recently, there was significant equipoise regarding the use of right heart catheterization in the management of patients with heart failure. In some centers, right heart catheterization was used routinely in patients admitted with significantly worsening heart failure requiring inotrope or vasodilator therapy, while in other centers, right heart catheters were used far more judiciously. Fortunately, the recent Evaluation Study of Congestive Heart Failure and Pulmonary Artery Catheterization Effectiveness (ESCAPE) trial has provided substantive data regarding the usefulness of right heart catheterization in a large clinical study. Surprisingly, treatment guided by right heart catheterization did not surpass the effectiveness of traditional clinical observation in managing heart failure patients. However, patients were considered eligible for the study only if there was equipoise regarding the need for hemodynamic evaluation in any given patient. For example, a cohort of patients still exists, including those in cardiogenic shock and those in whom the cause of hemodynamic collapse remains undefined who require the placement of a right heart catheterization either for diagnostic purposes or for more effective management. Similarly, impedance cardiography also provides useful information for the clinician; however, its role in the day-to-day management of patients with heart failure has not yet been proven. Impedance measures that are now being incorporated into pacemaker and ICD devices may add interesting opportunities in the future; however, studies must be undertaken to evaluate how to use these data in the most appropriate and useful way.

Several companies are now developing implantable monitors to provide daily or even real-time measures of either left- or right-sided cardiac hemodynamics. These devices provide a novel means of collecting relevant data regarding a patient's cardiac status; however, the role of these devices in improving both short- and long-term outcomes in heart failure patients still remains to be defined. Indeed, some studies suggest that simply providing each patient with a scale and a diary to record daily weights and an algorithm for when to call the outpatient clinical nurse might provide actionable measurements that are the equivalent of invasive technologies.

Recently, we evaluated whether a scale that was linked telephonically with a central monitoring facility could provide information that was more useful than that provided by a scale alone. Although the scale that was linked to a centralized facility provided the physician with trend lines for an individual patient over time as well, patient education and nurse-managed telephone conversations to insure that patients were weighing themselves at the same time of the day and with the same amount of clothing, the outcome of the group randomized to a simple scale was identical to that of the group that was randomized to ongoing monitoring. Thus, in the case of daily monitoring, simple devices may be adequate and more complex and expensive monitoring systems must be tested against a simple scale or against less costly nurse-managed wellness programs.

One of the most exciting uses of a nonimplanted diagnostic device is the role of echocardiography in assessing both the need for and the effectiveness of resynchronization therapy. Echocardiography has moved from a technology that provides two-dimensional images of cardiac function and structure to Doppler flow and tissue Doppler technologies that can provide far more information about cardiac function and hemodynamics. For example, novel programs can provide non-load-dependent assessment of left ventricular function, measurement of diastolic dysfunction, as well as highly technological assessments of valve function. Novel algorithms can also help assess the presence of cardiac dyssynchrony even in the presence of a narrow QRS complex as well as evaluating the success of resynchronization therapy in an individual patient. Sophisticated echocardiographic imaging using color flow Doppler, tissue Doppler, and pressure-dimension analysis can also help cardiologists to evaluate the function of both the mitral and aortic valve while exercise echocardiography can be useful in assessing cardiac reserve.

New devices that have been developed for the treatment of acute cardiac decompensation must also be evaluated based on the needs of an individual patient. For example, as discussed in the preceding chapters, some patients with coronary artery disease and heart failure may benefit from coronary revascularization either by bypass surgery or by percutaneous coronary intervention. While there is considerable recognition that patients with symptoms of angina can have enhanced quality of life after revascularization, there is only anecdotal data regarding the effects of revascularization on patients with heart failure and no symptoms of angina. Important information will be available in approximately two years when the long-term follow-up of Hypothesis 1 of the Surgical Treatment for Ischemic Heart Failure (STICH) trial is completed. Hypothesis 1 of the STICH trial randomized patients either to surgical revascularization alone or to the combination of revascularization therapy and left ventricular reconstruction. Surprisingly, revascularization with left ventricular reconstruction appeared to have no advantage over revascularization alone when assessing the primary endpoint of death or hospitalization. Thus, it is difficult to guess whether revascularization will surpass medical therapy in the treatment of patients with coronary artery disease and diminished left ventricular dysfunction but without angina. However, new percutaneous left ventricular support systems provide an opportunity to more safely and effectively perform catheter-based revascularization in patients with severe left ventricular dysfunction.

Percutaneous left ventricular support systems also provide an opportunity to support cardiac function for a brief period of time and to bridge patients to more definitive therapy or potentially to recovery. These support devices can be placed percutaneously through either the combination of access lines in both lower extremities or an arterial access line in the femoral artery and a venous access line placed into the left atrium through a transvenous approach. Simple instrumentation allows for easy modulation of flow. These devices have great utility when there is an urgent need to support the left ventricle and there is neither time nor the technical capabilities to surgically implant a traditional assist device; there is an expectation that the device will only be used for a short period of time as a bridge to an implanted ventricular assist device, or as a bridge to recovery. For example, a percutaneous assist device might be useful in a patient with acute myocarditis in whom there is an expectation that recovery might occur over a relatively short period of time. Percutaneous assist devices can also be useful during high-risk angioplasty or valve repair or placement in patients with significant left ventricular dysfunction or may simply provide physicians with time to plan or evaluate more definitive surgical strategies.

In the same group of patients, i.e. those with acute cardiac decompensation, the use of ultrafiltration might be helpful in the acute management and support of the patient or alternatively to remove fluid in a patient that is hemodynamically stable but who has an excessive amount of fluid accumulation. Finally, aortic counterpulsation may be helpful in patients in need of a short period of cardiac support. External counterpulsation can benefit patients with coronary artery disease and angina that cannot be mitigated by either coronary artery bypass grafting or percutaneous coronary intervention and can be used safely even in patients with cardiac dysfunction. However, its role in patients with heart failure in the absence of coronary artery disease and angina has not been demonstrated. Unfortunately, data do not exist as to whether a given patient will be better served by receiving ultrafiltration or left ventricular support; however, the presence of significant fluid accumulation in the absence of hypotension might favor ultrafiltration whereas cardiogenic shock and/or signs of significant hypoperfusion would favor the use of a support device.

In this text we have presented a balanced view of the many new devices – implantable and nonimplantable – that have been developed for the treatment of patients with heart failure. In the case of ICDs and biventricular pacemakers, there is a general consensus regarding the appropriate patient populations that will benefit from these devices. However, even in the case of ICDs and biventricular pacers, there are important questions that need to be answered since these devices clearly do not work in every patient. For the other diagnostic and therapeutic devices presented in this text, careful assessments must be made to understand the ideal patient for each device. In addition, investigators must continue to evaluate the usefulness of these devices in selective patient populations in order that recommendations can guide the physician in determining the most effective approach in any given patient. It is hoped that this text will serve as a starting point for clinicians to understand the relevance of these new and novel technologies in the care of patients with heart failure. The chapters in this textbook clearly illustrate that we have come a long way in the 30 years since the first successful implantation of a device in a patient with heart failure.

Index

Note: Italicized page numbers refer to figures and tables

(Conflict of Interest Table)

Author	Employment	Research grant	Other research support	Speakers bureau/ honoraria	Expert witness	Ownership interest	Consultant/ advisory board	Other
Aggarwal	Jefferson Medical College	None	None	None	None	None	None	None
Ardehali	UCLA	None	None	None	None	None	None	None
Bernal	Massachusetts General Hospital	None	None	None	None	None	None	None
Borggrefe	University Hospital Mannheim	None	None	Impulse Dynamics* Medtronic* St Jude Medical* AstraZeneca* Pfizer* Biotronic* Essex Pharma* Sanofi Aventis*	None	None	Immere Pluse* CV Therapeutiks* Boehringer Ingelheim* Medtronic*	None
Burkhoff	CircuLite, Inc.	None	None	Impulse Dynamics +	None	None	None	None
Butter	Heart Centre Brandenburg in Bernau	None	None	None	None	None	None	None
Cohen	Lenox Hill Hospital	None	None	None	None	Cardiac Assist Inc*	Cardiac Assist Inc*	None
Costanzo	Edward Heart Hospital	None	None	Chf solutions*	None	None	Chf solutions*	None
Drazner	UT Southwestern Medical Centre	None	None	None	None	None	None	None
Farmer	Baylor College of Medicine	None	None	None	None	None	Merek* Pfizer*	None
Feldman	Jefferson Medical College	None	None	None	None	Cardiokine, Inc. equity, board of directors	None	None
Greenspoon	Thomas Jefferson University	Medtronic* St Jude Medical* Boston Scientific* Biotronik*	None	Medtronic* St Jude Medical* Boston Scientific* Biotronik*	None	None	None	None

Author	Employment	Research grant	Other research support	Speakers bureau/ honoraria	Expert witness	Ownership interest	Consultant/ advisory board	Other
Gorcsan	University of Pittsburgh	Biotronik + GE* Toshiba* Medtronic* St. Jude*	None	None	None	None	GE* Biotronik* Toshiba* Medtronic* St. Jude*	None
Ho	Thomas Jefferson University Hospital	None	None	None	None	None	None	None
Kamath	Baylor University Medical Centre	None	None	None	None	None	None	None
Kiernan	Massachusetts General Hospital	None	None	None	None	None	None	None
Lawson	Sunny, Stony Brook	None	None	None	None	None	None	None
Mann	Washington University	None	None	None	None	Miragen*	Medtronic* Nile Therapeutics* Miragen* Armgo* Pericor Therapeutics*	None
Marelli	Bay Health Medical Centre	None	None	None	None	None	ABiomed Inc.*	None
Mather	Jefferson medical College	None	None	None	None	None	None	None
Mulukutla	University of Pittsburgh	None	None	None	None	None	ABiomed Inc.+	None
Palacios	Massachusetts General Hospital	None	None	None	None	None	None	None
Parvathaneni	University Hospitals Case Medical Center	University Hospitals Case Medical Center+	None	None	None	None	None	None

Name	Institution	1	2	3	4	5	6	7
Pavri	Thomas Jefferson University Hospital	None	None	Boston Scientific,* Medtronic* St. Jude Medical* Biotronik*	None	None	Boston Scientific, Medtronic* St. Jude Medical* Biotronik*	None
Piña	Case Western Reserve University	NIH-HF-ACTION SubStudy*	None	AZ, Novartis* Merck, Solvay* Sanofi-Aventis*	None	None	FDA*	None
Popescu	Christiana Cart	None	None	None	None	None	None	None
Ruggiero	Massachusetts General Hospital	None	None	None	None	None	None	None
Sabbah	IMPULSE DYNAMICS USA, INC	Impulse Dynamics*	None	None	None	None	Impulse Dynamics*	None
Schneider	None	None	None	None	None	None	None	None
Silver	Advocate Health Care and Univeristy of Illinois.	None	None	None	None	None	None	None
Stein	Jefferson Medical College.	None	None	None	None	None	None	None
Whellan	Thomas Jefferson University	Medtronic +	None	Medtronic*	None	None	Medtronic*	None

*Modest

+Significant

This table represents the relationships of writing group members that may be perceived as actual or reasonably perceived conflicts of interest as reported on the Disclosure Questionnaire which all writing group members are required to complete and submit. A relationship is considered to be "Significant" if (a) the person receives $10,000 or more during any 12 month period, or 5% or more of the person's gross income; or (b) the person owns 5% or more of the voting stock or share of the entity, or owns $10,000 or more of the fair market value of the entity. A relationship is considered to be "Modest" if it is less than "Significant" under the preceding definition.